Tumor Immunology

The Tumor Immunology and Immunotherapy Series
A series of books exploring the multidisciplinary nature of the field of tumor immunology.
Edited by ***Giorgio Parmiani***, *National Cancer Institute, Milan, Italy* and ***Michael T. Lotze***, *University of Pittsburgh Cancer Institute, Pittsburgh, USA.*

Volume One
Tumor Immunology: Molecularly Defined Antigens and Clinical Applications
Edited by *Giorgio Parmiani* and *Michael T. Lotze*

Volumes in Preparation

Mechanisms of Tumor Escape from the Immune Response
Edited by *Augusto C. Ochoa*

Tumor Antigens Recognised by T Cells and Antibodies
Edited by *Hans Stauss* and *Yutaka Kawakami*

TUMOR IMMUNOLOGY
MOLECULARLY DEFINED ANTIGENS AND CLINICAL APPLICATIONS

Edited by

Giorgio Parmiani
National Cancer Institute
Milan, Italy

and

Michael T. Lotze
University of Pittsburgh Cancer Institute
Pittsburgh, USA

London and New York

First published 2002
by Taylor and Francis
11 New Fetter Lane, London EC4P 4EE

Simultaneously published in the USA and Canada
by Taylor and Francis Inc,
29 West 35th Street, New York, NY 10001

Taylor and Francis is an imprint of the Taylor & Francis Group

Typeset in Times by Expo Holdings, Malaysia
Printed and bound in Singapore by Stamford Press Pte Ltd

British Library Cataloguing in Publication Data
A catalogue record for this book is available from the British Library

Library of Congress Cataloging in Publication Data
A catalogue record has been requested

ISBN: 0–415–27216–5

Contents

Series Preface

Tumor immunology has been a conflicting area of investigation for several decades, and has been characterized by a succession of excitements and disappointments. However, three major discoveries have been instrumental in causing a resurgence of interest in the field. First, the understanding of molecular steps of antigen recognition, processing and presentation for both HLA classes I and II restricted antigens; second, the milestone event of cloning genes encoding the T-cell recognized human melanoma antigens; and third, the identification of stimulatory and now inhibitory receptors of NK and T lymphocytes. Furthermore, the availability of vectors that allow the genetic engineering of most immune cells and of tumor cells significantly widened the possibility of understanding mechanisms of immune recognition and of manipulating, for therapeutic purposes, the immune system of tumor-bearing individuals. But also previous reagents, like monoclonal antibodies, apparently inefficient as a magic bullet in early therapeutic approaches, have now found new applications and remain the focus of intensive research in tumor immunology.

Tumor immunology is therefore, once again, enjoying a remarkable popularity and could lead to future successes in the immunotherapy of cancer, though several crucial questions need to be answered that require a concomitant effort of both pre-clinical and clinical investigators. We are not only continuing our quest for molecules that make tumor cells diverse from normal counterparts and foreign to the body but we have now to face the unexpected finding and understand how normal proteins and peptides can be recognized by the immune system and whether they can serve as targets of the immune response against growing neoplastic cells.

This new series of books in tumor immunology reflects the increased interest in this area which requires a multidisciplinary approach. It will attract the attention of molecular biologists, immunologists, gene therapists, and experimental and clinical oncologists. It intends to offer a forum of discussion in tumor immunology covering the latest results in the field.

Giorgio Parmiani and Michael T. Lotze

Contributors

Andrea Anichini
Unit of Immunobiology of Human Tumors
Istituto Nazionale Tumori
Via G. Venezian, 1
20133 Milan
Italy

Federico Garrido
Servicio de Análisis Clínicos
Hospital Universitario Virgen de las Nieves
Universidad de Granada
18014 Granada
Spain

Vicky Gunther
Department of Biological Sciences
University of Maryland
1000 Hilltop Circle
Baltimore, MD 21250
USA

Peter Hersey
Conjoint Professor in Oncology
University of Newcastle
Room 443, David Maddison Clinical Sciences Building
Newcastle, NSW 2300
Australia

Philip O. Livingston
Clinical Immunology Service
Department of Medicine
Memorial Sloan-Kettering Cancer Center
1275 York Avenue
New York, NY 10021
USA

Michael T. Lotze
Department of Surgery
University of Pittsburgh Medical Center
Pittsburgh Cancer Institute
Montefiore University Hospital
Pittsburgh, PA 15213-3241,
USA

Francesco M. Marincola
Surgery Branch, National Cancer Institute
Building 10, Room 2B42
10 Center Drive
Bethesda, MD 20892-1502
USA

Roberta Mortarini
Unit of Immunobiology of Human Tumors
Istituto Nazionale Tumori
Via G. Venezian, 1
20133 Milan
Italy

Suzanne Ostrand-Rosenberg
Department of Biological Sciences
University of Maryland
1000 Hilltop Circle
Baltimore, MD 21250
USA

Giorgio Parmiani
Unit of Immunobiology of Human Tumors
Istituto Nazionale Tumori
Via G. Venezian, 1
20133 Milan
Italy

Beth A. Pulaski
Department of Biological Sciences
University of Maryland
1000 Hilltop Circle
Baltimore, MD 21250
USA

Paul F. Robbins
Surgery Branch, National Cancer Institute
Building 10, Room 2B42
10 Center Drive
Bethesda, MD 20892-1502
USA

Francisco Ruiz-Cabello
Servicio de Análisis Clínicos
Hospital Universitario Virgen de las Nieves
Universidad de Granada
18014 Granada
Spain

Introduction

Giorgio Parmiani and Michael T. Lotze

The origin of modern tumor immunology dates back to the 1950s, when several groups of investigators in the USA and Europe demonstrated a) that the immune system of inbred mice and rats can recognize antigens expressed by tumor cells induced by chemical carcinogens; b) that such recognition results in rejection of a subsequent challenge of the same tumor in previously immunized animals; and c) that immune cells but not antibodies can mediate this reaction (Baldwin, 1955; Prehn and Main, 1957; Klein *et al.*, 1960; Old *et al.*, 1962). In the classical papers by Prehn, Klein and Old, most of the problems that pervaded the field in the following years (some of which are still to be solved) were clearly identified, with the possible exception of the escape of tumors from the immune response that became apparent later on, when tumor-infiltrating T lymphocytes could be functionally studied *in vitro* (Whiteside *et al.*, 1986).

The lack of quantitative *in vitro* techniques and the limited availability of molecular tools, however, prevented testing of the different hypotheses put forward to explain the nature of tumor antigens, the antigenic heterogeneity, the difficulty in triggering antitumor immunity, etc. The only available *in vitro* techniques were based on antibody reactions and, as such, were of limited use for the understanding of the lymphocyte-mediated mechanisms of antitumor activity. Therefore, most of these early tumor immunology studies were carried out on mouse models – at that time, inbred mouse strains became available thanks to the work of several pioneers of mouse genetics. Tumors could be induced in such animals by chemical carcinogens, radiation or viruses and transplanted from one genetically identical individual to another, an enormous step forward in the history of cancer research. These *in vivo* transplantation studies paved the way to understanding certain immunological aspects of the tumor–host interaction, as transplanted tumors have a predictable behavior in a given mouse strain in terms of growth, progression and induction of immune response.

The work of Prehn and subsequently of North showed that during tumor growth an eclipse occurs in the specific antitumor immunity which can be passively transferred by the host's lymphocytes. In addition, these *in vivo* studies made it clear that more than one antigen can be expressed by a single neoplasm, and that there is heterogeneity in the expression of tumor antigens both quantitatively and qualitatively, not only among different tumors induced by the same carcinogen and in the same strain of inbred mice, but also within a single neoplasm, as first shown by Prehn (1970). Meanwhile, serological techniques were already sophisticated enough to allow the study of the sera of mice that were either tumor bearing or immunized by a variety of procedures. However, antibodies with a clear and reproducible specificity against antigens different from those of endogenous mouse retroviruses of syngeneic tumors could not be detected in the overwhelming majority of cases and an effective antitumor immunity could not be transferred by antibodies.

Thus almost 10 years elapsed before *in vitro* systems were devised that could measure in quantitative terms the cytotoxic and proliferating activity of lymphocytes against syngeneic tumors (Brunner *et al.*, 1968). These techniques, which were essentially based on the ability to label target tumor cells with chromium 51 or other isotopes and lymphocytes with tritiated thymidine, allowed exploration of the reactions of the cellular arm of the immune system against different types of tumors in humans as such (Hellström and Hellström, 1969). Technology without new hypotheses, however, cannot solve scientific problems. It was the discovery of the mechanism of recognition by T cells in 1974, i.e. the MHC restriction for which Doherty and Zinkernagel won the Nobel prize, that led to the understanding of some of the fundamental mechanisms by which tumor cells can be specifically recognized and destroyed by the immune system. In fact, it was soon realized that tumor antigens can also be recognized by T cells in an MHC-restricted fashion (Trinchieri *et al.*, 1976). The rapid development of basic immunology, thanks to the introduction of molecular techniques, subsequently made it possible to define mechanisms by which antigens are presented as peptides to either T helper or T cytotoxic lymphocytes and to understand the function of antigen presenting cells (APC).

Serology has also played an important role in the brief history of tumor immunology. In fact, the search for antitumor antibodies was the major focus of the early studies aimed at assessing the *in vivo* response of animals bearing different types of neoplasms or deliberately immunized against syngeneic tumors. However, with few but important exceptions, the antibody response to tumors was usually restricted to proteins encoded by retroviruses commensal to mouse tumors or to differentiation antigens expressed by normal tissues as well. The important exception was the mouse tumor MethA whose individual antigen(s) could be biochemically defined after painstaking experiments thanks to the use of an antibody. Likewise, the outstanding work carried out by Old's group, aimed at evaluating the presence of tumor-specific antibodies in sera of hundreds of patients with different types of cancers, resulted in the identification and molecular characterization of only a handful of tumor-specific antigens, particularly in melanomas, due to the low frequency of such antibodies and their relatively low affinity. The availability of monoclonal antibody technology did not solve the problem. In fact, a plethora of monoclonal antibodies were raised against different human tumors but all of them only recognized differentiation molecules expressed in normal tissues too, albeit with a lower density. This effort, however, provided a wealth of data on the biological function of molecules associated with the differentiation pathway and/or with the neoplastic state, information that proved to be of great value in the subsequent investigations into the biology of human malignancies. During the last few years, however, serology has made a comeback thanks to phage display technology and the use of patient immune sera in the SEREX approach (see below).

Three major issues can be identified that have played a key role in the history of tumor immunology during the following years: 1) the expression and the molecular nature of tumor-specific antigens recognized by T cells on ''spontaneous'' mouse and human neoplasms; 2) the type of immune response (if any) that cancer patients can raise against growing autologous tumors; 3) the possible clinical application of the knowledge gained in the preclinical models of tumor immunology.

In the early 1980s the fundamental issue of tumor immunology still remained the **existence** and **molecular nature of tumor antigens** in cancers not deliberately induced in the laboratory under artificial conditions such as administration of high doses of carcinogens or radiation. However, thanks again to molecular techniques and to the cumbersome and skillful work of Thierry Boon's group, the first gene coding for a tumor antigen of a chemically induced murine tumor was cloned and the antigen characterized (De Plaen *et al.*, 1988). It took three more years before the genetic approach devised by Boon resulted in the cloning of the first gene encoding a human melanoma antigen (MAGE-1) recognized by HLA class I-restricted T cells (van der Bruggen *et al.*, 1991). This was a major achievement since it provided the basis for the establishment of tumor immunology as a discipline, although still more biologically than clinically oriented.

In the last few years many more human tumor antigens have been molecularly characterized by different groups in the United States and Europe. Surprisingly, however, the majority of human melanoma antigens (but also several mouse tumor antigens) recognized by T cells, particularly by cytotoxic T lymphocytes (CTL), turned out to be normal proteins expressed either by normal melanocytes (differentiation or lineage-related antigens) (Anichini *et al.*, 1993) or by tumors of different histologic origin and by a few normal cells present in specific tissues such as testis and placenta (see Boon and van der Bruggen, 1996). More recently, using a novel serological approach called SEREX (serological analysis of antigens by recombinant expression cloning with patient antibodies), it was found that such antigens could also be recognized by patient antibodies (Sahin *et al.*, 1995); this would imply a convergent recognition of identical antigens by the B and T cell systems, the difference being that B cells recognize proteins while T cells can only see protein fragments in the form of short peptides sitting in the groove of the MHC molecules of the plasma membrane.

Meanwhile, some antigens of unique type, namely those known to be usually involved in rejection of mouse tumors, were molecularly defined and found to be composed of different proteins bearing a point mutation that resulted in the generation of new peptide sequences recognized by CTL as ''foreign epitopes'' expressed by cancer cells. Only in the last few years have unique antigens been described in human tumors too; these antigens are also due to point mutations of biologically relevant proteins including β-catenin and CDK4 in melanoma, HLA in renal carcinoma, and also oncogenic proteins such as p53 or RAS in other epithelial tumors (review by Boon and van der Bruggen, 1996).

The **second central question** of tumor immunology is: are tumor antigens recognized during *in vivo* growth of the neoplasm and, if so, what is the kinetics of the host's immune response and by which component of the immune system is such a reaction activated (T cells, B cells, macrophages, NK cells)? Numerous articles in the scientific literature have been devoted to this issue. However, only now – thanks to molecular techniques – do we begin to understand the complex and dynamic interplay of soluble factors, host cells and tumor cells that takes place during the process of oncogenesis and subsequent tumor growth and progression. Evidence that the recognition and destruction of early tumor cells by the host (immunosurveillance) may occur in certain conditions has been accumulating during recent decades. This is based on the observation of a) spontaneous cancer regression; b) increased cancer incidence in immunosuppressed, organ transplanted patients; c) development of tumors in patients affected by primary immunodeficiency disorders and, more recently, HIV infection. The many articles published on these topics, however, only provide indirect evidence supporting the immunosurveillance hypothesis and, for some of the most common malignancies (breast, colon and lung cancers), even such indirect evidence is lacking.

In fact, "spontaneous regression" of human tumors has been reported by different authors but such regressions are usually difficult to document; in particular, it is almost impossible to reach the conclusion that they can be attributed to the immune system since none of these patients has been sufficiently studied from this point of view. Findings from "organ transplanted patients" undergoing chronic immunosuppressive therapy to prevent transplant rejection are more convincing and have been well documented and collected in specific registries thanks mainly to the work of Israel Penn (1991). They indicate an increase in a subset of neoplasms, in particular B cell-derived lymphomas, skin cancer, cervical cancer and Kaposi's sarcoma (all of which have a suspected viral origin), but not in other epithelial tumors including colon, lung and breast carcinoma. The increased incidence of skin tumors is heavily dependent on sun exposure, which is a well-known etiological agent. This may suggest that only tumors whose cells uniformly express strong antigens (i.e. those encoded by oncogenic viruses), which may play an essential role in maintaining the neoplastic condition, are efficiently dealt with by the immune system. Conversely, epithelial cancers may express no antigens or weak antigens or antigens that can be easily selected by the immune system without impairing the growth capacity of cancer cells. In a subgroup of these patients who received immunosuppressive drugs (e.g. azathioprine) in the early days of organ transplantation, however, it cannot be excluded that some tumors were directly induced by these chemicals. Moreover, recent studies indicate that cyclosporin, a widely used immunosuppressive drug, may in itself promote tumor growth.

Patients with *primary (congenital) immunodeficiencies* are another case in point, since some of them now live long enough to allow tumor development. In some of these individuals the risk of developing cancer is increased up to 100-fold, with approximately 10% of them being affected by tumor growth. Also, this group develops neoplasms that mostly involve the lymphoid system, including NHL, leukemias and Hodgkin's lymphoma, while there is no increased incidence of Kaposi's sarcoma (KS). Gastric carcinoma is the most frequent epithelial cancer reported in these patients, a finding that may imply a role of *Helicobacter pylori* in its genesis.

In *HIV-infected individuals* several types of malignancies may occur, but the predominant types are B cell lymphomas (NHL) and KS. The incidence of both tumors is increased several fold, particularly that of KS in males with advanced AIDS. It is hypothesized that NHL may develop due to a chronic stimulation of B cells by the HIV proteins gp120 and gp41 and/or the presence of B cell growth-stimulatory cytokines released into the blood of these patients. It is now known that the most likely culprit of KS is a new herpes virus (HHV-8) that shares sequences with EBV and is present also in KS of organ transplanted patients. The lack of T cell-mediated control of B cell growth allows their chronic proliferation, thereby increasing the chance of neoplastic transformation. However, a recent study of cancer deaths in HIV-infected individuals has shown a significant increase also of lung cancer and, to a lesser extent, of melanoma.

Overall, the evidence gathered from immunosuppressed individuals indicates that the immune system appears to be able to cope with incipient tumors that are likely to be induced by oncogenic viruses such as HPV (skin and cervical cancer), HHV-8 (KS), EBV (Hodgkin's lymphoma and NHL), since they confer a strong immunogenicity on such neoplastic cells; NHL may also be induced by an immunologically uncontrolled, polyclonal chronic stimulation of the B cell system. However, the immune control over the most common neoplasms (particularly epithelial cancers, with the possible exception of lung tumors) appears poor in such patients.

In recent years *in vivo* analysis of T cells was made possible by molecular techniques and immunohistochemistry. Several investigations reported that, at least in a certain subset of patients, tumor-infiltrating or peripheral blood T cells bearing a TCR which specifically recognized antigens of the autologous tumor *in vitro* could be isolated and characterized. In addition, melanoma antigen-specific T lymphocytes with a memory phenotype were found to be expanded in a limited proportion of melanoma patients both in the tumor lesions and in the blood (Romero *et al.*, 1998, Anichini *et al.*, 1999). Furthermore, vaccination studies revealed that the immune system can select antigen-negative tumor cells by destroying those cancer cells that show a high expression of HLA/peptide complexes (Jager *et al.*, 1996). Moreover, antibodies directed to oncoproteins (Her2-neu) overexpressed by tumor cells were also found in a large fraction of breast cancer patients. Taken together, these data indicate that *in vivo* recognition of tumor antigens occurs frequently, possibly in the early stages of tumor growth, although the result of such recognition may often be the selection of a subpopulation of antigen-negative melanoma cells rather than a complete destruction of the neoplasm.

The **third central issue** of modern tumor immunology is the **clinical application** of information obtained from preclinical studies. Since the early days of tumor immunology attempts have been made to translate the new information obtained in preclinical studies into the clinic. An outstanding example is that of Coley, a surgeon who treated local tumors with extracts of bacteria to cause an inflammatory reaction that would eventually induce a regression of the tumor mass, albeit in only a few patients. This regression was due to the release of different cytokines at the tumor site. This pioneering approach can be considered the precursor of the treatment with recombinant cytokines used today. Then came the non-specific immunotherapy in the form of vaccination (an inappropriate definition!) with BCG or other bacterial products; the enthusiasm for the use of these products was generated by George Mathé, who reported cure or prevention of relapse in leukemia patients given BCG by scarification. A plethora of studies followed, the rationale of which was rather confused, although animal models of mice and Guinea pigs did show that BCG could be effective in certain therapeutic settings (Zbar *et al.*, 1972); however, these results were clearly attributable to the strong immunogenicity of the transplanted tumors used in these experiments, with BCG serving as an adjuvant. The extensive use of this product in man was not justified at that time since no clear evidence existed that human tumors expressed antigens similar to those of tumors induced in inbred animals. A randomized phase III prospective clinical trial carried out at the National Tumor Institute of Milan by Veronesi and coworkers definitely excluded that BCG may increase the survival of stage III melanoma patients (Veronesi *et al.*, 1982). Vaccinations were then resumed by several groups, in particular in metastatic melanoma (stage III or stage IV) by using autologous or allogeneic irradiated melanoma cells administered alone or admixed with adjuvants such as BCG, bacterial extracts or haptens (see Mitchell *et al.*, 1996). The rationale behind those studies was based on the evidence that antibodies reacting specifically with melanoma cells can be found in a fraction of melanoma patients, these reactions being directed against differentiation-type antigens such as mono- or di-sialogangliosides (e.g. GM2, GD2, GD3). Given the lack of knowledge on the expression of tumor antigens and how to detect them, however, these studies were flawed by ignorance of which antigens were administered and whether any specific cell-mediated immune response was generated. Despite the considerable effort made by several groups in performing such clinical protocols, the information gained was negligible. In fact, the only immune response that could be evaluated was antibody production against well-known differentiation antigens of melanoma and other tumors, a reaction whose clinical significance remains to be established. Along these lines, however, more recent data, obtained from melanoma patients vaccinated with well-defined gangliosides (e.g. GM2) conjugated to the T helper-inducing protein KLH and admixed with an adjuvant, indicate a possible association with a better prognosis in patients who developed antibodies to the vaccine (Livingston *et al.*, 1994). This hypothesis is now under investigation in appropriate phase III randomized trials. A turning point in the history of immunotherapy was the advent of the recombinant form of the lymphocyte growth factor, interleukin-2 (IL-2) (Morgan *et al.*, 1976). In fact, IL-2 availability enabled the growth of lymphocytes *in vitro*. Thanks to the work of Eva Klein and Farkas Vanky, it was thus possible to isolate T lymphocytes from neoplastic lesions and keep them *in vitro* for a time sufficient to assess their antitumor activity (Klein *et al.*, 1976).

But IL-2 could also be administered *in vivo* to activate lymphocytes and promote their growth. The possibility of keeping T and NK cells activated *in vitro* allowed the use of this cytokine to be treated in cancer therapy. This approach was devised by Steven Rosenberg and Michael Lotze at the Surgery Branch of the NCI in the mid-1980s. Several hundred patients, particularly those with metastatic melanoma or kidney cancer, were treated either with a high dose of IL-2 alone (Lotze *et al.*, 1986) or with the combination of IL-2 and lymphokine-activated lymphocytes (LAK) or tumor-infiltrating lymphocytes (TIL) (Rosenberg *et al.*, 1994). Such treatment, which may be associated with toxicity in different organs, resulted in partial or complete regressions even of large tumor masses in visceral organs like the liver and lung and represented the first evidence that manipulation of the immune system may result in the cure of metastatic disease, albeit in a limited number of cases.

In recent years exciting new information has been obtained on how to devise new, more promising approaches both in active and adoptive immunotherapy for cancer. New vaccines are being constructed a) by genetic manipulation of tumor cells that are modified to increase their immunogenicity, or b) by the use of patients' own dendritic cells, the most potent APCs, expressing well-defined antigens provided by virus vectors, by pulsing with proteins/peptides or even in the form of nucleic acids (Tuting *et al.*, 1998). Viral or non-viral (liposomes, bacteria) vectors of genes encoding well-defined antigens are also being used to vaccinate patients affected by different malignancies. Clinical trials aimed at assessing the immunogenicity and antitumor activity of such vaccines are ongoing and at least some of them have already provided encouraging results (Nestle *et al.*, 1998; Rosenberg *et al.*, 1998). For adoptive transfer, lymphocytes can now be guided to target tumor cells either by bi-specific antibodies or by transfecting these immune effectors with chimeric receptors that couple the targeting specificity of an antibody to a given tumor antigen with the domain of the TCR necessary to trigger tumor cell killing by the activated lymphocytes. It is also of note that, more than 20 years since their discovery (Koheler and Milstein, 1973), monoclonal antibodies have found their place in the therapeutic setting, particularly in colon and breast cancer and in B cell lymphomas. In fact, anti-Her2-neu and anti-CD20 are now in phase III clinical trials after having shown a significant therapeutic effect in phase II studies, while the 171A antibody has been tested in a phase III adjuvant trial (Riethmuller *et al.*, 1999). All these topics will be covered in the different chapters of this volume.

Tumor Immunology is intended to provide a general introduction to the forthcoming volumes in the series on Tumor Immunology and Immunotherapy that will be published by Taylor and Francis and co-edited by ourselves. The present volume is designed for clinicians or scientists who need a general update on the basic principles in this field. Non-oncological immunologists may wish to extend their knowledge by reading one or more volumes of the series devoted to single hot topics in tumor immunology.

BASIC REFERENCES

Anichini, A., Maccalli, C., Mortarini, R., Salvi, S., Mazzocchi, A., Squarcina, P., Herlyn, M., and Parmiani G. (1993) Melanoma cells and normal melanocytes share antigens recognized by HLA-A2-restricted cytotoxic T cells from melanoma patients. *J. Exp. Med.*, **177**, 989–998.

The first description of differentiation, lineage-related antigens recognized by T cells in human melanomas and normal melanocytes.

Brunner, K.T., Mauel, J., Cerottini, J.C., and Chapuis, B. (1968) Quantitative assay of the lytic action of immune lymphoid cells on 51-Cr-labelled allogeneic target cells *in vitro*, inhibition by isoantibody and by drugs. *Immunology*, **14**, 181–196.

First clear evidence of quantitative evaluation of the lytic activity of immune lymphocytes.

Grabbe, S., Bruvers, S., Gallo, R.L., Knisely, T.L., Nazarenos, R., and Granstein, R.D. (1991) Tumor antigen presentation by murine epidermal cells. *J. Immunol.*, **146**, 3656–3661.

A paper which provides clear evidence that epidermal antigen-presenting cells are necessary for the presentation of tumor antigens.

Huang, A.Y.C., Golumbek, P., Ahmadzadeh, M., Jaffee, E., Pardoll, D., and Levitsky, H. (1994) Role of bone marrow-derived cells in presenting MHC class I-restricted tumor antigens. *Science*, **264**, 961–966.

This paper demonstrates that tumor antigens are primarily presented to the immune system of immunologically naive animals by the host's antigen-presenting cells (dendritic cells) deriving from the bone marrow and only marginally by the tumor cells that carry the antigen.

Kiessling, R., Klein, E., Pross, H., and Wigzell, H. (1975) ''Natural'' killer cells in the mouse. II. Cytotoxic cells with specificity for mouse Moloney leukemia cells. Characteristics of the killer cells. *Eur. J. Immunol.*, **5**, 117–121.

The first description of NK with a partial characterization of their function.

Klein, E., Becker, S., Svedmyr, E., Jondal, M., and Vanky, F. (1976) Tumor infiltrating lymphocytes. *Ann. N.Y. Acad. Sci.*, **276**, 207–216.

The first account of a series of experiments that show the antitumor activity of TILs evaluated *in vitro*.

Livingston, P.O., Wong, G.Y.C., Adluri, S., Tao, Y., Padavan, M., Parente, R., Hanlon, C., Calves, M.J., Helling, F., Ritter, G., Oettgen, H.F., and Old, L.J. (1994) Improved survival in AJCC stage III melanoma patients with GM2 antibodies: A randomized trial of adjuvant vaccination with GM2 ganglioside. *J. Clin. Oncol.*, **12**, 1036–1044.

Patients vaccinated with the ganglioside GM2 develop antibodies that apparently give a survival advantage.

Prehn, R.T., and Main, J.M. (1957) Immunity to methylcholanthrene-induced sarcomas. *J. Natl. Cancer Inst. USA*, **18**, 759–778.

The definitive demonstration that chemically induced fibrosarcomas in inbred mice express antigens that elicit a transplantation immunity against the tumor via antigens that are not expressed by normal cells.

Riethmüller, G., Holz, E., Schlimok, G., Schmiegel, W., Raab, R., Höffken, K., Gruber, R., Funke, I., Pichlmaier, H., Hirche, H., Buggisch, P., Witte, J., and Pichlmayr, R. (1998) Monoclonal antibody therapy for resected Dukes' C colorectal cancer: seven-year outcome of a multicenter randomized trial. *J. Clin Oncol.* **16**, 1788–1794.

Strong evidence that a monoclonal antibody can increase the overall survival of cancer patients when given in an adjuvant setting.

Romero, P., Dunbar, P.R., Valmori, D., Pittet, M., Ogg, G., Rimoldi, D., Chen, J.-L., Liénard, D., Cerottini, J.-C., and Cerundolo, V. (1998) *Ex vivo* staining of metastatic lymph nodes by class I major histocompatibility complex tetramers reveals high numbers of antigen-experienced tumor-specific cytolytic lymphocytes. *J. Exp. Med.*, **188**, 1641–1650.

This paper describes strong *in vivo* evidence that a specific T cell response to melanoma occurs in the invaded lymph nodes of some tumor patients and that the reactive cytotoxic T cells have a substantial proliferative and tumoricidal potential.

Rosenberg, S.A., Yannelli, J.R., Yang, J.C., Topalian, S.L., Schwartzentruber, D., Weber, J.S., Parkinson, D.R., Seipp, C.A., Einhorn, J.H., and White, D.E. (1994) Treatment of patients with metastatic melanoma with autologous tumor-infiltrating lymphocytes and interleukin-2. *J. Natl. Cancer Inst. USA*, **86**, 1159–1166.

Infusion of TIL and IL-2 may result in objective clinical responses in at least one-third of metastatic melanoma patients; such responses are associated with the *in vitro* antitumor activity of these effectors. In this study there was, however, substantial toxicity due to the high dose of IL-2.

Trinchieri, G., Aden, D.P., and Knowles, B.B. (1976) Cell mediated cytotoxicity to SV40 specific tumor associated antigens. *Nature*, **261**, 312–314.

The first evidence that tumor antigens, represented here by the antigens of a SV40 induced tumor, are recognized by T cells in an MHC class I-restricted fashion.

van der Bruggen, P., Traversari, C., Chomez, P., Lurquin, C., De Plaen, E., Van den Eynde, B., Knuth, A., and Boon, T. (1991) A gene encoding an antigen recognized by cytolytic T lymphocytes on a human melanoma. *Science*, **254**, 1643–1647.

The first report of the cloning of a gene encoding a human melanoma antigen recognized by autologous T cells on melanomas. This paper established that such antigens exist also in human neoplasms.

Whiteside, T.L., Miescher, S., Hurliman, J., Moretta, L., and Von Fliender, V. (1986) Separation, phenotyping and limiting dilution analysis of T-lymphocytes infiltrating human solid tumors. *Int. J. Cancer*, **37**, 803–811.

This work shows that T lymphocytes obtained from tumor tissue are functionally crippled and require *in vitro* stimulation to restore their potential antitumor activity.

ADDITIONAL REFERENCES

Anichini, A., Molla, A., Mortarini, R., Tragni, G., Bersani, I., Di Nicola, M., Gianni, M., Pilotti, S., Dunbar, R., Cerundolo, V., Parmiani, G. (1999) An expanded peripheral T cell population to a cytotoxic T lymphocyte (CTL)-defined, melanocyte-specific antigen in metastatic melanoma patients impacts on generation of peptide-specific CTL, but does not overcome tumor escape from immune surveillance in metastatic lesions. *J. Exp. Med.*, **190**, 651–668.

Baldwin, R.W. (1955) Immunity to methylcholanthrene-induced tumors in inbred rats following atrophy and regression of implanted tumors. *Br. J. Cancer*, **9**, 652–656.

Boon, T., and van der Bruggen, P. (1996) Human tumor antigens recognized by T lymphocytes. *J. Exp. Med.*, **183**, 725–729.

DePlaen, E., Lurquin, C., Van Pel, A., Mariame, B., Szikora, J.-P., Wölfel, T., Sibille, C., Chomez, P., and Boon, T. (1988) Immunogenic (tum-) variants of mouse tumor P815: cloning of the gene of tumor-antigen P91A and identification of the tummutation. *Proc. Natl. Acad. Sci. USA*, **85**, 2274–2278.

Hellström, K.E., and Hellström, I. (1969) Cellular immunity against tumor antigens. *Adv. Cancer Res.*, **12**, 167–223.

Jäger, E., Heike, M., Bernhard, H., Klein, O., Bernhard, G., Lautz, D., Michaelis, J., Meyer zum Buschenfelde, K.H., Knuth, A. (1996) Weekly high-dose leucovorin versus low-dose leucovorin combined with fluorouracil in advanced colorectal cancer: results of a randomized multicenter trial. Study Group for Palliative Treatment of Metastatic Colorectal Cancer Study Protocol 1. *J. Clin. Oncol.*, **14**, 2274–2279.

Klein, G., Sjogren, H.O., Klein, E., and Hellström, K.E. (1960) Demonstration of resistance against methylcholanthrene-induced sarcomas in the primary autochtonous host. *Cancer Res.*, **20**, 1561–1572.

Lotze, M.T., Chang, A.E., Seipp, C.A., Simpson, C., Vetto, J.T., and Rosenberg, S.A. (1986) High-dose recombinant interleukin-2 in the treatment of patients with disseminated cancer. *JAMA*, **256**, 3117–3124.

Mitchell, M. (1996) Immunotherapy of melanoma. *J. Invest. Dermatol. Symp. Proc.* **1**, 215–218.

Morgan, D.A., Ruscetti, F.W., and Gallo, R.C. (1976) Selective *in vitro* growth of T-lymphocytes from normal bone marrow. *Science*, **193**, 1007–1008.

Old, L.J., Boyse, E.A., Clarke, D.A., and Carswell, E.A. (1962) Antigenic properties of chemically induced tumors. *Ann. N. Y. Acad. Sci.*, **101**, 80–106.

Penn, I. (1991) Principles of tumor immunity: immunocompetence and cancer. In V. De Vita Jr., S. Hellmann, S.A. Rosenberg, (eds.), *Biologic Therapy of Cancer*, J.B. Lippincott Co., pp. 53–66.

Prehn, R.T. (1970) Analysis of antigenic heterogeneity within individual 3-methylcholanthrene-induced mouse sarcomas. *J. Natl. Cancer Inst. USA*, **45**, 1039–1045.

Sahin, U., Tureci, O., Schmitt, B., Cochlovius, T., Johannes, T., Schmits, R., Stenner, F., Luo, G., Schobert, I., and Pfreundschuh, M. (1995) Human neoplasms elicit multiple specific immune responses in the autologous host. *Proc. Natl. Acad. Sci. USA*, **92**, 11810–11813.

Tuting, T., Wilson, C.C., Martin, D.M., Kasamon, Y.L., Rowles, J., Ma, D.I., Slingluff, C.L. Jr., Wagner, S.N., van der Bruggen, P., Baar, J., Lotze, M.T., and Storkus, W.J. (1998) Autologous human monocyte-derived dendritic cells genetically modified to express melanoma antigens elicit primary cytotoxic T cell response *in vitro*: enhancement by cotransfection of genes encoding the Th1-biasing cytokines IL-12 and IFN-alfa. *J. Immunol.*, **160**, 1139–1147.

Veronesi, U., Adamus, J., Aubert, C., Bajetta, E., Beretta, G., Bonadonna, G., Bufalino, R., Cascinelli, N., Cocconi, G., Durand, J., De Marsillac, J., Ikonopisov, R.L., Kiss, B., Lejeune, F., MacKie, R., Madej, G., Mulder, H., Mechl, Z., Milton, G.W., Morabito, A., Peter, H., Priario, J., Paul, E., Rumke, P., Sertoli, R., and Tomin, R. (1982) A randomized trial of adjuvant chemotherapy and immunotherapy in cutaneous melanoma. *N. Engl. J. Med.*, **307**, 913–916.

Zbar, B., Bernstein, I.D., Bartlett, G.L., Hanna, M.G. Jr., and Rapp, H.-J., (1972) Immunotherapy of cancer: regression of intradermal tumors and prevention of growth of lymph node metastases after intralesional injection of living *Mycobacterium bovis*. *J. Natl. Cancer Inst. USA*, **49**, 119–130.

1 Immune Recognition of Cancer – Tumor Antigens

Paul F. Robbins

ABBREVIATIONS

APC	Antigen-presenting cells
CLA	Cutaneous lymphocyte-associated antigen
CTL	Cytotoxic T lymphocytes
DTH	Delayed type hypersensitivity
GM-CSF	Granulocyte-monocyte colony-stimulating-factor
HPV	Human papillomavirus
IFA	Incomplete Freund's adjuvant
IFN-γ	Interferon gamma
IL-2, -12	Interleukin-2, -12
LAK	Lymphokine activated killer
MC1R	Melanocortin 1 receptor
PBL	Peripheral blood lymphocytes
PBMC	Peripheral blood mononuclear cells
PCR	Polymerase chain reaction
RT-PCR	Reverse transcriptase polymerase chain reaction
TAL	Tumor associated lymphocytes
TCR(s)	T cell receptor(s)
TIL	Tumor-infiltrating lymphocytes
TNF-α	Tumor necrosis factor alpha

Tumor antigens

1. **Many tumor antigens are now molecularly characterized.**
2. **These antigens are expressed by histologically different human neoplasms.**
3. **Tumor antigens are recognized by T cells (either CD4 Th or CD8 CTL) and by B cells (antibodies).**
4. **According to tissue distribution, tumor antigens include: a) normal differentiation proteins, b) normal proteins preferentially expressed by tumor cells (e.g. MAGE), c) widely expressed normal antigens, d) unique antigens.**
5. **Tumor antigens are heterogeneously expressed among tumors and even within a single neoplastic lesion.**
6. **Tumor antigen epitopes are presented as short (8–10 mers) or longer (13–23 mers) peptides by MHC class I and II molecules respectively to naive T cells.**
7. **Tumor antigens have a different immunogenicity (often low) both *in vitro* and *in vivo*.**
8. **Peptide/protein tumor antigens, either alone or in combination, are being used to vaccinate cancer patients.**

INTRODUCTION

Observations initially made in the early 1980s indicated that lymphoid cells activated with IL-2 (LAK) could lyse tumor cells and mediate tumor regression in mice. Human clinical trials demonstrated tumor regression in 15–20% melanoma and renal cancer patients treated with IL-2 as well as LAK plus IL-2. Subsequent studies demonstrated that the *in vitro* stimulation of lymphocytes from tumor-bearing hosts with specific tumor cells as well as the expansion of TIL in the presence of IL-2 could result in the generation of tumor-reactive T cells. Cultured $CD8^+$ lymphocytes could be isolated from patients with a variety of malignancies that recognized autologous as well as allogeneic tumor cells expressing shared class I MHC restriction elements (Darrow *et al.*, 1989; Hom *et al.*, 1991; Ioannides *et al.*, 1991; Finke *et al.*, 1992). These T cells generally failed to recognize autologous or allogeneic normal cells, and thus appeared to recognize specific tumor antigens in a conventional class I restricted manner, as previously demonstrated in responses against viruses and other foreign antigens (Yewdell and Bennink, 1992). Tumor-reactive T cells were found to release IFN-γ, TNF-α and GM-CSF in response to tumor stimulation and mediated tumor cell lysis (Schwartzentruber *et al.*, 1991). In addition, class II restricted $CD4^+$ T cells were identified that released the same set of cytokines as well as IL-2 in response to specific tumor stimulation. Although these cells were more effective than LAK cells at mediating tumor regressions in human clinical trials, complete long-term cures were found in only a small percentage of treated patients.

Over the past decade, efforts of a number of laboratories have focused on the identification of the antigens recognized by tumor-reactive T cells, with the hope that this will lead to the development of more effective antitumor therapies. A variety of methods

TABLE 1.1
Methods used to identify tumor antigens

A. Class I antigens

CDNA library expression cloning

- Generate cDNA library from tumor cells in eukaryotic expression vector
- Transfect cDNA pools into non-tumor target cells expressing appropriate MHC
- Add T cells to transfectants, measure cytokine release
- Isolate individual cDNA clones, retest

Identification of peptides recognized by tumor reactive T cells

- Purify MHC molecules from tumor cells
- Fractionate peptides using HPLC
- Pulse on target cells, measure cytokine release
- Synthesize candidate peptides, test for recognition

Identify candidate antigens with a limited or tissue specific expression pattern
Identify candidate peptides bound to tumor cell surface class I molecules
Test candidate antigens/peptides for recognition by tumor-reactive T cells
Generate tumor-reactive T cells using candidate class I binding peptides

B. Class II antigens

Protein isolation

- Purify proteins from tumor cells
- Test for recognition following pulsing on antigen presenting cells

Identify candidate peptides bound to tumor cell surface class II molecules
CDNA library expression cloning

- Class I approach – transfect class II+ antigen-presenting cells with cDNA pools

C. B cell antigens

CDNA library expression cloning (SEREX)

- Generate cDNA library in λ phage expression vector
- Identify individual phage plaques that react with patient antisera

have been employed to identify tumor antigen gene products (Table 1.1). The majority of tumor antigens have been isolated using a genetic approach (see Figure 1.1), which initially involves the generation of a cDNA library from tumor cell mRNA in a eukaryotic expression vector. Pools of cDNAs, generally containing between 100 and 200 individual cDNA clones, have been produced and introduced into highly transfectable cell lines expressing the appropriate class I MHC gene product. Transfected cells have then been assayed for their ability to stimulate cytokine release from tumor-reactive T cells. In another approach (see Figure 1.2), peptides have been eluted from cell surface MHC molecules, fractionated using reversed phase HPLC columns, and used to sensitize target cells for recognition by T cells. Positive pools of peptides have then been successively fractionated, and individual peptides identified by mass spectrometry have then been synthesized and tested for their ability to sensitize targets for recognition by specific T cells. In another approach tissue-specific molecules, representing candidate antigen, have either been tested for recognition by tumor-reactive T cells or used for T cell sensitizations. Use of sera from cancer patients to screen bacterial expression libraries, a technique that

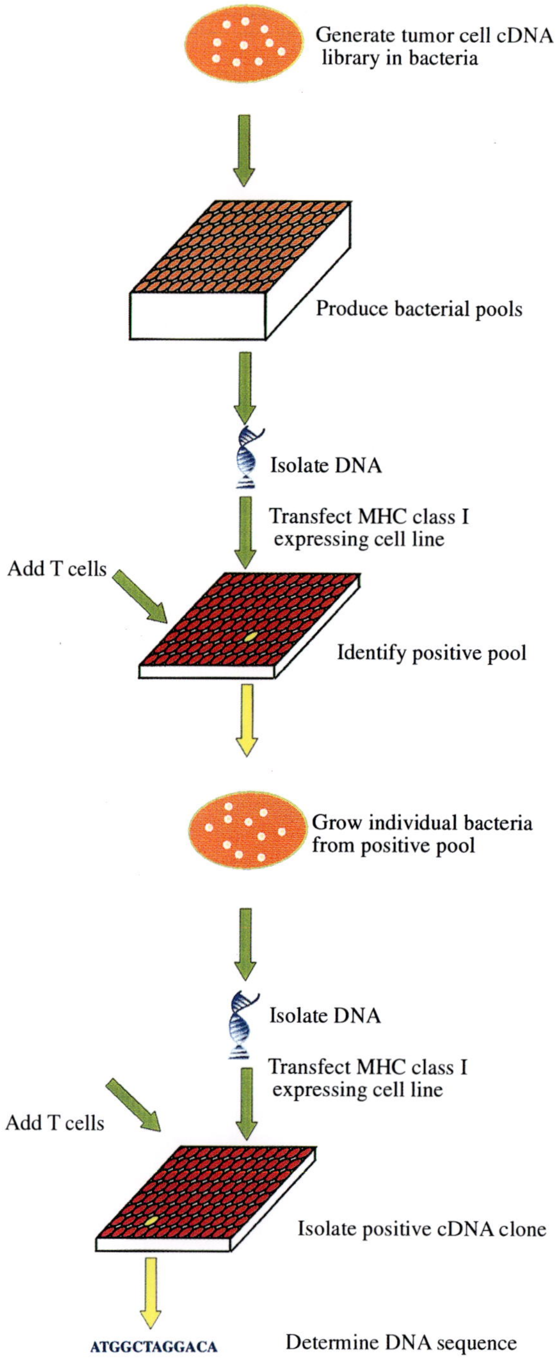

Figure 1.1 Genetic approach to the identification of molecularly defined tumor antigens.

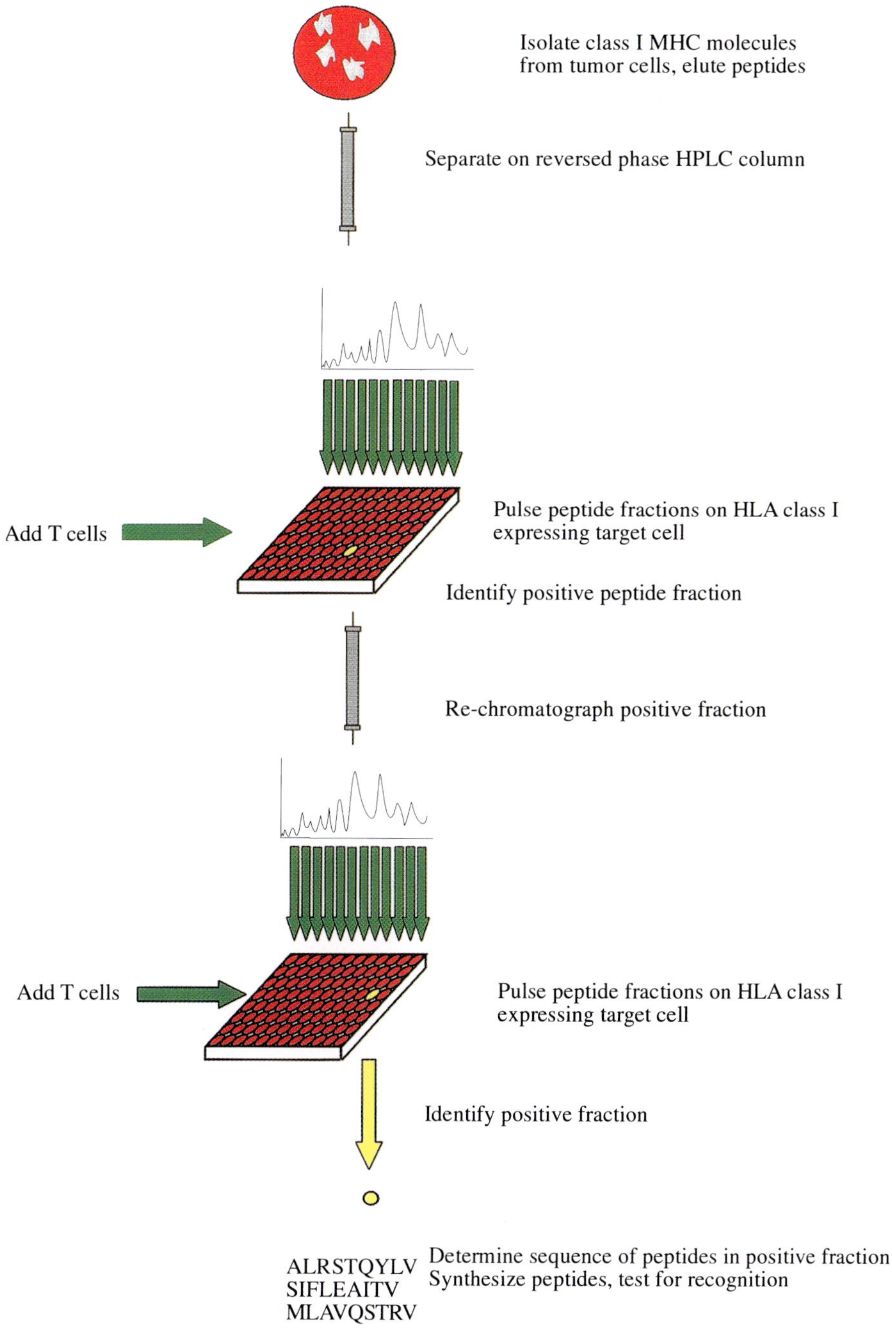

Figure 1.2 Biochemical approach to the identification of molecularly defined tumor antigens.

has been termed SEREX, has resulted in the identification of a number of products that are also recognized by $CD8^+$, tumor-reactive T cells.

Identification of the peptide epitopes recognized by $CD8^+$ tumor-reactive T cells has been carried out through the use of peptide binding motifs. Analysis of the sequences of peptides that have been independently identified in a variety of antigens, as well as the sequences of peptides eluted from class I MHC molecules, have revealed that a limited number of amino acids are found at particular positions, termed anchor residues, in these peptides. These anchor residues are critically important for binding to class I MHC molecules, and consensus sequences have been identified for a large number of class I molecules (Rammensee *et al.*, 1995). These findings have allowed the generation of algorithms that can be used to predict potential class I MHC binding peptides (Parker *et al.*, 1995), which can then be synthesized and directly tested for their ability to bind to the appropriate class I MHC molecules. Peptides can then be screened for their ability to sensitize targets for recognition by tumor-reactive T cells.

As a result of these studies, a variety of antigens restricted by MHC class I have been identified in human cancers, primarily in melanoma. These antigens can be grouped in a number of categories, based upon their patterns of expression in tumor and normal tissues (Tables 1.2–1.5). In addition, a number of antigens have been identified in mouse tumors, providing a basis for the evaluation of tumor therapies in mouse model systems. The efficacy of specific tumor antigen immunization is now being evaluated in a variety of

TABLE 1.2
Class I HLA-restricted cancer/testis antigens

Gene	*HLA allele*	*Peptide epitope*	*Reference*
MAGE-1	A1	EADPTGHSY	Traversari *et al.*, 1992
MAGE-1	A3	SLFRAVITK	Chaux *et al.*, 1999
MAGE-1	A24	NYKHCFPEI	Fujie *et al.*, 1999
MAGE-1	A28	EVYDGREHSA	Chaux *et al.*, 1999
MAGE-1	B53	DPARYEFLW	Chaux *et al.*, 1999
MAGE-1	Cw2	SAFPTTINF	Chaux *et al.*, 1999
MAGE-1	Cw3	SAYGEPRKL	Chaux *et al.*, 1999
MAGE-1	Cw16	SAYGEPRKL	van der Bruggen *et al.*, 1994b
MAGE-2	A2	KMVELVHFL YLQLVFGIEV	Visseren *et al.*, 1997
MAGE-2	A24	EYLQLVFGI	Tahara *et al.*, 1999
MAGE-3	A1	EADPIGHLY	Gaugler *et al.*, 1994
MAGE-3	A2	FLWGPRALV	van der Bruggen *et al.*, 1994a
MAGE-3	A24	TFPDLESEF	Oiso *et al.*, 1999
MAGE-3	B44	MEVDPIGHLY	Herman *et al.*, 1996
MAGE-6	A34	MVKISGGPR	Zorn and Hercend, 1999
MAGE-A4	A2	GVYDGREHTV	Duffour *et al.*, 1999
MAGE-A10	A2	GLYDGMEHL	Huang *et al.*, 1999
BAGE	Cw16	AARAVFLAL	Boel *et al.*, 1995
DAM	A2	FLWGPRAYA	Fleischhauer *et al.*, 1998
GAGE-1/2	Cw6	YRPRPRRY	Van den Eynde *et al.*, 1995
RAGE	B7	SPSSNRIRNT	Gaugler *et al.*, 1996
NY-ESO-1	A2	SLLMWITQCFL	Jäger *et al.*, 1998
NY-ESO-1	A2	SLLMWITQC	Jäger *et al.*, 1998
NY-ESO-1	A2	QLSLLMWIT	Jäger *et al.*, 1998
NY-ESO-1a (CAG-3)	A31	ASGPGGGAPR	Wang *et al.*, 1998b

clinical protocols. Peptides that have been identified from tumor antigens have been administered either singly or as peptide mixtures. In addition, a variety of recombinant viral constructs encoding these antigens, including vaccinia, fowlpox and adenovirus, have been administered to cancer patients. As discussed below, modified peptides with increased binding to MHC class I alleles are also being evaluated in clinical vaccine trials. These studies, which have begun to provide some insight into the nature of immune responses, should hopefully lead to the development of effective cancer vaccines that are capable of mediating tumor regression in the majority of cancer patients.

CANCER-TESTIS ANTIGENS

The first human tumor antigen was identified using T cells from patient MZ2, who had been immunized with multiple injections of autologous irradiated tumor (van der Bruggen *et al.*, 1991). This gene, termed MAGE-1, was isolated following the screening of cells that were stable transfected with an autologous melanoma genomic library with a T cell clone

TABLE 1.3
Class I HLA-restricted melanocyte differentiation antigens

Gene	*HLA allele*	*Peptide epitope*	*Reference*
MART-1	A2	AAGIGILTV	Kawakami *et al.*, 1994c
MART-1	A2	EAAGIGILTV	Kawakami *et al.*, 1994c
MART-1	A2	AAGIGILTVA	Kawakami *et al.*, 1994c
MART-1	A2	ILTVILGVL	Castelli *et al.*, 1995
MART-1	B45	AEEAAGIGILT	Schneider *et al.*, 1998
MART-1	B45	AEEAAGIGIL	Schneider *et al.*, 1998)
MCIR	A2	TILLGIFFL	Salazar-Onfray *et al.*, 1997
		FLALIICNA	Salazar-Onfray *et al.*, 1997
Gp100	A2	KTWGQYWQV	Kawakami *et al.*, 1995
Gp100	A2	ITDQVPFSV	Kawakami *et al.*, 1995
Gp100	A2	YLEPGPVTA	Kawakami *et al.*, 1995
Gp100	A2	LLDGTATLRL	Kawakami *et al.*, 1995
Gp100	A2	VLYRYGFSV	Kawakami *et al.*, 1995
Gp100	A2	RLMKQDFSV	Kawakami *et al.*, 1995
Gp100	A2	RLPRIFCSC	Kawakami *et al.*, 1995
Gp100	A2	RLMKQDDFSV	Kawakami *et al.*, 1998
Gp100	A3	SLIYRRRLMK	Kawakami *et al.*, 1998
Gp100	A3	ALLAVGATK	Skipper *et al.*, 1996b
Gp100	A24	VYFFLPDHL (intron)	Robbins *et al.*, 1997
Gp100	Cw8	SNDGPTLI	Castelli *et al.*, 1999
Tyrosinase	A1	KCDICTDEY	Kittlesen *et al.*, 1998
Tyrosinase	A1	SSDYVIPIGTY	Kawakami, 1998
Tyrosinase	A2	MLLAVLYCL	Wölfel *et al.*, 1994
Tyrosinase	A2	YMDGTMSQV	Wölfel *et al.*, 1994
Tyrosinase	A24	AFLPWHRLF	Kang *et al.*, 1995
Tyrosinase	B44	SEIWRDIDF	Brichard *et al.*, 1996
TRP-1	A31	MSLQRQFLR	Wang *et al.*, 1996b
TRP-2	A31	LLPGGRPYR	Wang *et al.*, 1996a
TRP-2	A2	SVYDFFVWL	Parkhurst *et al.*, 1998
TRP-2	A3, 33	LLGPGRPYK	Wang *et al.*, 1998a
TRP-2	Cw8	ANDPIFVVL	Castelli *et al.*, 1999

TABLE 1.4
Class I HLA-restricted widely expressed antigens

Gene	*HLA allele*	*Peptide epitope*	*Reference*
HER2/neu	A2	VVLGVVFGI	Rongcun *et al.*, 1999
		RLLQETELV	Rongcun *et al.*, 1999
HER2/neu	A2	KIFGSLAFL	Fisk *et al.*, 1995
HER2/neu	A2	IISAVVGIL	Peoples *et al.*, 1995
iCE*	B7	SPRWWPTCL	Ronsin *et al.*, 1999
PRAME	A24	LYVDSLFFL	Ikeda *et al.*, 1997
P15	A24	AYGLDFYIL	Robbins *et al.*, 1995
SART-1	A24	EYRGFTQDF	Kikuchi *et al.*, 1999
SART-1	A*2601	KGSGKMKTE	Shichijo *et al.*, 1998
SART-3	A24	VYDYNCHVDL	Yang *et al.*, 1999
		AYIDFEMKI	Yang *et al.*, 1999

*iCE, intestinal carboxyl esterase.

TABLE 1.5
Class I HLA-restricted tumor-specific antigens*

Gene	*HLA allele*	*Peptide epitope*	*Reference*
AFP	A2	GVALQTMKQ	Butterfield *et al.*, 1999
β-catenin	A24	SYLDSGIHF	Rubinfeld *et al.*, 1997
CAMEL	A2	MLMAQEALAFL	Aarnoudse *et al.*, 1999
Caspase-8	B35	FPSDSWCYF	Mandruzzato *et al.*, 1997
CDK-4	A2	ACDPHSGHFV	Wölfel *et al.*, 1995
ELF2M	A68	ETVSEQSNV	Hogan *et al.*, 1998
GnT-V	A2	VLPDVFIRC(V)†	Guilloux *et al.*, 1996
G250	A2	HLSTAFARV	Vissers *et al.*, 1999
HSP70-2M	A2	SLFEGIDIY	Gaudin *et al.*, 1999
HA-A*0201-R170I	A2	CVEWLRIYLENGK	Brändle *et al.*, 1996
HST-2	A31	YSWMDISCWI	Suzuki *et al.*, 1999
hTERT	A2	ILAKFLHWL	Vonderheide *et al.*, 1999
KIAA0205	B44*03	AEPINIQTV	Gueguen *et al.*, 1998
MUM-1	B44	EEKLIVVLF	Coulie *et al.*, 1994
MUM-2	B44	SELFRSGLDY	Chiari *et al.*, 1999
MUM-2	Cw6	FRSGLDSYV	Chiari *et al.*, 1999
Myosin-m	A3	KINKNPKYK	Zorn and Hercend, 1999
TRP-2/INT2	A68	EVISCKLIKR	Lupetti *et al.*, 1998

* Include both unique (CDK-4, MUM-1, MUM-2, β-catenin, HLA-A2-R170I, ELF2m, myosin-m, caspase-8, KIAA0205, HSP70-2 m) and shared (CAMEL, TRP-2/INT2, GnT-V, G 250) antigens.
† Nonamer and decamer peptides are both recognized by CTLs.

from this patient. This gene was found to belong to a multi-gene family containing at least 12 genes (De Plaen *et al.*, 1994). Members of this gene family have been found to be expressed in male germ cells in the testis, which lack expression of class I and class II gene products, but not other normal tissues (Takahashi *et al.*, 1995). Expression of six members of the MAGE gene family, MAGE-1, 2, 3, 4, 6 and 12, has been seen in tumors derived from a variety of additional tissue including neuroblastoma, glioblastoma, prostate, mammary, ovarian, colorectal and esophageal carcinomas (Van den Eynde and van der

Bruggen, 1997). The MAGE-3 gene appears to be expressed in a higher percentage of tumors than other members of the gene family, being found in about two-thirds of all melanomas and about half of head and neck squamous carcinomas (Gaugler *et al.*, 1994). The BAGE (Boel *et al.*, 1995) and GAGE (Van den Eynde *et al.*, 1995) genes, which appear to be representatives of multi-gene families with a similar expression pattern to the genes of the MAGE family, were isolated by screening a cDNA library from patient MZ2 with autologous T cell clones (see Table 1.2).

A single peptide was identified from MAGE-1 that was recognized in the context of HLA-A1 (Traversari *et al.*, 1992). The HLA-A1 restricted MAGE-3 epitope was found to be encoded by the same region encoding the MAGE-1 HLA-A1 epitope, differing at 2 of the 9 amino acid residues within the epitope (Gaugler *et al.*, 1994). Both of the peptides conformed to the consensus for binding to HLA-A1 (D or E at position 3, Y at position 9). A CTL clone has also been found to recognize a peptide from MAGE-1 in the context of HLA-Cw16 (van der Bruggen *et al.*, 1994b).

A number of attempts have been made to identify epitopes from MAGE family genes that are recognized in the context of additional HLA alleles (Table 1.2). Candidate peptides from MAGE-1 and -3, identified using consensus HLA binding motifs in conjunction with HLA binding assays, have been used to carry out PBL stimulations. Using this approach, T cells that recognize peptides from MAGE-3 in the context of HLA-A2 (van der Bruggen *et al.*, 1994a), HLA-B44 (Fleischhauer *et al.*, 1996), and HLA-A24 (Tanaka *et al.*, 1997) have been generated. Additional studies may be required to verify that T cells generated using these peptides can recognize endogenously processed epitopes from this gene product.

Another approach that has been used to identify T cell epitopes has been to immunize transgenic mice expressing the human HLA-A2 class I molecule with candidate peptides from the human MAGE-2 gene. Two out of three HLA-A2-binding MAGE-2 peptides that elicited peptide-specific CTL in HLA-A2 transgenic mice also appeared to generate T cells that recognized tumor cells expressing HLA-A2 and MAGE-3 (Visseren *et al.*, 1997). Although the results indicated that these epitopes are endogenously processed and presented in tumor cell lines, it is not clear that these peptides can induce immune responses in human cancer patients. To identify CTL epitopes that are naturally processed and can be found on tumor cells, DC were infected with a recombinant canary poxvirus (ALVA C) containing the entire MAGE-A1 gene. These DC were used to stimulate donors' PBL, which were then cloned using autologous cells transduced with a retrovirus coding for MAGE-A1. This strategy led to generation of cloned CTL that recognized several new MAGE-A1 epitopes on MAGE-A1-positive target cells (Caux *et al.*, 1999). Additional epitopes of the MAGE family (MAGE-2, -3, -4, -6 and -10) have also recently been identified (Table 1.2) (Duffour *et al.*, 1999; Huang *et al.*, 1999; Oiso *et al.*, 1999; Tahara *et al.*, 1999; Zorn and Hercend, 1999).

RAGE is an antigen that was first found to be expressed in a renal cancer but not in another 57 fresh renal cell carcinomas examined, while 37% of renal cell carcinoma lines tested positive (Gaugler *et al.*, 1996). Several other types of fresh tumors (bladder cancer, sarcoma), including a small percentage of melanomas (8/177) and breast cancers (3/128), were positive. Once again, RAGE was more frequently expressed in cultured lines. The only normal tissue that expressed RAGE was retina, and thus RAGE appears to represent an antigen with a unique expression pattern (Gaugler *et al.*, 1996).

The use of this antigen in cancer vaccination, however, remains questionable due to its limited expression in fresh tumors.

Additional members of the cancer/testis family of genes have been isolated through the screening of bacterial expression libraries with serum from cancer patients (SEREX). A previously unidentified gene termed NY-ESO-1 was recently isolated using the SEREX technique from a patient with a squamous carcinoma of the head and neck (Chen *et al.*, 1997). Expression of this gene appeared to be limited in normal tissues to testis and ovary, but a wide variety of tumors including melanomas, breast, prostate, ovarian and bladder cancers were found to express this gene product. Approximately 10% of patients with melanoma, ovarian, breast and lung cancer develop anti-ESO-1 antibodies (Stockert *et al.*, 1998), indicating that this represented a highly immunogenic protein. Expression of NY-ESO-1 has been found in 1/4 to 1/3 of all melanoma, breast and ovarian cancers (Chen *et al.*, 1997) ; thus, anti-NY-ESO-1 antibodies are present in about one-third of the patients containing tumors that expressed this antigen.

Further studies revealed that a melanoma patient with a high titer of anti-NY-ESO-1 antibodies also contained HLA-A2 restricted CTL that reacted with this antigen (Jäger *et al.*, 1998). When peptides that fit the HLA-A2 binding motif were examined for their ability to be recognized by the CTL line, it appeared that three partially overlapping peptides, SLLMWITQC, SLLMWITQCFL and QLSLLMWIT, that loosely fit the HLA-A2 binding motif were found to be recognized when pulsed on HLA-A2 expressing target cells. Several peptides containing these non-consensus anchor residues have now been identified, primarily from tumor antigens. Recognition of the NY-ESO-1 gene product has also been observed by several HLA-A31 restricted T cell clones (Wang *et al.*, 1998b). Certain CTL clones failed to recognize any peptides derived from the normal NY-ESO-1 open reading frame; instead, these clones recognized peptides that were translated from a novel product generated by the use of an alternative methionine start site. Use of this start site would result in the translation of a short product in a different open reading frame from the 180 amino acid open reading frame that is presumed to represent the normal NY-ESO-1 protein product. Additional HLA-A31 restricted T cell clones recognized a peptide epitope derived from the long NY-ESO-1 open reading frame. Analysis of T cell responses indicated that products derived from both open reading frames were expressed in melanomas as well as breast tumor cells (Wang *et al.*, 1998b).

DIFFERENTIATION ANTIGENS

The finding that some melanoma reactive CTL recognized normal melanocytes suggested that tissue-specific antigens might serve as the targets of tumor-reactive T cells (Anichini *et al.*, 1993). This was confirmed by the isolation of a gene that was termed MART-1 (Kawakami *et al.*, 1994a) or Melan-A (Coulie *et al.*, 1994) following the screening of a cDNA library with HLA-A2 restricted TIL or CTL clones, respectively. The MART-1 gene product was expressed in retinal tissue, which contains melanocytes, as well as in normal skin melanocytes. This gene encodes a 108 amino acid protein of unknown function, and contains a hydrophobic region between amino acids 27 and 47 that may represent a transmembrane region. Preliminary evidence also indicates that MART-1 is expressed in melanosomes (Kawakami *et al.*, 1997).

Twenty-three peptides within this sequence that fit the HLA-A2 binding motif were then synthesized and tested for reactivity with MART-1 reactive TIL (Kawakami *et al.*, 1994c). Ten out of 10 MART-1 reactive TIL as well as a MART-1 reactive T cell clone all reacted with a single nanomer peptide, AAGIGILTV (MART-1_{27-35}), as well as decamer peptides that contain 1 amino acid on the amino (EAAGIGILTV) and carboxy (AAGIGILTVI) terminus of MART-1_{27-35}. This appears to represent a dominant T cell epitope in patients expressing this class I MHC haplotype, since 22 out of 30 HLA-A2 restricted TIL recognized this peptide (Kawakami *et al.*, 1999). Another partially overlapping peptide, ILTVILGVL, was reported to be recognized by HLA-A2 restricted, MART-1 reactive T cells (Castelli *et al.*, 1995), but the majority of MART-1 reactive T cells do not appear to react with this peptide (Valmori *et al.*, 1998 ; Y. Kawakami, personal communication). A melanoma reactive T cell has also been found to recognize MART-1 in the context of HLA-B45 (Schneider *et al.*, 1998). Curiously, the optimal epitopes recognized by two HLA-B45 restricted MART-1 reactive T cell clones, AEEAAGIGILT and AEEAAGIGIL, partially overlapped with the MART-1 HLA-A2 epitope (Table 1.3).

Responses to MART-1 appear to be immunodominant in HLA-A2 individuals, and responses can readily be elicited in HLA-A2+ normal as well as melanoma patients. One possible explanation for these findings is that the MART-1 peptide represents an epitope mimic. In one study, evidence was obtained indicating that MART-1 reactive T cells reacted with peptides derived from a variety of sources, including viral proteins (Loftus *et al.*, 1998). Thus, T cells reactive with exogenous antigens such as viral epitopes may cross-react with the MART-1 epitope, thereby leading to the relatively high precursor frequency of T cells reactive with this epitope.

Another interesting source of differentiation-like antigens is the melanocyte-stimulating hormone receptor MC1R. In fact, this receptor is expressed on cells of melanocytic lineage and can generate peptides which stimulate HLA-A2-restricted CTLs (Salazar-Onfray *et al.*, 1997).

The gene encoding a 661 amino acid melanocyte differentiation antigen, gp100, was also isolated by screening a cDNA expression library with a melanoma reactive CTL (Kawakami *et al.*, 1994b). This gene had previously been isolated and shown to encode a protein recognized by a number of monoclonal anti-melanoma antibodies (Adema *et al.*, 1993). The gp100 protein was found to be expressed in the melanosomal matrix and was shown to represent an enzyme that is involved in melanin synthesis (Lee *et al.*, 1996).

The screening of candidate peptides from gp100 with 4 TIL resulted in the initial identification of 3 nanomer peptides, gp100:154–162, 209–217 and 280–288 and 2 decamer peptides, gp100:457–466 and 476–485 as peptide epitopes (Kawakami *et al.*, 1995). The gp100:280-288 peptide was also identified by fractionating HLA-A2 binding peptides isolated from melanoma cells and testing for reactivity with melanoma-reactive CTL lines (Cox *et al.*, 1994). In this study, 5 out the 5 CTL lines tested reacted with the gp100:280–288 peptide. Responses against this epitope were not as predominant in TIL, since approximately 20% of HLA-A2 restricted, melanoma-reactive TIL reacted with each of the peptide epitopes gp100:154–162, 209–217, and 280–288 (Kawakami *et al.*, 1999).

Two additional gp100 epitopes have recently been shown to be recognized by HLA-A2 restricted melanoma-reactive T cells. One peptide, gp100:619-627, was recently found to be recognized by an HLA-A2 restricted CTL clone, but was not recognized by a number of bulk, uncloned TIL lines (Kawakami *et al.*, 1998). A second gp100 epitope, gp100:639-647 (RLPRIFCSC), was unusual in that it contained 2 cysteine residues, one at position 7 and one at the C terminal anchor position (Kawakami *et al.*, 1998). In order to better understand the chemical nature of the naturally processed epitopes, peptides were synthesized in which the cysteine residues were replaced with α-aminobutyric acid, an amino acid that cannot be oxidized but that contains a side chain similar in size to the cysteine side chain. Replacement of the cysteines at either position individually or at both positions with amino acids containing side chains of a similar length to cysteine but lacking the sulfhydryl group appeared to significantly enhance T cell recognition. These results may indicate that the formation of disulfide bonds, either with a second cysteine residue or another sulfhydryl compound, may inhibit binding of the peptide to class I. Interactions with amino acids in the HLA-A2 binding pocket may prevent modification of cysteine residue side chains in this peptide; however, the data do not exclude the possibility that cysteine residues present in the natural epitope may contain unknown modifications that interfere with disulfide bond formation.

The intronic region of the gp100 gene has also been shown to encode an antigenic epitope recognized by an HLA-A24 restricted CTL clone (Robbins *et al.*, 1997). The insert that was isolated by screening a melanoma cDNA library had retained a sequence corresponding to the fourth intron of the gp100 gene. The intronic region, which encoded 35 additional amino acids in the normal open reading frame, was found to encode the peptide epitope. This transcript was expressed at relatively low levels in melanomas, but was also expressed in melanocytes, since an HLA-A24 melanocyte cell line was recognized by this CTL. Additional gp100 epitopes were recently described that are recognized by HLA-A3 and HLA-Cw8-restricted CTLs on melanoma targets (Skipper *et al.*, 1996b; Castelli *et al.*, 1999).

A number of T cell epitopes have also been identified in tyrosinase, a critical enzyme involved in the first steps of melanin synthesis. The gene encoding tyrosinase, which was first isolated in 1987 (Kwon *et al.*, 1987) , was subsequently shown to be recognized by 2 HLA-A2 restricted, melanoma reactive T cell clones (Brichard *et al.*, 1993). These clones recognized 2 distinct epitopes of tyrosinase, one starting with the amino terminal methionine of the tyrosinase signal sequence (MLLAVLYCL, tyr:1–9) and a second beginning with amino acid residue 369 (YMNGTMSQV, tyr:369–377) (Wölfel *et al.*, 1994). The naturally processed tyr:369–377 peptide epitope has been shown to contain a substitution of an aspartic acid for an asparagine residue at the third position that results from post-translational modification (Skipper *et al.*, 1996a). This modification, which was found at an asparagine residue that is part of an N-linked glycosylation site, may result from the activity of a mammalian enzyme that removes N-linked oligosaccharide side chains from glycopeptides (Suzuki *et al.*, 1993).

Distinct epitopes of tyrosinase recognized in the context of HLA-A24 (Robbins *et al.*, 1994; Kang *et al.*, 1995), HLA-B44 (Brichard *et al.*, 1996) as well as HLA-A1 (Kittlesen *et al.*, 1998) have been identified. In addition, 5 out of 6 HLA-A1 restricted CTL lines isolated from melanoma patients appeared to recognize the tyrosinase nanomer KCDICTDEY as well as the overlapping dodecamer DAEKCDICTDEY. Altered peptides containing either a serine or alanine residue at position 2 of the nanomer as well as the corresponding residue in the dodecamer were recognized at concentrations that were 100 to 1000-fold lower than the unmodified peptide. These results, which are similar to those discussed above for the gp100:639-647 epitope, indicate that N terminal cysteine present in the naturally processed T cell epitope may be protected from modification through binding to the HLA-A1 molecule. Modification of the downstream cysteine residue, however, may occur in the naturally processed HLA-A1 tyrosinase epitope.

Studies have also demonstrated that melanoma reactive T cells recognize the melanosomal proteins TRP-1(gp75) (Wang *et al.*, 1995) and TRP-2 (Wang *et al.*, 1996a). The gp75 protein, which has been found to be recognized by IgG antibodies in the serum of a patient with melanoma (Mattes *et al.*, 1983), represents one of the most abundant intracellular glycoproteins in melanocyte-lineage cells. A gp75 epitope recognized by HLA-A31 restricted melanoma reactive T cells was subsequently shown to be encoded at the amino terminus of a short, 24 amino acid alternative open reading frame (Wang *et al.*, 1996b). In addition to the epitope encoded by an alternative open reading frame of the NY-ESO-1 gene described above (Wang *et al.*, 1998b), T cell epitopes encoded by alternative open reading frames of a gene encoding a normal self protein (Malarkannan *et al.*, 1995) as well as a retroviral product (Mayrand *et al.*, 1998) have been observed. Thus, the translation of alternative open reading frames appears to represent a general mechanism for generating T cell epitopes.

Attempts have also been made to determine if T cell epitopes from TRP-1 and TRP-2 are recognized in the context of additional class I alleles. Both the TRP-1 and TRP-2 peptides were found to bind to HLA-A3, -A11, -A31, -A33 and -A68, and a TRP-2 peptide was recognized by T cells in the context of HLA-A31 and -A33 (Wang *et al.*, 1998a). These HLA types possess similar structures as well as similar binding motifs and fit into what has been termed the HLA-A3 like ''supertype'' (Sidney *et al.*, 1996). Thus, it may be possible to identify peptides that can be used to immunize patients expressing one of the class I alleles in the HLA-A3 superfamily. In an attempt to identify TRP-2 peptides that are recognized in the context of HLA-A2, peptides from this protein that fit the HLA-A2 binding motif were initially tested for binding to this class I molecule using a standard competitive inhibition assay (Sette *et al.*, 1994a). Twenty-one peptides that inhibited the binding of a standard peptide at a concentration of 2 μM or below were then used to generate CTL *in vitro* using PBL from HLA-A2 melanoma patients. One out of 21 HLA-A2 binding peptides that were tested, SVYDFFVWL, (TRP2:180-188) elicited CTL from patient PBL that recognized T2 cells pulsed with this peptide as well as HLA-A2+, TRP-2+ melanomas (Parkhurst *et al.*, 1998). Previously, the TRP-2:181-188 peptide, which is identical in the human and mouse TRP-2 proteins, was found to represent an immunodominant epitope recognized in the context of H-2K^b by B16-reactive CTL (Bloom *et al.*, 1997). Regression of established B16 lung metastases was observed following adoptive transfer of a CTL line generated by stimulation with this peptide. Subsequent studies demonstrated that the TRP-2:180–188 represented the optimal peptide recognized by mouse TRP-2 reactive CTL (J. Yang, personal communication). Thus, therapeutic strategies can be evaluated in a mouse model systems using the identical epitope recognized by human tumor-reactive T cells.

WIDELY EXPRESSED PROTEINS

Tumor antigens that appear to be expressed in a variety of normal tissues have been also been described (see Table 1.4). One example of this type of antigen is represented by the PRAME antigen (Ikeda *et al.*, 1997). A tumor derived from melanoma patient LB33, termed LB33.MEL.A, appeared to express multiple antigens that were recognized by autologous CTL in the context of the HLA-A28, B13, B44 and Cw6 class I genes (Lehmann *et al.*, 1995). A cell line derived from a tumor recurrence that was not recognized by these CTL, termed MEL.B, had lost the expression of all HLA class I alleles with the exception of HLA-A24. A CTL line generated against the MEL.B tumor, however, failed to recognize the MEL.A tumor. Using a conventional cDNA library approach, an antigen was isolated that appeared to be expressed at relative high levels in the testis and endometrium, and at lower but significant levels in other normal tissues such as ovary, adrenals, kidney, brain and skin. Expression of an NK inhibitory receptor molecule on the PRAME-reactive T cells prevented the recognition of the original tumor, and possibly normal tissues, due to recognition of the HLA-Cw7 class I molecule.

In other cases where expression has been found at relatively high levels in normal tissues, such as the p15 antigen, it is not clear what mechanism is responsible for the ability of T cells to discriminate tumor from normal tissues (Robbins *et al.*, 1995). A previously undescribed antigen termed SART-1 has also recently been cloned using a CTL line that was generated by stimulation with an autologous **squamous cell carcinoma** (Shichijo *et al.*, 1998). Expression of this gene was observed in **lung adenocarcinomas** as well as lung and **esophageal squamous cell carcinomas**. Preliminary results indicated that a second translated product that initiated within the central portion of this gene was expressed in the cytoplasm of tumor cells but not normal cells, and recognition of this product might account for the tumor specificity of T cell responses against this antigen (Yang *et al.*, 1999). Widely expressed antigens were also recently found in renal cell cancer as derived from intestinal carboxyl esterase (Ronsin *et al.*, 1999), while overexpression of the oncoproteion HER2/neu has been shown to provide epitopes recognized by T cells after DC presentation in several tumors, including ovarian and breast cancers and melanoma (Rongcun *et al.*, 1999).

TUMOR-SPECIFIC ANTIGENS

A number of antigens that have a more limited pattern of expression than the cancer/testis or melanocyte differentiation antigens have been isolated. Certain somatic mutations have only been identified in a single tumor; however, other mutations appear to be expressed in multiple tumors, implying that these mutations may play a role in tumorogenesis. In a few cases, transcripts that appear to be limited in their expression to tumor cells have been shown to encode tumor antigens. Mutated class I epitopes have been identified from a number of mouse tumors, and appear to represent potent tumor rejection antigens (Lurquin *et al.*, 1989; Mandelboim *et al.*, 1995; Dubey *et al.*, 1997). The restricted expression pattern of these products, however, clearly limits their use in tumor vaccines at the present time. Nevertheless, these studies have provided insights into the biology of tumor cells that may lead to the development of anti-cancer agents. The following is a summary of the main features of the tumor-restricted antigens (Table 1.5).

A previously undescribed gene termed MUM-1 was isolated using HLA-B44 restricted T cells of a melanoma patient (Coulie *et al.*, 1995). This cDNA clone appeared to contain an intronic sequence that had been retained within the mRNA transcript, and the region that spanned the intron/exon boundary encoded the T cell epitope. The cDNA clone also contained a single base pair mutation that altered a T cell contact residue, since both the normal and mutated peptides appeared to bind equivalently to HLA-B44.

A mutated HLA-A2 molecule has been identified using T cells that recognize a **renal carcinoma** (Brandle *et al.*, 1996). This mutation, which was present in the α helix region of the HLA-A2 $\alpha 2$ domain, effectively resulted in the generation of an allogeneic MHC molecule in this tumor. This represents the first observation of a somatic mutation in a tumor that alters the amino acid sequence of an MHC molecule. Mutations that alter MHC molecules expressed in tumors may generally result in the rejection of tumors that express these products and thus may only rarely be observed.

More recently, several peptide epitopes that bound to HLA-A2 were isolated in a renal cell carcinoma expressing the G250 molecules. At least one of these peptides was able to induce HLA-A2-restricted CTL that recognize renal tumor cells endogeneously expressing the peptide (Vissers *et al.*, 1999). It is of interest that G250 is found in 85% of renal cancer cells but not in normal kidney.

A mutated product of the cyclin-dependent kinase 4 (CDK4) gene, a gene involved in cell cycle progression, was isolated using an HLA-A2 restricted CTL clone (Wölfel *et al.*, 1995). The region encoding the minimal T cell epitope, ACDPHSGHFV, contained a single base pair change resulting in a substitution of cysteine for arginine at the second position in this peptide. Target cells could be sensitized for lysis by CDK4 reactive T cell clones using approximately 100-fold lower concentrations of the mutant than the normal peptide, but antigen processing may also be affected by this mutation. Significantly, binding of the normal CDK4 inhibitor, $p16^{INK4a}$, appeared to be partially disrupted by the CDK4 mutation. The $p16^{INK4a}$ gene was found to be frequently mutated in a variety of cancers including melanomas, and genetic susceptibility to melanoma is associated with mutations of the $p16^{INK4a}$ locus (Sherr, 1996). Thus, disruption of this interaction either through inactivation of the p16 gene product or mutation of particular key residues in the CDK4 gene product may lead to unregulated tumor cell growth. This mutation was also observed in 1 out of 28 additional melanomas that were examined, providing further support for the role of this mutation in carcinogenesis.

Use of tumor reactive T cells that recognized a **bladder carcinoma** in the context of HLA-B44 also resulted in the isolation of a previously undescribed gene containing a single point mutation (Gueguen *et al.*, 1998). A point mutation in this gene resulted in the substitution of an asparagine for an aspartic acid residue at position 5 of the peptide epitope. This residue appeared to represent a T cell contact residue, since binding of this peptide to HLA-B*4403 was unaffected by this alteration. This mutation was expressed in the tumor cell line as well as a fresh tumor sample that was isolated from the autologous patient, but not in over 100 additional tumors that were examined. It is not clear if this mutation has any effect on tumor cells, since the function of this gene product is unknown.

A cDNA clone encoding a mutated caspase-8 (CASP-8) gene product was recently isolated by carrying out expression cloning using HLA-B35 restricted T cells reactive with a **squamous cell carcinoma** (Mandruzzato *et al.*, 1997). This cDNA contained a single point mutation within that resulted in the substitution of a serine residue for the normal stop codon of the CASP-8 gene product. This change resulted in a carboxy terminal extension of the normal open reading frame by 88 amino acids, and the T cell epitope was encoded within this region. Preliminary evidence indicated that the CASP-8 mutation interfered with the apoptotic activity of this protein; this mutation was not, however, found in 150 additional tumors that were analyzed. Thus, it is not clear if alterations in the apoptotic pathway plays a role any role in tumorogenesis.

A mutated β-catenin gene product was isolated by screening a cDNA library using an HLA-A24 restricted tumor reactive CTL line (Robbins *et al.*, 1996). The peptide epitope that was identified, corresponding to amino acids 29 to 37 of the β-catenin molecule (SYLDSGIHF), contained a single point mutation in codon 37 that changed a serine to a phenylalanine residue. The mutated peptide was recognized at a 10^6 fold lower concentration than the normal peptide, and binding studies indicated that the mutated peptide had a significantly higher binding affinity for HLA-A24 than the normal peptide. The identical mutation has now been found in **melanomas** isolated from a total of 4 out of the 45 patients that were examined (Rubinfeld *et al.*, 1997; P. Robbins, unpublished observations). In addition, melanomas containing a mutation of the serine residue at position 45 of β-catenin as well as deletions encompassing this region, which contains several serine residues that appear to represent phosphorylation sites, were isolated from additional patients (Rubinfeld *et al.*, 1997). Mutations in this region of β-catenin have been observed in a variety of tumor types including colon (Korinek *et al.*, 1997; Morin *et al.*, 1997) and hepatocellular carcinomas (de La Coste *et al.*, 1998). These mutations appear to stabilize the β-catenin molecule and to promote formation of complexes with members of the Tcf family of DNA binding proteins, which could potentially activate target genes involved in tumorogenesis.

Aberrant gene transcripts whose expression appears to be limited to tumor cells have also been identified. A product of the N-acetylglucosaminyltransferase V (GnT-V) gene was isolated by expression cloning techniques using an HLA-A2 restricted tumor reactive T cell clone (Guilloux *et al.*, 1996). Activation of a cryptic promoter present within one of the introns of the GnT-V gene resulted in the generation of an aberrant transcript, and the T cell epitope was encoded by sequences within a short open reading frame of 74 amino acids encoded within this region. The intronic transcript appeared to be expressed in about 50% of the melanomas that were examined but not in the majority of other tumor types tested. In addition, semi-quantitative RT-PCR analysis indicated that this product was not expressed in normal skin. Cultured melanocytes appeared to express this product; however, this may represent a tissue culture artifact. The GnT-V transcript identified in this report may represent one of only a few examples of a truly tumor-specific product.

Results reported in a recent study indicate that a retained intronic sequence from the TRP-2 gene may also represent a tumor-specific product (Lupetti *et al.*, 1998). A partial cDNA clone that was isolated using an HLA-A68 restricted, melanoma reactive T cell clone was found to contain the second intron of the TRP-2 gene as well as a portion of the fourth intron of this gene. Translation of the normal TRP-2 open reading frame, which extended through part of the second intron before a stop codon was encountered, would result in the production of a protein of 227 amino acids, 39 of which would be encoded by the intronic sequence. A T cell epitope that conformed to the HLA-A68 binding motif, EVISCKLIKR, was encoded within the region derived from the second intron (Rammensee *et al.*, 1995). The results of RT-PCR analysis indicated that transcripts containing the second intron were either undetectable or were expressed at very low levels in melanocytes, whereas this transcript was readily detected in melanomas that expressed TRP-2. These T cells failed to recognize melanocytes expressing HLA-A68, as expected on the basis of these findings. In contrast, comparable levels of a gp100 gene transcript containing the fourth intron of this gene were found in melanocytes and melanomas. As noted above, T cells that recognized a gp100 epitope encoded within the fourth intron of gp100 in the context of HLA-A24 had previously been found to react with melanoma cells as well as normal melanocytes expressing this class I allele (Robbins *et al.*, 1997). Thus, it appears that epitopes derived from introns can represent either tumor-specific or normal differentiation antigens.

Additional recently reported tumor-specific antigens that are generated either by point mutations or other less defined mechanisms resulting into new unique or shared antigens, respectively. A TIL line obtained from a primary regressing melanoma was shown to recognize a point mutated form of myosin (Zorn and Hercend, 1999), while mutation of HSP70-2 generated a high affinity epitope in a renal cell carcinoma recognized by HLA-A2-restricted CTL (Gaudin *et al.*, 1999). The list of new antigens generated by mutation in melanoma also includes two epitopes recognized either by HLA-B44 or HLA-Cw6-restricted CTLs on melanoma cells of a patient who enjoyed an unusually favorable clinical evaluation associated with strong and sustained antitumor CTL response (Chiari *et al.*, 1999). It is of interest that even lung cancers may express unique antigens, like that isolated by immunoaffinity chromatography, reverse phase HPLC and mass spectrometry from a tumor line, which turned out to be a mutated form of the elongation factor 2 recognized by HLA-A68-restricted CTLs (Hogan *et al.*, 1998). This work emphasizes the biochemical approach to characterization of natural antigens in tumor different from melanoma. By a similar approach a new antigen, whose tissue distribution however remains to be determined, has been isolated from a gastric signal ring carcinoma (Suzuky *et al.*, 1999). Antigens which are expressed in tumor cells but not in normal counterparts can be generated by a variety of mechanisms (see above). Peptide epitopes that are derived from α-fetoprotein, a protein known to be overexpressed in several liver tumors, are recognized by CTLs generated by exploiting the potent antigen presentation function of DC. Evidence that such effectors can target naturally processed peptides is still, however, lacking (Butterfield *et al.*, 1999).

A remarkable new finding in terms of tumor-specific antigens is that reported by Vonderheide and co-workers (1999), who found that the telomerase catalytic subunit (hTERT) can provide peptide epitopes recognized by T cells in more than 85% of human tumor tested, but not on normal tissues with the possible exception of activated B cells. Though some tumors may lack hTERT activity and further studies are needed, hTERT represents a promising antigen to be tested *in vivo* (Table 1.5).

Viruses have been shown to be involved with the development of certain human tumor types, and viral proteins represent tumor-specific molecules that can be used as targets for T cell vaccines. The HPV has been shown to play a role in the development of cervical carcinomas, and T cell epitopes have been identified in the HPV E7 gene (Alexander *et al.*, 1996; Ressing *et al.*, 1996). Endogenous retroviral sequences, which have been found in the genome of both mice and man, have also been shown to be recognized by tumor reactive T cells. A CTL line generated by immunization with a GM-CSF transduced CT26 mouse colon tumor cell line was capable of mediating tumor regression upon adoptive transfer (Huang *et al.*, 1996). The T cell epitope, identified by elution of peptides from the tumor cell surface, was derived from an endogenous retroviral envelope sequence. Expression of this antigen, which was found in a variety of tumors but not in normal tissues, may have resulted from the transformation process. Antigens derived from endogenous retroviruses, if identified in human tumors, would represent additional targets for the development of antitumor therapies.

Thus, the search for widely expressed, common tumor-specific antigens has resulted in a number of new candidate antigens that can now be further characterized and, used for vaccination of cancer patients.

CLASS II MHC RESTRICTED TUMOR ANTIGENS

Studies carried out in mouse model systems have demonstrated that class II restricted T cells can in some cases mediate tumor regression. Although it is not clear what role they play in these responses, cytokine production in the tumor microenvironment by $CD4^+$ cells may be involved in the activation of tumor-reactive $CD8^+$ T cells. Observations suggest, however, that $CD4^+$ T cells may play a critical role in activating APC to facilitate efficient stimulation of naïve $CD8^+$ T cells (Bennett *et al.*, 1997; Bennett *et al.*, 1998; Schoenberger *et al.*, 1998). In addition, recruitment of inflammatory cells such as neutrophils by tumor-reactive $CD4^+$ T cells may play a role in tumor rejection (Cavallo *et al.*, 1992).

A number of class II antigens have now been identified in mouse tumor model systems. Studies carried out with murine leukemias have demonstrated a clear role for class II restricted T cells that recognize an antigen derived from an endogenous retroviral envelope in mediating antitumor immune responses (Iwashiro *et al.*, 1993). A mutated gene encoding the L9 ribosomal protein isolated from a murine sarcoma has been shown to be recognized by tumor-specific, class II restricted T cells (Monach *et al.*, 1995). Adoptive transfer of T cell clones directed against the mutated L9 peptide epitope has been shown to mediate tumor regression.

Class II restricted T cells have been identified that recognize a wide variety of human tumor types (Schwartzentruber *et al.*, 1992; Topalian *et al.*, 1994a, 1994b; Heike *et al.*, 1996; Nakao *et al.*, 1997). A $CD4^+$ melanoma reactive TIL has been shown to recognize the non-mutated tyrosinase gene product after screening transfectants expressing candidate melanoma antigens (Topalian *et al.*, 1994a) and two peptide epitopes of tyrosinase that are recognized in the context of HLA-DRB1*0401 have been identified (Topalian *et al.*, 1996), while $CD4^+$ T cell clones recognizing additional tyrosinase peptides were obtained from a patient PBLs (Kobayashi *et al.*, 1998) (see Table 1.6). Recently, genes that encode

TABLE 1.6
Class II HLA-restricted antigens

Gene	*HLA-DRB1 allele*	*Peptide epitope*	*Reference*
Epitopes from normal protein antigens			
Gp100	*0401	p44–59	Li *et al.*, 1998
MAGE-3	*1101	TSYVKVLHHMVKISG	Manici *et al.*, 1999
MAGE-3	*1301	AELVHFLLLKYRAR	Chaux *et al.*, 1999
MAGE-1, -2, -3, -6	*1301	LLKYRAREPVTKAE	Chaux *et al.*, 1999
Tyrosinase	*0401	QNILLSNAPLGPQFP	Topalian *et al.*, 1994a
		DYSYLQDSDPDSFQD	Topalian *et al.*, 1996
Tyrosinase	*1501	p386–406	Kobayashi *et al.*, 1998
Epitopes from mutated protein antigens			
CDC27m	*0401	FSWAMDLDPKGA	Wang *et al.*, 1999a
TPI*m	*0101	GELIGILNAAKVPAD	Pieper *et al.*, 1999
Epitopes resulting from a fused protein			
LDLR/FUT†	*0101	GGAPPVTWRRAPAPG	Wang *et al.*, 1999b
		WRRAPAPGAKAMAPG	Wang *et al.*, 1999b

* Triosephosphate isomerase.
† Low density lipid receptor/GDP-L-fucose: β-D-galactosidase 2-α-L-fucosyltrasferase.

antigens recognized by class II restricted, melanoma reactive T cells have also been identified using a modification of the cDNA library cloning approach used to isolate class I antigens (Wang *et al.*, 1999a) or other approaches (Chaux *et al.*, 1999; Manici *et al.*, 1999; Pieper *et al.*, 1999). It is remarkable that two of these antigens were the result of a mutation (Wang *et al.*, 1999a; Pieper *et al.*, 1999), while a third one resulted from a fusion between a gene coding for a low density lipid receptor (LDLR) and a gene encoding the GDP-L-fucose:β-D-galactosidase 2-α-L-fucosyltrasferase (FUT) (Wang *et al.*, 1999b). Two additional antigens are shared determinants of the MAGE family (Chaux *et al.*, 1999; Manici *et al.*, 1999).

Additional efforts have focused on the generation of responses against candidate antigens. *In vitro* stimulation with peptides derived from the junction of the bcr-abl fusion protein resulted in the generation of T cells that recognize APC that had been pulsed with tumor cell lysates (Manering *et al.*, 1997). Class II restricted $CD4^+$ responses have also been elicited *in vitro* using peptides derived from the HPV E7 protein (De Gruji *et al.*, 1998).

The identification of peptides that are bound to class II MHC molecules isolated from tumor cells represents another method for identifying candidate epitopes. A number of peptides have recently been identified in peptide pools isolated from melanoma cell derived class II molecules, including peptides from annexin and gp100 (Halder *et al.*, 1997). Use of a gp100 peptide isolated from the melanoma for *in vitro* sensitization appeared to result in the generation of peptide reactive, but not tumor-reactive T cells.

The observation that a number of tumor antigens elicit IgG antibodies indicates that the molecules may also contain $CD4^+$ T cell epitopes. Antibodies directed against a number of antigens that are recognized by class I restricted T cells, including NY-ESO-1, which was originally discovered using this technique, tyrosinase, TRP-1, MAGE-1 and MAGE-3, have been found in the serum of melanoma, ovarian, lung and breast cancer patients (Stockert *et al.*, 1998). Further exploration of the nature of these antigens using purified recombinant proteins as well as class II binding peptides derived from these molecules may provide additional targets for immunotherapy.

IDENTIFICATION OF EPITOPES ON CANDIDATE ANTIGENS

A number of potential approaches to identify new tumor antigen peptide epitopes have been reported, including *in vitro* sensitization with HLA binding peptides as well as the immunization of transgenic mice expressing human MHC alleles. The identification of candidate epitopes that are naturally processed and presented in tumor cells could be carried out by sequencing peptides that have been eluted from the tumor cell surface. An attempt has recently been made to generate tumor-reactive T cells using HLA-A2 binding peptides from gp100 that had not previously been shown to be recognized by HLA-A2 restricted T cells (Tsai *et al.*, 1997). Three out of 6 gp100 peptides that had been identified on the basis of their high to moderate affinity for HLA-A2 appeared to elicit melanoma reactive CTL *in vitro*. In contrast, 2 of the 6 peptides were capable of generating peptide-reactive T cells that failed to recognize tumor targets. Subsequent studies have resulted in the demonstration that the gp100:619-627 peptide was recognized by CTL clones isolated from a melanoma patient (Kawakami *et al.*, 1998). In the study cited above (Tsai *et al.*, 1997), the gp100:619-627 peptide appeared to induce peptide-reactive T cells; however, clear tumor reactivity could not be demonstrated using T cells stimulated using this peptide. Stimulation with peptide pulsed targets expressing relatively high levels of class I MHC complexes may, however, result in the generation of low affinity T cells that cannot recognize tumor cell targets expressing relatively low levels of endogenously processed antigens. In contrast, T cells that arise following *in vitro* or *in vivo* stimulation with tumor, such as TIL, presumably express high affinity receptors that are capable of recognizing naturally processed epitopes. T cell tolerance may also play a role in skewing the repertoire of T cells that respond to peptides derived from self-antigens such as gp100 towards cells that bind these epitopes with a relatively low affinity. The relatively large pool of T cells with low affinity for peptides may overgrow a small population of high affinity T cells that can recognize tumor cells expressing low levels of endogenously processed epitopes.

Peptides derived from the MC1R have been tested for their ability to stimulate melanoma-reactive T cells (Salazar-Onfray *et al.*, 1997). This protein, which appears to be expressed primarily in cells of the melanocyte lineage, is a member of a family of G-protein-coupled receptors that bind melanocyte-stimulating hormone. Stimulations of PBMC from normal donors carried out using three peptides derived from the MC1R protein with either high or intermediate affinity for HLA-A2 appeared to result in the generation of T cells that recognized HLA-A2+, M1CR+ melanomas.

The Her2/neu protein, which is a member of the tyrosinase kinase family of receptors, has been frequently found to be amplified and over-expressed in a variety of tumors including breast, ovarian and colorectal tumors (see Table 4) (Slamon *et al.*, 1987). In addition, some studies have suggested that overexpression of this protein may influence the tumorogenicity of cancer cells (Katsumata *et al.*, 1995; Schlegel *et al.*, 1997), thus making this an attractive target for the development of anti-cancer therapies. Studies of the specificity of Tumor Associated Lymphocytes (TAL) that had been isolated from malignant ascites and cultured in the presence of IL-2 indicated that they recognized several HLA-A2 binding peptides derived from Her2/neu (Fisk *et al.*, 1995). Four out of 4 TAL lines appeared to recognize the HER-2/neu:369-377 peptide, indicating that this represented an immunodominant peptide epitope. It has been reported that the HER-2/neu:654-662 peptide was recognized by breast and ovarian cancer TIL (Peoples *et al.*, 1995), and additional peptides derived from this protein that appear to represent T cell epitopes have been identified by immunizing double transgenic mice expressing the human HLA-A2 and CD8 molecules (Lustgarten *et al.*, 1997), as well as by stimulating normal PBL with peptide pulsed dendritic cells (Kawashima *et al.*, 1998).

Antigen-presenting cells that have been either directly transfected with constructs encoding target molecules or infected with recombinant viral constructs have also been used to stimulate tumor-reactive T cells. Stimulation with autologous adherent cells isolated from peripheral blood that had been infected with a recombinant vaccinia virus encoding tyrosinase has been shown to result in the generation of tumor-reactive T cells that recognize tyrosinase in association with a variety of MHC restriction elements (Yee *et al.*, 1996). In addition, tumor-reactive T cells appeared to be generated following stimulation with dendritic cells that had been transfected with genes encoding MART-1 and gp100, tyrosinase, MAGE-1 or MAGE-3 in conjunction with IL-12 or IFN-α (Tuting *et al.*, 1998).

A number of studies have been carried out in an attempt to generate responses against peptides derived from the p53 tumor suppressor protein. Initial studies carried out in HLA-A2 transgenic mice utilized immunization with a number of peptides from the human p53 protein (Theobald *et al.*, 1995). Human p53 peptides that differed from the mouse p53 sequence were found to generate T cells that were capable of recognizing human tumors that overexpressed p53 but not non-transformed human cells. In a subsequent study, T cells responses of normal HLA-A2 transgenic mice were compared with A2 transgenic mice that lacked expression of p53 in any normal tissues (p53 knock out mice) (Theobald *et al.*, 1997). A wild type peptide, p53:187–197, was found to elicit an immune response in p53 knock-out mice but not normal mice, indicating that expression of this peptide in normal tissues may result in T cell tolerance. Another p53 peptide, mouse p53:261–269, which is identical to the human p53:264–272 peptide, could stimulate response in both normal and knock-out mice; however, T cells derived from normal mice appeared to have a significantly lower affinity for this peptide than knock-out mice. The CTL that were generated from normal mice appeared to recognize peptide pulsed targets but failed to recognize tumor cells that overexpressed p53, whereas those generated in the knock-out mice recognized tumor cells. Immunization of p53 knock-out mice with syngeneic tumor cells that overexpressed p53 has also been shown to result in stimulation of T cells that recognized p53 peptides (Vierboom *et al.*, 1997). Transfer of these T cells into p53+ tumor-bearing nude as well as normal mice was found to result in tumor regression, but no adverse effects on normal mouse tissues were observed.

The results of some studies carried out with human PBL have indicated that stimulation with the human p53:264–272 peptide may result in the generation of tumor-reactive T cells. A CTL clone generated by *in vitro* stimulation with this peptide appeared to recognize 2 squamous carcinoma cell lines (Ropke *et al.*, 1996). There appeared to be a lack of correlation between recognition and overexpression of p53, since one of the cell lines that was recognized did not overexpress p53, whereas an HLA-A2+ squamous carcinoma cell line that overexpressed p53 was not recognized. Thus, there may be additional factors that influence the recognition of these cell lines. In a separate investigation, CTL lines generated from a healthy donor with the p53:264–272 peptide were shown to recognize peptide pulsed targets as well as one melanoma and 2 breast cancer cell lines (Gnjatic *et al.*, 1998). The tumor cell lines that were recognized overexpressed p53, although one of the breast cancer cell lines that was recognized did not express a mutated p53 gene product.

A number of molecules that represent potential T cell targets have been identified through the use of the SEREX technique (Chen *et al.*, 1998; Scanlan *et al.*, 1998; Tureci *et al.*, 1998). Representational difference analysis, a genetic technique that relies on differences in the expression in various tissues, has been used to isolate other potential T cell targets. These include a new member of the MAGE gene family (Lucas *et al.*, 1998) as well as LAGE (Lethe *et al.*, 1998) , a gene that is highly homologous to NY-ESO-1. The development of efficient methods for stimulating T cell responses against candidate antigens such as these may facilitate the development of new therapeutic reagents.

MODULATION OF T CELL RECOGNITION

Studies carried out *in vitro* have indicated that a number of factors may influence T cell recognition of peptide/MHC complexes. Analysis of the expression of MAGE-1 in melanomas using a quantitative PCR technique indicated that at least 10% of the level found in a reference melanoma MZ2-MEL.3.0 expressing a high level of the MAGE-1 gene transcript was required for recognition by specific CTL (Lethe *et al.*, 1997). An initial report indicated that tumor-reactive T cells could be generated by stimulating with lymphoblasts that had been pulsed with an HLA-A2-binding peptide from MAGE-3 (van der Bruggen *et al.*, 1994a). In a second study, however, T cells that were generated using peptide pulsed target cells could recognize cells that had been transfected with the MAGE-3 cDNA, but failed to recognize tumor cells expressing normal endogenous levels of this protein (Valmori *et al.*, 1997). The ability of T cell epitopes to be efficiently processed and presented on the cell surface has been shown to be influenced by sequences within the peptide epitope as well as sequences that flank the T cell epitope (Eisenlohr *et al.*, 1992; Ossendorp *et al.*, 1996). The level of expression of a particular tumor antigen gene product, as well as the levels of expression of adhesion molecules (Mortarini *et al.*, 1990), clearly can influence tumor cell recognition by T cells. Studies of tumor clones (Rivoltini *et al.*, 1995) as well as tumor cell lines selected *in vitro* for resistance to lysis by CTL (Kono *et al.*, 1997) have demonstrated a correlation between the level of class I gene expression and T cell recognition. Variations in the levels of MART-1 and gp100, as well as class I gene expression in melanoma cell lines derived from different patients, were also shown to significantly affect CTL recognition of those cell lines (Cormier *et al.*, 1999). In addition, the affinity of the TCR for the peptide-MHC complex might be influenced by self-tolerance, since peptides expressed on normal tissues such as melanocytes may anergize T cells bearing high affinity TCRs.

The affinity of peptide binding to an MHC class I product, as assessed in equilibrium binding assays (Sette *et al.*, 1994b), as well as in assays that measure the stability of peptide/MHC complexes, appears to be an important determinant of peptide immunogenicity (Parker *et al.*, 1995; van der Burg *et al.*, 1996). Nevertheless, a number of the dominant tumor antigen epitopes that have been identified from MART-1 and gp100 do not fit the optimal HLA-A2 binding motif and appear to bind to HLA-A2 with relatively low or intermediate affinities. It is not clear why responses directed against these epitopes are so predominant in HLA-A2 melanoma patients.

Several studies have now suggested that substitution of optimal for non-optimal anchor residues in peptide derived from gp100 and MART-1 can significantly enhance the immunogenicity of these peptides. Substitutions of either leucine or methionine for threonine at position 2 of the gp100:209–217 peptide appeared to enhance the HLA-A2 binding affinity by a factor of 52 and 9, respectively (Parkhurst *et al.*, 1996). Tumor-reactive T cells could be elicited more reliably after fewer *in vitro* stimulations when the modified peptide containing methionine at position 2 was used than when the native gp100:209–217 peptide was used. As described below, the results of clinical trials demonstrated that injection of modified gp100 peptides resulted in enhanced anti-peptide as well as anti-tumor responses (Rosenberg *et al.*, 1998a).

Alterations have also been made in the MART-1 HLA-A2 peptide in an attempt to enhance the immunogenicity of this peptide, which appears to possess a relatively low affinity for HLA-A2. The decamer peptide EAAGIGILTV (MART-1_{26-35}) appeared to be recognized at significantly lower concentrations than the nanomer peptide by several peptide reactive T cell clones (Romero *et al.*, 1997; Schneider *et al.*, 1998). Significant differences were observed when the recognition of MART-1 peptide-variants by peptide-reactive T cell clones was examined (Valmori *et al.*, 1998). Variants of the MART-1_{26-35} peptide that contained a substitution of leucine or methionine at position 2 appeared to possess more stable binding to HLA-A2 than the unmodified decamer and nanomer. Peptides containing substitution of tyrosinase or phenylalanine for glutamic acid at position 1 of the decamer also demonstrated enhanced binding to HLA-A2, but only the leucine-containing peptide appeared to be strongly recognized by all of the T cell clones. Recognition of the leucine-containing peptide by T cell clones appeared to be enhanced by between 100 and 20,000 fold in comparison to the native nanomer. This peptide was also found to generate tumor-reactive cells *in vitro* more readily than the native peptide, suggesting that this peptide might represent a more potent immunogen *in vivo*. A similar finding was obtained when the nonamer MART-1_{27-35} was modified by a single substitution with leucine at position 1 (Rivoltini *et al.*, 1999).

Self-tolerance mechanisms may also influence responses to antigens such as MART-1 and gp100. In a recent report, T cells isolated from patients with vitiligo, an autoimmune disease that appears to result from the destruction of normal skin melanocytes, were examined for their ability to recognize the MART-1 antigen using a class I MHC tetramer bound to an optimized MART-1 peptide (Ogg *et al.*, 1998). The PBMC from 7 out of 9 HLA-A2+ vitiligo patients appeared to contain a relatively high frequency of T cells reactive with the MART-1 peptide, when analyzed using this technique. These T cells expressed high levels of the skin homing receptor CLA antigen, a form of the P selectin-binding glycoprotein 1 (Fuhlbrigge *et al.*, 1997). In one out of six normal HLA-A2+ individuals, T cells reactive with MART-1 were found, but these cells did not appear to express CLA. Thus, expression of accessory molecules such as CLA may play a role in the maintenance of tolerance to normal tissue antigens.

T CELL RECEPTOR ANALYSIS

Some studies have demonstrated preferential usage of particular TCR α and β variable region sequences in responses to melanoma antigens (Sensi *et al.*, 1995). However, additional studies have demonstrated that recognition of a single antigenic epitope may be mediated by T cells expressing a diverse set of TCRs (Cole *et al.*, 1997). T cells that express certain TCRs have, however, been shown to be enriched in populations of TIL isolated from untreated melanoma patients (Clemente *et al.*, 1998) as well as from patients immunized with either dinitrophenyl modified tumor cells or the HLA-A1 MAGE-3 peptide epitope (Sensi *et al.*, 1998). The repertoire of TCRs expressed by tumor-reactive T cells may be quite varied in the peripheral blood of patients; nevertheless, a more restricted set of T cell clonotypes may be expanded *in vivo* at the tumor site or in tumor-involved lymph nodes. The generation of clonotypic markers based upon unique sequences present in the complementary determining regions of individual TCRs α or β chains may also facilitate monitoring of lymphocyte survival and trafficking at these sites *in vivo*.

CLINICAL APPLICATIONS

Clinical trials are now being carried out to evaluate the effect of immunization with specific peptides as well as recombinant viral constructs encoding tumor antigens, and the observations made in these trials may play an important role in the development of future therapies (Table 1.7). A critical feature of these trials is the use and development of assays that allow accurate monitoring of patient responses. The effects of immunization have been monitored using limiting dilution assays (Coulie *et al.*, 1992; Mazzocchi *et al.*, 1994) as

TABLE 1.7
Approaches to cancer immunotherapy based upon defined tumor antigens

1. Immunization with peptide epitopes
- Inject peptides with adjuvants
- Use cytokines such as IL-2 and IL-12
- Pulse peptides on antigen presenting cells such as dendritic cells
- Use modified peptides with increased binding to class I molecules

2. Immunization with viral constructs
- Vaccinia, fowlpox, adenoviral constructs encoding whole tumor antigen proteins
- Constructs encoding peptide epitope minigenes or modified peptide epitope minigenes

3. Immunization with "naked" DNA

4. Adoptive transfer of T cell clones directed against peptide epitopes
- Isolate tumor-reactive T cell clones from normal or immunized patients after *in vitro* sensitization

5. Immunization with whole protein

6. Immunization with combinations of class I and class II peptide epitopes

well as measurements of the ability of T cells to generate immune responses following one or a small number of *in vitro* stimulations. Assays that allow the individual tumor-reactive T cells to be directly enumerated, such as the ELISPOT assay, have also been used to characterize antitumor immune responses (Scheibenbogen *et al.*, 1997). The use of complexes of class I MHC tetramers bound to specific peptides has facilitated the detection as well as the direct isolation of peptide-specific T cells (Altman *et al.*, 1996; Dunbar *et al.*, 1998). In a recent study, T cell precursors reactive with the MART-1:26–35 peptide were detected in melanoma patients at frequencies between 1 in 50 and 1 in 500 in tumor-infiltrated lymph nodes, whereas the frequency of T cells at the same sites that were reactive with the tyrosinase 368–376 peptide was below the limit of detection (< 0.05%) (Romero *et al.*, 1998). The analysis of TCR expression can also be used to detect the presence of specific T cells. These assays can be carried out using cells isolated from tumor-involved lymph nodes as well as tumor and peripheral blood, which will allow monitoring of lymphocyte trafficking following immunization or adoptive transfer.

A number of clinical trials have been carried out using the HLA-A1 binding peptides derived from the MAGE-1 and MAGE-3 antigens as well as peptides from MART-1, gp100 and tyrosinase (see Chapter 5). Partial and complete tumor regressions were seen in 7 out of 25 patients immunized with the MAGE-3 peptide in soluble form (Marchand *et al.*, 1999). Immunization with autologous APC that had been pulsed with the MAGE-1 peptide appeared to result in some enhancement of the frequency of peptide-reactive T cells in the peripheral blood of immunized patients, but no significant clinical responses were observed (Hu *et al.*, 1996).

The efficacy of recombinant viral vaccines that encode melanoma antigens has also been evaluated in clinical trials. Objective clinical responses were only rarely observed in patients adenoviral or vaccinia and constructs encoding gp100 as well as MART-1, and *in vitro* responses to these antigens were not enhanced in immunized patients. One possible explanation for these findings is the observation that high titers of neutralizing antibodies were present in the majority of patients in these trials before vaccination with these constructs, presumably resulting from smallpox vaccination and environmental exposure to adenovirus (Rosenberg *et al.*, 1998b).

In an attempt to develop immunotherapies for patients with other tumors, a clinical trial involving immunization with the HER-2/neu:369–377 peptide has recently been carried out in the Surgery Branch, NCI. No clinical responses were seen in this trial, where patients were immunized with 1 mg of peptide in IFA. In an attempt to assess the ability of this peptide to immunize these patients, the CTL response of PBMC obtained from breast cancer patients, obtained either before or after multiple peptide immunizations, was examined following out a single *in vitro* stimulation with peptide for 7 to 10 days. A vigorous peptide-specific T cell response was elicited by *in vitro* stimulation of post-immunization PBMC isolated from 3 of the 4 patients that were examined, whereas a weak peptide-specific response could be generated from only 1 out of 4 patients prior to immunization (Zaks and Rosenberg, 1998). The CTL isolated from immunized patients could recognize targets pulsed with a minimum of approximately 1 ng/ml of peptide, in the range of the minimum concentration required for the recognition of targets pulsed with other tumor epitopes (Kawakami *et al.*, 1994b; Kawakami *et al.*, 1995). The peptide-reactive CTL that were generated from immunized patients, however, failed to react with either HLA-A2+ breast and ovarian tumor cell lines that naturally overexpressed HER-2/neu or with transfected cell lines expressing both of these gene products. In an *in vitro* study where the ability of a variety of peptides including the HER-2/neu:369-377 peptide to stimulate responses *in vitro* was examined, only 2 out of 29 peptide-reactive cultures appeared to recognize tumors that overexpressed this gene product (Kawashima *et al.*, 1998). The tumor cell lines used as targets in this study, however, had been treated with IFN-γ, and it is not clear how well these T cells would recognize unmanipulated targets. Thus, endogenous processing of Her-2/neu may not generally result in sufficient level of expression of this peptide epitope on the cell surface to allow recognition by peptide-reactive T cells.

Even in the case of well-characterized tumor antigens, differences in expression levels as well as heterogeneity in antigen expression *in vivo* may impact on the efficacy of immunotherapies. In several studies where antigen expression in tumor cells was examined using immunohistochemistry, melanoma cells appeared to express relatively homogenous levels of tyrosinase, whereas the levels of other antigens such as MART-1, gp100 or TRP-1 appeared to be more variable (Chen *et al.*, 1995; Cormier *et al.*, 1998). Treatment of cells with reagents that enhance tumor cell recognition by T cells represent one approach to this problem. Induction of MHC class I gene expression and enhanced recognition of small cell lung cancer cells by MAGE-3 reactive T cells were seen following treatment of tumor cells with IFN-γ (Traversari *et al.*, 1997) (see Chapter 5).

Immune responses directed against specific antigens may also result in the generation of antigen loss variants *in vivo*. As described above, autologous CTL recognized a melanoma cell line derived from patient LB33 in 1988 in the context of multiple class I restriction elements, but a subsequent metastasis isolated 3 years later from this patient had lost expression of all of class I alleles with the exception of HLA-A24 (Lehmann *et al.*, 1995). Evidence for the loss of antigen as well as HLA class I gene expression has been obtained by analyzing sequential biopsies from additional patients (Jäger *et al.*, 1997; Thurner *et al.*, 1999). In addition, it has been suggested that there may be an inverse correlation between the ability to generate peptide responses and the level of expression of the tumor antigens containing these epitopes *in vivo* (Jäger *et al.*, 1996). From these studies it is not clear if antigen loss represents a response to selective pressure provided by the immune response to tumor antigens or if these changes simply reflect the accumulation of genetic abnormalities in tumor cells over time. A more detailed analysis examining tumors taken before and after specific peptide vaccination suggests, however, that immunization may, in at least some patients, contribute to the outgrowth of tumor antigen loss variants (Riker *et al.*, 2000).

These studies have provided the basis for a number of ongoing as well as future clinical trials. In a clinical trial recently initiated in the Surgery Branch (NCI), melanoma patients have been immunized with peptides derived from MART-1, tyrosinase and gp100 in an attempt to prevent the outgrowth of tumor antigen loss variants. Additional vaccine candidates include recombinant viral constructs that encode optimized epitopes expressed either in the context of full length genes or as minigenes. The adoptive transfer of melanoma-reactive T cell clones generated by *in vitro* culture with peptide epitopes represents another strategy that is now being evaluated in clinical trials. The identification of additional shared antigens recognized by $CD4^+$ tumor-reactive T cells may also lead to the development of peptide as well as protein vaccines that target class II as well as class I antigens. Finally, some combination of these approaches may lead to the development of cancer vaccines that result in long-term cures in the majority of patients.

Unanswered Questions

1. **Are the available antigens representative of the full repertoire of human tumor antigens?**
2. **Which are the features of antigens that characterize a priori their immunogenicity?**
3. **Are unique, MHC class I-restricted antigens equivalent to the tumor-rejection antigens of mice?**
4. **Which are the most stable antigens i.e. those less prone to be selected *in vivo*?**
5. **Can MHC-class II restricted antigens be grouped like the class I-restricted counterparts?**
6. **Which is the role of MHC class II-restricted epitopes in the activation of patients' immune response?**
7. **Does tolerance play a role in the specificity or affinity of T cell responses to normal self antigens?**

REFERENCES

Aarnoudse, C.A., van den Doel, P.B., Heemskerk, B., and Schrier, P.I. (1999) Interleukin-2-induced, melanoma-specific T cells recognize camel, an unexpected translation product of LAGE-1. *Int. J. Cancer*, **82**, 442–448.

Adema, G.J., de Boer, A.J., van't Hullenaar, R., Denijn, M., Ruiter, D.J., Vogel, A.M., and Figdor, C.G. (1993) Melanocyte lineage-specific antigens recognized by monoclonal antibodies NKI-beteb, HMB-50, and HMB-45 are encoded by a single cDNA. *Am. J. Pathol.*, **143**, 1579–1585.

Alexander, M., Salgaller, M.L., Celis, E., Sette, A., Barnes, W.A., Rosenberg, S.A., and Steller, M.A. (1996) Generation of tumor-specific cytolytic T lymphocytes from peripheral blood of cervical cancer patients by *in vitro* stimulation with a synthetic human papillomavirus type 16 E7 epitope. *Am. J. Obstet. Gynecol.*, **175**, 1586–1593.

Altman, J.D., Moss, P.A.H., Goulder, P.J.R., Barouch, D.H., McHeyzer-Williams, M.G., Bell, J.I., McMichael, A.J., and Davis, M.M. (1996) Phenotypic analysis of antigen-specific T lymphocytes. *Science*, **274**, 94–96.

Anichini, A., Maccalli, C., Mortarini, R., Salvi, S., Mazzocchi, A., Squarcina, P., Herlyn, M., and Parmiani, G. (1993) Melanoma cells and normal melanocytes share antigens recognized by HLA-A2 restricted cytotoxic T cell clones from melanoma patients. *J. Exp. Med.*, **177**, 989–998.

Bennett, S.R., Carbone, F.R., Karamalis, F., Miller, J.F., and Heath, W.R. (1997) Induction of a CD8+ cytotoxic T lymphocyte response by cross-priming requires cognate CD4+ T cell help. *J. Exp. Med.*, **186**, 65–70.

Bennett, S.R., Carbone, F.R., Karamalis, F., Flavell, R.A., Miller, J.F., and Heath, W.R. (1998) Help for cytotoxic-T-cell responses is mediated by CD40 signalling. *Nature*, **393**, 478–480.

Bloom, M.B., Perry-Lalley, D., Robbins, P.F., Li, Y., el-Gamil, M., Rosenberg, S.A., and Yang, J.C. (1997) Identification of tyrosinase-related protein 2 as a tumor rejection antigen for the B16 melanoma. *J. Exp. Med.*, **185**, 453–459.

Boel, P., Wildmann, C., Sensi, M.L., Brasseur, R., Renauld, J.C., Coulie, P., Boon, T., and van der Bruggen, P. (1995) BAGE: a new gene encoding an antigen recognized on human melanomas by cytolytic T lymphocytes. *Immunity*, **2**, 167–175.

Brandle, D., Brasseur, F., Weynants, P., Boon, T., and Van den Eynde, B. (1996) A mutated HLA-A2 molecule recognized by autologous cytotoxic T lymphocytes on a human renal cell carcinoma. *J. Exp. Med.*, **183**, 2501–2508.

Brichard, V., Van Pel, A., Wölfel, T., Wölfel, C., De Plaen, E., Lethe, B., Coulie, P., and Boon, T. (1993) The tyrosinase gene codes for an antigen recognized by autologous cytolytic T lymphocytes on HLA-A2 melanomas. *J. Exp. Med.*, **178**, 489–495.

Brichard, V.G., Herman, J., Van Pel, A., Wildmann, C., Gaugler, B., Wölfel, T., Boon, T., and Lethe, B. (1996) A tyrosinase nonapeptide presented by HLA-B44 is recognized on a human melanoma by autologous cytolytic T lymphocytes. *Eur. J. Immunol.*, **26**, 224–230.

Butterfield, L.H., Koh, A., Meng, W., Vollmer, C.M., Ribas, A., Dissette, V., Lee, E., Glaspy, J.A., McBride, W.H., and Economou, J.S. (1999) Generation of human T-cells responses to an HLA-A2.1-restricted peptide epitope derived from (α-fetoprotein. *Cancer Res.*, **59**, 3134–3142.

Castelli, C., Storkus, W.J., Maeurer, M.J., Martin, D.M., Huang, E.C., Pramanik, B.N., Nagabhushan, T.L., Parmiani, G., and Lotze, M.T. (1995) Mass spectrometric identification of a naturally processed melanoma peptide recognized by CD8+ cytotoxic T lymphocytes. *J. Exp. Med.*, **181**, 363–368.

Castelli, C., Tarsini, P., Mazzocchi, A., Rini, F., Rivoltini, L., Ravagnani, F., Gallino, F., Belli, F., and Parmiani, G. (1999) Novel HLA-Cw8-restricted T cell epitopes derived from tyrosinase-related protein-2 and gp100 melanoma antigens. *J. Immunol.*, **162**, 1739–1748.

Cavallo, F., Giovarelli, M, Gulino, A., Vacca, A., Stoppacciaro, A., Modesti, A., and Forni, G. (1992) Role of neutrophils and CD4+ T lymphocytes in the primary and memory response to nonimmunogenic murine mammary adenocarcinoma made immunogenic by IL-2 gene. *J. Immunol.*, **149**, 3627–3635.

Chaux, P., Vantomme, V., Stroobant, V., Thielemans, K., Corthals, J., Luiten, R., Eggermont, A.M.M., Boon, T., and van der Bruggen, P. (1999) Identification of MAGE-3, epitopes presented by HLA-DR molecules to CD4+ T lymphocytes. *J. Exp. Med.*, **189**, 767–777.

Chen, Y.T., Stockert, E., Tsang, S., Coplan, K.A., and Old, L.J. (1995) Immunophenotyping of melanomas for tyrosinase: implications for vaccine development. *Proc. Natl. Acad. Sci. USA*, **92**, 8125–8129.

Chen, Y.T., Scanlan, M.J., Sahin, U., Tureci, O., Gure, A.O., Tsang, S., Williamson, B., Stockert, E., Pfreundschuh, M., and Old, L.J. (1997) A testicular antigen aberrantly expressed in human cancers detected by autologous antibody screening. *Proc. Natl. Acad. Sci. USA*, **94**, 1914–1918.

Chen, Y.T., Gure, A.O., Tsang, S., Stockert, E., Jäger, E., Knuth, A., and Old, L.J. (1998) Identification of multiple cancer/testis antigens by allogeneic antibody screening of a melanoma cell line library. *Proc. Natl. Acad. Sci. USA*, **95**, 6919–6923.

Chiari, R., Foury, F., De Plaen, E., Baurain, J.-F., Thonnard, J., and Coulie, P.G. (1999) Two antigens recognized by autologous cytolytic T lymphocytes on a melanoma result from a single point mutation in an essential housekeeping gene. *Cancer Res.*, **59**, 5785–5792.

Clemente, C., Rao, S., Lupetti, R., Tragni, G., Pisarra, P., Bersani, I., Parmiani, G., Mihm, M.C. Jr., and Sensi, M. (1998) Immunohistochemical analysis of the T-cell receptor beta-chain variable regions expressed by T lymphocytes infiltrating primary human melanoma. *Lab. Invest.*, **78**, 619–627.

Cole, D.J., Wilson, M.C., Rivoltini, L., Custer, M., and Nishimura, M.I. (1997) T-cell receptor repertoire in matched MART-1 peptide-stimulated peripheral blood lymphocytes and tumor-infiltrating lymphocytes. *Cancer Res.*, **57**, 5320–5327.

Cormier, J.N., Abati, A., Fetsch, P., Hijazi, Y.M., Rosenberg, S.A., Marincola, F.M., and Topalian, S.L. (1998) Comparative analysis of the *in vivo* expression of tyrosinase, MART-1/Melan-A, and gp100 in metastatic melanoma lesions: implications for immunotherapy. *J. Immunother.*, **21**, 27–31.

Cormier, J.N., Panelli, M., Hackett, J.A., Betinotti, M.P., Mixon, A., Wunderlich, J., Parker, L.L., Restifo, N.P., Ferrone, S., and Marincola, F.M. (1999) Natural variation of the expression of HLA and endogenous antigen modulates CTL recognition in an *in vitro* melanoma model. *Int. J. Cancer*, **80**, 781–790.

Coulie, P.G., Somville, M., Lehmann, F., Hainaut, P., Brasseur, F., Devos, R., and Boon, T. (1992) Precursor frequency analysis of human cytolytic T lymphocytes directed against autologous melanoma cells. *Int. J. Cancer*, **50**, 289–297.

Coulie, P.G., Brichard, V., Van Pel, A., Wölfel, T., Schneider, J., Traversari, C., Mattei, S., De Plaen, E., Lurquin, C., Szikora, J.P., and *et al.* (1994) A new gene coding for a differentiation antigen recognized by autologous cytolytic T lymphocytes on HLA-A2 melanomas. *J. Exp. Med.*, **180**, 35–42.

Coulie, P.G., Lehmann, F., Lethe, B., Herman, J., Lurquin, C., Andrawiss, M., and Boon, T. (1995) A mutated intron sequence codes for an antigenic peptide recognized by cytolytic T lymphocytes on a human melanoma. *Proc. Natl. Acad. Sci. USA*, **92**, 7976–7980.

Cox, A.L., Skipper, J., Chen, Y., Henderson, R.A., Darrow, T.L., Shabanowitz, J., Engelhard, V.H., Hunt, D.F., and Slingluff, C.L. Jr. (1994) Identification of a peptide recognized by five melanoma-specific human cytotoxic T cell lines. *Science*, **264**, 716–719.

Darrow, T.L., Slingluff, C.L., and Seigler, H.F. (1989) The role of HLA class I antigens in recognition of melanoma cells by tumor-specific cytotoxic T lymphocytes: evidence for shared tumor antigens. *J. Immunol.*, **142**, 3329–3335.

De Grujil, T.D., Bontkes, H.J., Walboomers, J.M.M., Stukart, M.J., Doekhie, F.S., Remmink, A.J., Helmerhorst, T.J.M., Verheijen, R.H.M., Duggan-Keen, M.F., Stern, P.L., Meijer, C.I., and Scheper, R.J. (1998) Differential T helper cell responses to human papillomavirus type 16 E7 related to viral clearance or persistence in patients with cervical neoplasia: a longitudinal study. *Cancer Res.*, **58**, 1700–1706.

de La Coste, A., Romagnolo, B., Billuart, P., Renard, C.A., Buendia, M. A., Soubrane, O., Fabre, M., Chelly, J., Beldjord, C., Kahn, A., and Perret, C. (1998) Somatic mutations of the beta-catenin gene are frequent in mouse and human hepatocellular carcinomas. *Proc. Natl. Acad. Sci. USA*, **95**, 8847–8851.

De Plaen, E., Arden, K., Traversari, C., Gaforio, J.J., Szikora, J.P., De Smet, C., Brasseur, F., van der Bruggen, P., Lethe, B., Lurquin, C., and Boon, T. (1994) Structure, chromosomal localization, and expression of 12 genes of the MAGE family. *Immunogenetics*, **40**, 360–369.

Dubey, P., Hendrickson, R.C., Meredith, S.C., Siegel, C.T., Shabanowitz, J., Skipper, J.C., Engelhard, V.H., Hunt, D.F., and Schreiber, H. (1997) The immunodominant antigen of an ultraviolet-induced regressor tumor is generated by a somatic point mutation in the DEAD box helicase p68. *J. Exp. Med.*, **185**, 695–705.

Duffour, M.-T., Chaux, P., Lurquin, C., Cornelis, G., Boon, T., and van der Bruggen, P. (1999) A MAGE-A4 peptide presented by HLA-A2 is recognized by cytolytic T lymphocyte. *Eur. J. Cancer*, **29**, 3329–3337.

Dunbar, P.R., Ogg, G.S., Chen, J., Rust, N., van der Bruggen, P., and Cerundolo, V. (1998) Direct isolation, phenotyping and cloning of low-frequency antigen-specific cytotoxic T lymphocytes from peripheral blood. *Curr. Biol.*, **8**, 413–416.

Eisenlohr, L.C., Yewdell, J.W., and Bennink, J.R. (1992) Flanking sequences influence the presentation of an endogenously synthesized peptide to cytotoxic T lymphocytes. *J. Exp. Med.*, **175**, 481–487.

Finke, J.H., Rayman, P., Edinger, M., Tubbs, R.R., Stanley, J., Kelin, E., and Bukowski, R. (1992) Characterization of a human renal-cell-carcinoma-specific cytotoxic CD8+ T-cell line. *J. Immunother.*, **11**, 1–11.

Fisk, B., Blevins, T.L., Wharton, J.T., and Ioannides, C.G. (1995) Identification of an immunodominant peptide of HER-2/neu protooncogene recognized by ovarian tumor-specific cytotoxic T lymphocyte lines. *J. Exp. Med.*, **181**, 2109–2117.

Fleischhauer, K., Fruci, D., Van Endert, P., Herman, J., Tanzarella, S., Wallny, H.J., Coulie, P., Bordignon, C., and Traversari, C. (1996) Characterization of antigenic peptides presented by HLA-B44 molecules on tumor cells expressing the gene MAGE-3. *Int. J. Cancer*, **68**, 622–628.

Fleischhauer, K., Gattinoni, L., Dalerba, P., Lauvau, G., Zanaria, E., Dabovic, B., van Endert, P.M., Bordignon, C., and Traversari, C. (1998) The *DAM* gene family encodes a new group of tumor-specific antigens recognized by human leukocyte antigen A2-restricted cytotoxic T lymphocytes. *Cancer Res.*, **58**, 2969–2972.

Fuhlbrigge, R.C., Kieffer, J.D., Armerding, D., and Kupper, T.S. (1997) Cutaneous lymphocyte antigen is a specialized form of PSGL-1 expressed on skin-homing T cells. *Nature*, **389**, 978–981.

Fujie, T., Tahara, K., Tanaka, K., Mori, M., Takesako, K., and Akiyoshi, T. (1999) A MAGE-1-encoded HLA-A24-binding synthetic peptide induces specific anti-tumor cytotoxic T lymphocytes. *Int. J. Cancer*, **80**, 169–172.

Gaudin, C., Kremer, F., Angevin, E., Scott, V., and Triebel, F. (1999) A HSP70-2 mutation recognized by CTL on a human renal cell carcinoma. *J. Immunol.*, **162**, 1730–1738.

Gaugler, B., Van den Eynde, B., van der Bruggen, P., Romero, P., Gaforio, J.J., De Plaen, E., Lethe, B., Brasseur, F., and Boon, T. (1994) Human gene MAGE-3 codes for an antigen recognized on a melanoma by autologous cytolytic T lymphocytes. *J. Exp. Med.*, **179**, 921–930.

Gaugler, B., Brouwenstijn, N., Vantomme, V., Szikora, J.P., Van der Spek, C.W., Patard, J.J., Boon, T., Schrier, P., and Van den Eynde, B.J. (1996) A new gene coding for an antigen recognized by autologous cytolytic T lymphocytes on a human renal carcinoma. *Immunogenetics*, **44**, 323–330.

Gnjatic, S., Cai, Z., Viguier, M., Chouaib, S., Guillet, J.G., and Choppin, J. (1998) Accumulation of the p53 protein allows recognition by human CTL of a wild-type p53 epitope presented by breast carcinomas and melanomas. *J. Immunol.*, **160**, 328–333.

Gueguen, M., Patard, J.J., Gaugler, B., Brasseur, F., Renauld, J.C., Van Cangh, P.J., Boon, T., and Van den Eynde, B.J. (1998) An antigen recognized by autologous CTLs on a human bladder carcinoma. *J. Immunol.*, **160**, 6188–6194.

Guilloux, Y., Lucas, S., Brichard, V.G., Van Pel, A., Viret, C., De Plaen, E., Brasseur, F., Lethe, B., Jotereau, F., and Boon, T. (1996) A peptide recognized by human cytolytic T lymphocytes on HLA-A2 melanomas is encoded by an intron sequence of the N-acetylglucosaminyltransferase V gene. *J. Exp. Med.*, **183**, 1173–1183.

Halder, T., Pawelec, G., Kirkin, A.F., Zeuthen, J., Meyer, H.E., Kun, L., and Kalbacher, H. (1997) Isolation of novel HLA-DR restricted potential tumor-associated antigens from the melanoma cell line FM3. *Cancer Res.*, **57**, 3238–3244.

Heike, M., Schlaak, J., Schulze-Bergkamen, H., Heyl, S., Herr, W., Schmitt, U., Schneider, P.M., and Meyer zum Buschenfelde, K.H. (1996) Specificities and functions of CD4+ HLA class II-restricted T cell clones against a human sarcoma. *J. Immunol.*, **156**, 2205–2213.

Herman, J., van der Bruggen, P., Luescher, I.F., Mandruzzato, S., Romero, P., Thonnard, J., Fleischhauer, K., Boon, T., and Coulie, P.G. (1996) A peptide encoded by the human MAGE3 gene and presented by HLA-B44 induces cytolytic T lymphocytes that recognize tumor cells expressing MAGE3. *Immunogenetics*, **43**, 377–383.

Hogan, K.T., Eisinger, D.P., Cupp, S.B. III, Lekstrom, K.J., Deacon, D.D., Shabanowitz, J., Hunt, D.F., Engelhard, V.H., Slingluff, C.L. Jr, and Ross, M.M. (1998) The peptide recognized by HLA-A68.2-restricted, squamous cell carcinoma of the lung-specific cytotoxic T lymphocytes is derived from a mutated elongation factor 2 gene. *Cancer Res.*, **58**, 5144–5150.

Hom, S.S., Topalian, S.L., Simoni, S.T., Mancini, M.J., and Rosenberg, S.A. (1991) Common expression of melanoma tumor-associated antigens recognized by human tumor-infiltrating lymphocytes: Analysis by human lymphocyte antigen restriction. *J. Immunother.*, **10**, 153–164.

Hu, X., Chakraborty, N.G., Sporn, J.R., Kurtzman, S.H., Ergin, M.T., and Mukherji, B. (1996) Enhancement of cytolytic T lymphocyte precursor frequency in melanoma patients following immunization with the MAGE-1 peptide loaded antigen presenting cell-based vaccine. *Cancer Res.*, **56**, 2479–2483.

Huang, A.Y., Gulden, P.H., Woods, A.S., Thomas, M.C., Tong, C.D., Wang, W., Engelhard, V.H., Pasternack, G., Cotter, R., Hunt, D., Pardoll, D.M., and Jaffee, E.M. (1996) The immunodominant major histocompatibility complex class I-restricted antigen of a murine colon tumor derives from an endogenous retroviral gene product. *Proc. Natl. Acad. Sci. USA*, **93**, 9730–9735.

Huang, L.-Q., Brasseur, F., Serrano, A., De Plaen, E., van der Bruggen, P., Boon, T., and Van Pel, A. (1999) Cytolytic T lymphocytes recognize an antigen encoded by MAGE-A10 on a human melanoma. *J. Immunol.*, **162**, 6849–6854.

Ikeda, H., Lethe, B., Lehmann, F., van Baren, N., Baurain, J.F., de Smet, C., Chambost, H., Vitale, M., Moretta, A., Boon, T., and Coulie, P.G. (1997) Characterization of an antigen that is recognized on a melanoma showing partial HLA loss by CTL expressing an NK inhibitory receptor. *Immunity*, **6**, 199–208.

Ioannides, C.G., Platsoucas, C.D., Rashed, S., Wharton, J.T., Edwards, C.L., and Freedman, R.S. (1991) Tumor cytolysis by lymphocytes infiltrating ovarian malignant ascites. *Cancer Res.*, **51**, 4257–4265.

Iwashiro, M., Kondo, T., Shimizu, T., Yamagishi, H., Takahashi, K., Matsubayashi, Y., Masuda, T., Otaka, A., Fujii, N., Ishimoto, A., and *et al.* (1993) Multiplicity of virus-encoded helper T-cell epitopes expressed on FBL-3 tumor cells. *J. Virol.*, **67**, 4533–4542.

Jäger, E., Ringhoffer, M., Karbach, J., Arand, M., Oesch, F., and Knuth, A. (1996) Inverse relationship of melanocyte differentiation antigen expression in melanoma tissues and CD8+ cytotoxic-T-cell responses: evidence for immunoselection of antigen-loss variants *in vivo*. *Int. J. Cancer*, **66**, 470–476.

Jäger, E., Ringhoffer, M., Altmannsberger, M., Arand, M., Karbach, J., Jäger, D., Oesch, F., and Knuth, A. (1997) Immunoselection *in vivo*: independent loss of MHC class I and melanocyte differentiation antigen expression in metastatic melanoma. *Int. J. Cancer*, **71**, 142–147.

Jäger, E., Chen, Y.T., Drijfhout, J.W., Karbach, J., Ringhoffer, M., Jäger, D., Arand, M., Wada, H., Noguchi, Y., Stockert, E., Old, L.J., and Knuth, A. (1998) Simultaneous humoral and cellular immune response against cancer-testis antigen NY-ESO-1: definition of human histocompatibility leukocyte antigen (HLA)-A2-binding peptide epitopes. *J. Exp. Med.*, **187**, 265–270.

Kang, X.-Q., Kawakami, Y., Sakaguchi, K., El-Gamil, M., Wang, R.-F., Yannelli, J.R., Appella, E., Rosenberg, S.A., and Robbins, P.F. (1995) Identification of a tyrosinase epitope reocognized by HLA-A24 restricted tumor-infiltrating lymphocytes. *J. Immunol.*, **155**, 1343–1348.

Katsumata, M., Okudaira, T., Samanta, A., Clark, D.P., Drebin, J.A., Jolicouer, P., and Greene, M.I. (1995) Prevention of breast tumor development *in vivo* by downregulation of the p185neu receptor. *Nature Med.*, **1**, 644–648.

Kawakami, Y., Eliyahu, S., Delgado, C.H., Robbins, P.F., Rivoltini, L., Topalian, S.L., Miki, T., and Rosenberg, S.A. (1994a) Cloning of the gene coding for a shared human melanoma antigen recognized by autologous T cells infiltrating into tumor. *Proc. Natl. Acad. Sci. USA*, **91**, 3515–3519.

Kawakami, Y., Eliyahu, S., Delgado, C.H., Robbins, P.F., Sakaguchi, K., Appella, E., Yannelli, J.R., Adema, G.J., Miki, T., and Rosenberg, S.A. (1994b) Identification of a human melanoma antigen recognized by tumor infiltrating lymphocytes associated with *in vivo* tumor rejection. *Proc. Natl. Acad. Sci. USA*, **91**, 6458–6462.

Kawakami, Y., Eliyahu, S., Sakaguchi, K., Robbins, P.F., Rivoltini, L., Yannelli, J.B., Appella, E., and Rosenberg, S.A. (1994c) Identification of the immunodominant peptides of the MART-1 human melanoma antigen recognized by the majority of HLA-A2 restricted tumor infiltrating lymphocytes. *J. Exp. Med.*, **180**, 347–352.

Kawakami, Y., Eliyahu, S., Jennings, C., Sakaguchi, K., Kang, X.-Q., Southwood, S., Robbins, P.F., Sette, A., Appella, E., and Rosenberg, S.A. (1995) Recognition of multiple epitopes in the human melanoma antigen gp100 associated with *in vivo* tumor regression. *J. Immunol.*, **154**, 3961–3968.

Kawakami, Y., Battles, J.K., Kobayashi, T., Ennis, W., Wang, X., Tupesis, J.P., Marincola, F.M., Robbins, P.F., Hearing, V.J., Gonda, M.A., and Rosenberg, S.A. (1997) Production of recombinant MART-1 proteins and specific antiMART-1 polyclonal and monoclonal antibodies: use in the characterization of the human melanoma antigen MART-1. *J. Immunol. Methods*, **202**, 13–25.

Kawakami, Y., P.F. Robbins, X. Wang, J.P. Tupesis, M.R. Parkhurst, X. Kang, K. Sakaguchi, E. Appella, and S.A. Rosenberg (1998) Identification of new melanoma epitopes on melanosomal proteins recognized by tumor infiltrating lymphocytes restricted by HLA-A1, -A2 and -A3 alleles. *J. Immunol.*, **161**, 6985–6992.

Kawakami, Y., Dang, N., Wang, X., Tupesis, J., Robbins, P.F., Wang, R.-F., Wunderlich, J.R., Yannelli, J.R., and Rosenberg, S.A. (1999) Recognition of shared melanoma antigens in association with major HLA-A alleles by tumor infiltrating lymphocytes from 123 patients with melanoma. *J. Immunother.*, in press.

Kawashima, I., Hudson, S.J., Tsai, V., Southwood, S., Takesako, K., Appella, E., Sette, A., and Celis, E. (1998) The multi-epitope approach for immunotherapy for cancer: identification of several CTL epitopes from various tumor-associated antigens expressed on solid epithelial tumors. *Hum. Immunol.*, **59**, 1–14.

Kikuchi, M., Nakao, M., Inoue, Y., Matsunaga, K., Shichijo, S., Yamana, H., and Itoh, K. (1999) Identification of a SART-1-derived peptide capable of inducing HLA-A24-restricted and tumor-specific cytotoxic T lymphocytes. *Int. J. Cancer*, **81**, 459–466.

Kittlesen, D.J., Thompson, L.W., Gulden, P.H., Skipper, J.C., Colella, T.A., Shabanowitz, J.A., Hunt, D.F., Engelhard, V.H., and Slingluff, C.L. Jr. (1998) Human melanoma patients recognize an HLA-A1-restricted CTL epitope from tyrosinase containing two cysteine residues: implications for tumor vaccine development. *J. Immunol.*, **160**, 2099–2106.

Kobayashi, H., Kosubo, T., Sato, K., Kimura, S., Asano, K., Takahashi, H., Iizuka, H., Miyokawa, N., and Katagiri, M. (1998) CD4+ T cells from peripheral blood of a melanoma patient recognize peptides derived fromn onmutated tyrosinase. *Cancer Res.*, **58**, 296–301.

Kono, K., Halapi, E., Hising, C., Petersson, M., Gerdin, E., Vanky, F., and Kiessling, R. (1997) Mechanisms of escape from CD8+ T-cell clones specific for the HER-2/neu proto-oncogene expressed in ovarian carcinomas: related and unrelated to decreased MHC class 1 expression. *Int. J. Cancer*, **70**, 112–119.

Korinek, V., Barker, N., Morin, P.J., van Wichen, D., de Weger, R., Kinzler, K.W., Vogelstein, B., and Clevers, H. (1997) Constitutive transcriptional activation by a beta-catenin-Tcf complex in APC-/- colon carcinoma. *Science*, **275**, 1784–1787.

Kwon, B.S., Haq, A.K., Pomerantz, S.H., and Halaban, R. (1987) Isolation and sequence of a cDNA clone for human tyrosinase that maps at the mouse c-albino locus. *Proc. Natl. Acad. Sci. USA*, **84**, 7473–7477.

Lee, Z.H., Hou, L., Moellmann, G., Kuklinska, E., Antol, K., Fraser, M., Halaban, R., and Kwon, B.S. (1996) Characterization and subcellular localization of human Pmel 17/silver, a 110-kDa (pre)melanosomal membrane protein associated with 5,6,-dihydroxyindole-2-carboxylic acid (DHICA) converting activity. *J. Invest. Dermatol.*, **106**, 605–610.

Lehmann, F., Marchand, M., Hainaut, P., Pouillart, P., Sastre, X., Ikeda, H., Boon, T., and Coulie, P.G. (1995) Differences in the antigens recognized by cytolytic T cells on two successive metastases of a melanoma patient are consistent with immune selection. *Eur. J. Immunol.*, **25**, 340–347.

Lethe, B., van der Bruggen, P., Brasseur, F., and Boon, T. (1997) MAGE-1 expression threshold for the lysis of melanoma cell lines by a specific cytotoxic T lymphocyte. *Melanoma Res.*, **7**, S83–S88.

Lethe, B., Lucas, S., Michaux, L., De Smet, C., Godelaine, D., Serrano, A., De Plaen, E., and Boon, T. (1998) LAGE-1, a new gene with tumor specificity. *Int. J. Cancer*, **76**, 903–908.

Li, K., Adibzadeh, M., Holder, T., Kolbacher, H., Heinzel, S., Müller, C., Zeuthen, J., and Pawelec, G. (1998) Tumour-specific MHC-class-II-restricted responses after *in vitro* sensitization to synthetic peptides corresponding to gp100 and annexin II eluted from melanoma cells. *Cancer Immunol. Immunother.*, **47**, 32–38.

Loftus, D.J., Squarcina, P., Nielsen, M.B., Geisler, C., Castelli, C., Odum, N., Appella, E., Parmiani, G., and Rivoltini, L. (1998) Peptides derived from self-proteins as partial agonists and antagonists of human CD8+ T-cell clones reactive to melanoma/melanocyte epitope MART1(27–35). *Cancer Res.*, **58**, 2433–2439.

Lucas, S., De Smet, C., Arden, K.C., Viars, C.S., Lethe, B., Lurquin, C., and Boon, T. (1998) Identification of a new MAGE gene with tumor-specific expression by representational difference analysis. *Cancer Res.*, **58**, 743–752.

Lupetti, R., Pisarra, P., Verrecchia, A., Farina, C., Nicolini, G., Anichini, A., Bordignon, C., Sensi, M., Parmiani, G., and Traversari, C. (1998) Translation of a retained intron in tyrosinase-related protein (TRP) 2 mRNA generates a new cytotoxic T lymphocyte (CTL)-defined and shared human melanoma antigen not expressed in normal cells of the melanocytic lineage. *J. Exp. Med.*, **188**, 1005–1016.

Lurquin, C., Van Pel, A., Mariame, B., De Plaen, E., Szikora, J.P., Janssens, C., Reddehase, M.J., Lejeune, J., and Boon, T. (1989) Structure of the gene of tum-transplantation antigen P91A: the mutated exon encodes a peptide recognized with Ld by cytolytic T cells. *Cell*, **58**, 293–303.

Lustgarten, J., Theobald, M., Labadie, C., LaFace, D., Peterson, P., Disis, M.L., Cheever, M.A., and Sherman, L.A. (1997) Identification of Her-2/Neu CTL epitopes using double transgenic mice expressing HLA-A2.1 and human CD.8. *Hum. Immunol.*, **52**, 109–118.

Malarkannan, S., Afkarian, M., and Shastri, N. (1995) A rare cryptic translation product is presented by Kb major histocompatibility complex class I molecule to alloreactive T cells. *J. Exp. Med.*, **182**, 1739–1750.

Mandelboim, O., Vadai, E., Fridkin, M., Katz-Hillel, A., Feldman, M., Berke, G., and Eisenbach, L. (1995) Regression of established murine carcinoma metastases following vaccination with tumour-associated antigen peptides. *Nature Med.*, **1**, 1179–1183.

Mandruzzato, S., Brasseur, F., Andry, G., Boon, T., and van der Bruggen, P. (1997) A CASP-8 mutation recognized by cytolytic T lymphocytes on a human head and neck carcinoma. *J. Exp. Med.*, **186**, 785–793.

Manering, S.I., McKenzie, J.L., Fearnley, d.B., and Hart, D.N.J. (1997) HLA-DR1-restricted bcr-abl (b3a2)-specific CD4+ T lymphocytes respond to dendritic cells pulsed with b3a2 peptide and antigen-presenting cells exposed to b3a2 containing cell lysates. *Blood*, **90**, 290–297.

Manici, S., Sturniolo, T., Imro, M.A., Hammer, J., Sinigaglia, F., Noppen, C., Spagnoli, G., Mazzi, B., Bellone, M., Dellabona P., and Protti, M.P. (1999) Melanoma cells present a MAGE-3 epitope to CD4+ cytotoxic T cells in association with histocompatibility leukocyte antigen DR11. *J. Exp. Med.*, **189**, 871–876.

Marchand, M., van Baren, N., Weynants, P., Brichard, V., Dreno, B., Tessier, M.H., Rankin, E., Parmiani, G., Arienti, F., Humblet, Y., Bourlond, A., Vanwijck, R., Lienard, D., Beauduin, M., Dietrich, P.Y., Russo, V., Kerger, J., Masucci, G., Jäger, E., De Greve, J., Atzpodien, J., Brasseur, F., Coulie, P.G., van der Bruggen, P., and Boon, T. (1999) Tumor regressions observed in patients with metastatic melanoma treated with an antigenic peptide encoded by gene MAGE-3 and presented by HLA-A1. *Int. J. Cancer*, **80**, 219–230.

Mattes, M.J., Thomson, T.M., Old, L.J., and Lloyd, K.O. (1983) A pigmentation-associated, differentiation antigen of human melanoma defined by a precipitating antibody in human serum. *Int. J. Cancer*, **32**, 717–721.

Mayrand, S.M., Schwarz, D.A., and Green, W.R. (1998) An alternative translational reading frame encodes an immunodominant retroviral CTL determinant expressed by an immunodeficiency-causing retrovirus. *J. Immunol.*, **160**, 39–50.

Mazzocchi, A., Belli, F., Mascheroni, L., Vegetti, C., Parmiani, G., and Anichini, A. (1994) Frequency of cytotoxic T lymphocyte precursors (CTLp) interacting with autologous tumor via the T-cell receptor: limiting dilution analysis of specific CTLp in peripheral blood and tumor-invaded lymph nodes of melanoma patients. *Int. J. Cancer*, **58**, **58**, 330–339.

Monach, P.A., Meredith, S.C., Siegel, C.T., and Schreiber, H. (1995) A unique tumor antigen produced by a single amino acid substitution. *Immunity*, **2**, 45–59.

Morin, P.J., Sparks, A.B., Korinek, V., Barker, N., Clevers, H., Vogelstein, B., and Kinzler, K.W. (1997) Activation of beta-catenin-Tcf signaling in colon cancer by mutations in beta-catenin or APC. *Science*, **275**, 1787–1790.

Mortarini, R., Belli, F., Parmiani, G., and Anichini, A. (1990) Cytokine-mediated modulation of HLA-class II, ICAM-1, LFA-3 and tumor-associated antigen profile of melanoma cells. Comparison with anti-proliferative activity by rIL1-beta, rTNF-alpha, rIFN-gamma, rIL4 and their combinations. *Int. J. Cancer*, **45**, 334–341.

Nakao, M., Sata, M., Saitsu, H., Yutani, S., Kawamoto, M., Kojiro, M., and Itoh, K. (1997) CD4+ hepatic cancer-specific cytotoxic T lymphocytes in patients with hepatocellular carcinoma. *Cell. Immunol.*, **177**, 35–48.

Ogg, G.S., Rod Dunbar, P., Romero, P., Chen, J.L., and Cerundolo, V. (1998) High frequency of skin-homing melanocyte-specific cytotoxic T lymphocytes in autoimmune vitiligo. *J. Exp. Med.*, **188**, 1203–1208.

Oiso, M., Eura, M., Katsura, F., Takiguchi, M., Sobao, Y., Masuyama, K., Nakashima, M., Itoh, K., and Ishikawa, T. (1999) A newly identified MAGE-3-derived epitope recognized by HLA-A24-restricted cytotoxic T lymphocytes. *Int. J. Cancer*, **81**, 387–394.

Ossendorp, F., Eggers, M., Neisig, A., Ruppert, T., Groettrup, M., Sijts, A., Mengede, E., Kloetzel, P.M., Neefjes, J., Koszinowski, U., and Melief, C. (1996) A single residue exchange within a viral CTL epitope alters proteasome-mediated degradation resulting in lack of antigen presentation. *Immunity*, **5**, 115–124.

Parker, K.C., Shields, M., DiBrino, M., Brooks, A., and Coligan, J.E. (1995) Peptide binding to MHC class I molecules: implications for antigenic peptide prediction. *Immunol. Res.*, **14**, 34–57.

Parkhurst, M.R., Salgaller, M., Southwood, S., Robbins, P., Sette, A., Rosenberg, S.A., and Kawakami, Y. (1996) Improved induction of melanoma reactive CTL with peptides from the melanoma antigen gp100 modified at HLA-A0201 binding residues. *J. Immunol.*, **157**, 2539–2548.

Parkhurst, M.R., Fitzgerald, E.B., Southwood, S., Sette, A., Rosenberg, S.A., and Kawakami, Y. (1998) Identification of a shared HLA-A*0201 restricted T cell epitope from the melanoma antigen tyrosinase related protein 2 (TRP-2). *Cancer Res.*, **58**, 4895–4901.

Peoples, G.E., Goedegebuure, P.S., Smith, R., Linehan, D.C., Yoshino, I., and Eberlein, T.J. (1995) Breast and ovarian cancer-specific cytotoxic T lymphocytes recognize the same HER2/neu-derived peptide. *Proc. Natl. Acad. Sci. USA*, **92**, 432–436.

Pieper, R., Christian, R.E., Gonzales, M.I., Nishimura, M.I., Gupta, G., Settlage, R.E., Shabanowitz, J., Rosenberg, S.A., Hunt, D.F., and Topalian, S.L. (1999) Biochemical identification of a mutated human melanoma antigen recognized by CD4+ T cells. *J. Exp. Med.*, **189**, 757–766.

Rammensee, H.G., Friede, T., and Stevanoviic, S. (1995) MHC ligands and peptide motifs: first listing. *Immunogenetics*, **41**, 178–228.

Ressing, M.E., van Driel, W.J., Celis, E., Sette, A., Brandt, M.P., Hartman, M., Anholts, J.D., Schreuder, G.M., ter Harmsel, W.B., Fleuren, G.J., Trimbos, B.J., Kast, W.M., and Melief, C.J. (1996) Occasional memory cytotoxic T-cell responses of patients with human papillomavirus type 16-positive cervical lesions against a human leukocyte antigen-A *0201-restricted E7-encoded epitope. *Cancer Res.*, **56**, 582–588.

Riker, A.I., Kammula, U.S., Panelli, M.C., Wang, E., Abati, A., Fetsch, P., Lee, K.-H., Steinberg, S.M., Rosenberg, S.A., and Marincola, F.M. (2000) Immune selection following antigen specific immunotherapy of melanoma. *Surgery*, in press.

Rivoltini, L., Barracchini, K.C., Viggiano, V., Kawakami, Y., Smith, A., Mixon, A., Restifo, N.P., Topalian, S.L., Simonis, T.B., Rosenberg, S.A., and Marincola, F.M. (1995) Quantitative correlation between HLA class I allele expression and recognition of melanoma cells by antigen-specific cytotoxic T lymphocytes. *Cancer Res.*, **55**, 3149–3157.

Rivoltini, L., Squarcina, P., Loftus, D.J., Castelli, C., Tarsini, P., Mazzocchi, A., Rini, F., Viggiano, V., Belli, F., and Parmiani, G. (1999) A superagonist variant of peptide MART1/Melan A_{27-35} elicits anti-melanoma CD8+ T cells with enhanced functional characteristics: implication for more effective immunotherapy. *Cancer Res.*, **59**, 301–306.

Robbins, P.F., El-Gamil, M., Kawakami, Y., Stevens, E., Yannelli, J., and Rosenberg, S.A. (1994) Recognition of tyrosinase by tumor infiltrating lymphocytes from a patient responding to immunotherapy. *Cancer Res.*, **54**, 3124–3126.

Robbins, P.F., El-Gamil, M., Li, Y.F., Topalian, S.L., Rivoltini, L., Sakaguchi, K., Appella, E., Kawakami, Y., and Rosenberg, S.A. (1995) Cloning of a new gene encoding an antigen recognized by melanoma-specific HLA-A24 restricted tumor-infiltrating lymphocytes. *J. Immunol.*, **154**, 5944–5950.

Robbins, P.F., El-Gamil, M., Li, Y.F., Kawakami, Y., Loftus, D., Appella, E., and Rosenberg, S.A. (1996) A mutated β-catenin gene encodes a melanoma-specific antigen recognized by tumor infiltrating lymphocytes. *J. Exp. Med.*, **183**, 1185–1192.

Robbins, P.F., El-Gamil, M., Li, Y.F., Fitzgerald, E.B., Kawakami, Y., and Rosenberg, S.A. (1997) The intronic region of an incompletely spliced gp100 gene transcript encodes an epitope recognized by melanoma-reactive tumor-infiltrating lymphocytes. *J. Immunol.*, **159**, 303–308.

Romero, P., Gervois, N., Schneider, J., Escobar, P., Valmori, D., Pannetier, C., Steinle, A., Wölfel, T., Lienard, D., Brichard, V., van Pel, A., Jotereau, F., and Cerottini, J.C. (1997) Cytolytic T lymphocyte recognition of the immunodominant HLA-A*0201-restricted Melan-A/MART-1 antigenic peptide in melanoma. *J. Immunol.*, **159**, 2366–2374.

Romero, P., Dunbar, P.R., Valmori, D., Pittet, M., Ogg, G.S., Rimoldi, D., Chen, J.-L., Lienard, D., Cerottini, J.-C., and Cerundolo, V. (1998) *Ex vivo* staining of metastatic lymph nodes by class I major histocompatibility complex tetramers reveals high numbers of antigen-experienced tumor-specific cytolytic T lymphocytes. *J. Exp. Med.*, **188**, 1641–1650.

Rongcun, Y., Salazar-Onfray, F., Charo, J., Malmberg, K.J., Evrin, K., Maes, H., Kono, K., Hising, C., Petersson, M., Larsson, O., Lan, L., Appella, E., Sette, A., Celis, E., and Kiessling, R. (1999) Identification of new HER2/neu-derived peptide epitopes that can elicit specific CTL against autologous and allogeneic carcinomas and melanomas. *J. Immunol.*, **163**, 1037–1044.

Ronsin, C., Chung-Scott, V., Poullion, I., Aknouche, N., Gaudin, C., and Triebel, F. (1999) A non-AUG-defined alternative open reading frame of the intestinal carboxyl esterase mRNA generates an epitope recognized by renal cell carcinoma-reactive tumor-infiltrating lymphocytes *in situ*. *J. Immunol.*, **163**, 483–490.

Ropke, M., Hald, J., Guldberg, P., Zeuthen, J., Norgaard, L., Fugger, L., Svejgaard, A., Van der Burg, S., Nijman, H.W., Melief, C.J., and Claesson, M.H. (1996) Spontaneous human squamous cell carcinomas are killed by a human cytotoxic T lymphocyte clone recognizing a wild-type p53-derived peptide. *Proc. Natl. Acad. Sci. USA*, **93**, 14704–14707.

Rosenberg, S.A., Yang, J.C., Schwartzentruber, D.J., Hwu, P., Marincola, F.M., Topalian, S.L., Restifo, N.P., Dudley, M.E., Schwarz, S.L., Spiess, P.J., Wunderlich, J.R., Parkhurst, M.R., Kawakami, Y., Seipp, C.A., Einhorn, J.H., and White, D.E. (1998a) Immunologic and therapeutic evaluation of a synthetic peptide vaccine for the treatment of patients with metastatic melanoma. *Nature Med.*, **4**, 321–327.

Rosenberg, S.A., Zhai, Y., Yang, J.C., Schwartzentruber, D.J., Hwu, P., Marincola, F.M., Topalian, S.L., Restifo, N.P., Seipp, C.A., Einhorn, J.H., Roberts, B., and White, D.E. (1998b) Immunizing patients with metastatic melanoma using recombinant adenoviruses encoding MART-1 or gp100 melanoma antigens. *J. Natl. Cancer Inst. USA*, **90**, 1894–1900.

Rubinfeld, B., Robbins, P., El-Gamil, M., Albert, I., Porfiri, E., and Polakis, P. (1997) Stabilization of beta-catenin by genetic defects in melanoma cell lines. *Science*, **275**, 1790–1792.

Salazar-Onfray, F., Nakazawa, T., Chhajlani, V., Petersson, M., Karre, K., Masucci, G., Celis, E., Sette, A., Southwood, S., Appella, E., and Kiessling, R. (1997) Synthetic peptides derived from the melanocyte-stimulating hormone receptor MC1R can stimulate HLA-A2-restricted cytotoxic T lymphocytes that recognize naturally processed peptides on human melanoma cells. *Cancer Res.*, **57**, 4348–4355.

Scanlan, M.J., Chen, Y.T., Williamson, B., Gure, A.O., Stockert, E., Gordan, J.D., Tureci, O., Sahin, U., Pfreundschuh, M., and Old, L.J. (1998) Characterization of human colon cancer antigens recognized by autologous antibodies. *Int. J. Cancer*, **76**, 652–658.

Scheibenbogen, C., Lee, K.H., Stevanovic, S., Witzens, M., Willhauck, M., Waldmann, V., Naeher, H., Rammensee, H.G., and Keilholz, U. (1997) Analysis of the T cell response to tumor and viral peptide antigens by an IFNgamma-ELISPOT assay. *Int. J. Cancer*, **71**, 932–936.

Schlegel, J., Trenkle, T., Stumm, G., and Kiessling, M. (1997) Growth inhibition by dominant-negative mutations of the neu-encoded oncoprotein. *Int. J. Cancer*, **70**, 78–83.

Schneider, J., Brichard, V., Boon, T., Meyer zum Buschenfelde, K.H., and Wölfel, T. (1998) Overlapping peptides of melanocyte differentiation antigen Melan-A/MART-1 recognized by autologous cytolytic T lymphocytes in association with HLA-B45.1 and HLA-A2.1. *Int. J. Cancer*, **75**, 451–458.

Schoenberger, S.P., Toes, R.E., van der Voort, E.L., Offringa, R., and Melief, C.J. (1998) T-cell help for cytotoxic T lymphocytes is mediated by CD40-CD40L interactions. *Nature*, **393**, 413–414.

Schwartzentruber, D.J., Topalian, S.L., Mancini, M.J., and Rosenberg, S.A. (1991) Specific release of granulocyte-macrophage colony-stimulating factor, tumor necrosis factor-α, and IFN-γ by human tumor-infiltrating lymphocytes after autologous tumor stimulation. *J. Immunol.*, **146**, 3674–3681.

Schwartzentruber, D.J., Solomon, D., Rosenberg, S.A., and Topalian, S.L. (1992) Characterization of lymphocytes infiltrating human breast cancer: specific immune reactivity detected by measuring cytokine secretion. *J. Immunother.*, **12**, 1–12.

Sensi, M., Traversari, C., Radrizzani, M., Salvi, S., Maccalli, C., Mortarini, R., Rivoltini, L., Farina, C., Nicolini, G., Wölfel, T., Brichard, V., Boon, T., Bordignon, C., Anichini, A., and Parmiani, G. (1995) Cytotoxic T lymphocyte clones from different patients display limited T-cell receptors variable gene usage in HLA-A2 restricted recognition of Melan/Mart-1 melanoma antigen. *Proc. Natl. Acad. Sci. USA.*, **92**, 5674–5678.

Sensi, M., Farina, C., Maccalli, C., Anichini, A., Berd, D., and Parmiani, G. (1998) Intralesional selection of T cell clonotypes in the immune response to melanoma antigens occurring during vaccination. *J. Immunother.*, **21**, 198–204.

Sette, A., Sidney, J., del Guercio, M.-F., Southwood, S., Ruppert, J., Dahlberg, C., Grey, H.M., and Kubo, R.T. (1994a) Peptide binding to the most frequent HLA-A class I alleles measured by quantitative molecular binding assays. *Mol. Immunol.*, **31**, 813–822.

Sette, A., Vitiello, A., Reherman, B., Fowler, P., Nayersina, R., Kast, W.M., Melief, C.J., Oseroff, C., Yuan, L., and Ruppert, J. (1994b) The relationship between class I binding affinity and immunogenicity of potential cytotoxic T cell epitopes. *J. Immunol.*, **153**, 5586–5592.

Sherr, C.J. (1996) Cancer cell cycles. *Science*, **274**, 1672–1677.

Shichijo, S., Nakao, M., Imai, Y., Takasu, H., Kawamoto, M., Niiya, F., Yang, D., Toh, Y., Yamana, H., and Itoh, K. (1998) A gene encoding antigenic peptides of human squamous cell carcinoma recognized by cytotoxic T lymphocytes. *J. Exp. Med.*, **187**, 277–288.

Sidney, J., Grey, H.M., Southwood, S., Celis, E., Wentworth, P.A., del Guercio, M.F., Kubo, R.T., Chesnut, R.W., and Sette, A. (1996) Definition of an HLA-A3-like supermotif demonstrates the overlapping peptide-binding repertoires of common HLA molecules. *Hum. Immunol.*, **45**, 79–93.

Skipper, J.C., Hendrickson, R.C., Gulden, P.H., Brichard, V., Van Pel, A., Chen, Y., Shabanowitz, J., Wölfel, T., Slingluff, C.L., Jr., Boon, T., Hunt, D.F., and Engelhard, V.H. (1996a) An HLA-A2-restricted tyrosinase antigen on melanoma cells results from posttranslational modification and suggests a novel pathway for processing of membrane proteins. *J. Exp. Med.*, **183**, 527–534.

Skipper, J.C., Kittlesen, D.J., Hendrickson, R.C., Deacon, D.D., Harthun, N.L., Wagner, S.N., Hunt, D.F., Engelhard, V.H., and Slingluff, C.L. Jr. (1996b) Shared epitopes for HLA-A3-restricted melanoma-reactive human CTL include a naturally processed epitope from Pmel-17/gp100. *J. Immunol.*, **157**, 5027–5033.

Slamon, D.J., Clark, G.M., Wong, S.G., Levin, W.J., Ulrich, A., and McGuire, W.L. (1987) Human breast cancer: correlation of relapse and survival with amplification of the HER-2/neu oncogene. *Science*, **235**, 177–182.

Stockert, E., Jäger, E., Chen, Y.T., Scanlan, M.J., Gout, I., Karbach, J., Arand, M., Knuth, A., and Old, L.J. (1998) A survey of the humoral immune response of cancer patients to a panel of human tumor antigen. *J. Exp. Med.*, **187**, 1349–1354.

Suzuki, T., Seko, A., Kitajima, K., Inoue, Y., and Inoue, S. (1993) Identification of peptide:N-glycanase activity in mammalian-derived cultured cells. *Biochem. Biophys. Res. Commun.*, **194**, 1124–1130.

Suzuki, K., Sahara, H., Okada, Y., Yososhima, T., Hirohashi, Y., Nabeta, Y., Hirai, I., Torigoe, T., Takahashi, S., Matsuura, A., Takahashi, N., Sasaki, A., Suzuki, M., Hamuro, J., Ikeda, H., Wada, Y., Hirata, K., Kikuchi, K., and Sato, N. (1999) Identification of natural antigenic peptides of a human gastric signet ring cell carcinoma recognized by HLA-A31-restricted cytotoxic T lymphocytes. *J. Immunol.*, **163**, 2783–2791.

Tahara, K., Takesako, K., Sette, A., Celis, E., Kitano, S., and Akiyoshi, T. (1999) Identification of a MAGE-2-encoded human leukocyte antigen-A24-binding synthetic peptide that induces specific antitumor cytotoxic T lymphocytes. *Clin. Cancer Res.*, **5**, 2236–2241.

Takahashi, K., Shichijo, S., Noguchi, M., Hirohata, M., and Itoh, K. (1995) Identification of MAGE-1 and MAGE-4 proteins in spermatogonia and primary spermatocytes of testis. *Cancer Res.*, **55**, 3478–3482.

Tanaka, F., Fujie, T., Tahara, K., Mori, M., Takesako, K., Sette, A., Celis, E., and Akiyoshi, T. (1997) Induction of antitumor cytotoxic T lymphocytes with a MAGE-3-encoded synthetic peptide presented by human leukocytes antigen-A24. *Cancer Res.*, **57**, 4465–4468.

Theobald, M., Biggs, J., Dittmer, D., Levine, A.J., and Sherman, L.A. (1995) Targeting p53 as a general tumor antigen. *Proc. Natl. Acad. Sci. USA*, **92**, 11993–11997.

Theobald, M., Biggs, J., Hernandez, J., Lustgarten, J., Labadie, C., and Sherman, L.A. (1997) Tolerance to p53 by A2.1-restricted cytotoxic T lymphocytes. *J. Exp. Med.*, **185**, 833–841.

Thurner, B., Haendle, I., Roder, C., Dieckmann, D., Keikavoussi, P., Jonuleit, H., Bender, A., Maczek, C., Schreiner, D., von den Driesch, P., Bröcker, E.B., Steinman, R.M., Enk, A., Kämpgen, E., and Schuler, G. (1999) Vaccination with Mage-3A1 peptide-pulsed mature, monocyte-derived dendritic cells expands specific cytotoxic T cells and induced regression of some metastases in advanced stage IV melanoma. *J. Exp. Med.*, **190**, 1669–1678.

Topalian, S.L., Rivoltini, L., Mancini, M., Markus, N.R., Robbins, P.F., Kawakami, Y., and Rosenberg, S.A. (1994a) Human CD4+ T cells specificaly recognize a shared melanoma-associated antigen encoded by the tyrosinase gene. *Proc. Natl. Acad. Sci. USA*, **91**, 9461–9465.

Topalian, S.L., Rivoltini, L., Mancini, M., Ng, J., Hartzman, R.J., and Rosenberg, S.A. (1994b) Melanoma-specific CD4+ T lymphocytes recognize human melanoma antigens processed and presented by Epstein-Barr-transformed B cells. *Int. J. Cancer*, **58**, 69–79.

Topalian, S.L., Gonzales, M.I., Parkhurst, M., Li, Y.F., Southwood, S., Sette, A., Rosenberg, S.A., and Robbins, P.F. (1996) Melanoma-specific CD4+ T cells recognize nonmutated HLA-DR-restricted tyrosinase epitopes. *J. Exp. Med.*, **183**, 1965–1971.

Traversari, C., van der Bruggen, P., Luescher, I.F., Lurquin, C., Chomez, P., Van Pel, A., De Plaen, E., Amar-Costesec, A., and Boon, T. (1992) A nonapeptide encoded by human gene MAGE-1 is recognized on HLA-A1 by cytolytic T lymphocytes directed against tumor antigen MZ2-E. *J. Exp. Med.*, **176**, 1453–1457.

Traversari, C., Meazza, R., Coppolecchia, M., Basso, S., Verrecchia, A., van der Bruggen, P., Ardizzoni, A., Gaggero, A., and Ferrini, S. (1997) IFN-gamma gene transfer restores HLA-class I expression and MAGE-3 antigen presentation to CTL in HLA-deficient small cell lung cancer. *Gene Ther.*, **4**, 1029–1035.

Tsai, V., Southwood, S., Sidney, J., Sakaguchi, K., Kawakami, Y., Appella, E., Sette, A., and Celis, E. (1997) Identification of subdominant CTL epitopes of the GP100 melanoma-associated tumor antigen by primary *in vitro* immunization with peptide-pulsed dendritic cells. *J. Immunol.*, **158**, 1796–1802.

Tureci, O., Chen, Y.T., Sahin, U., Gure, A.O., Zwick, C., Villena, C., Tsang, S., Seitz, G., Old, L.J., and Pfreundschuh, M. (1998) Expression of SSX genes in human tumors. *Int. J. Cancer*, **77**, 19–23.

Tuting, T., Wilson, C.C., Martin, D.M., Kasamon, Y.L., Rowles, J., Ma, D.I., Slingluff, C.L. Jr., Wagner, S.N., van der Bruggen, P., Baar, J., Lotze, M.T., and Storkus, W.J. (1998) Autologous human monocyte-derived dendritic cells genetically modified to express melanoma antigens elicit primary cytotoxic T cell responses *in vitro*: enhancement by cotransfection of genes encoding the Th1-biasing cytokines IL-12 and IFN-alpha. *J. Immunol.*, **160**, 1139–1147.

Valmori, D., Lienard, D., Waanders, G., Rimoldi, D., Cerottini, J.C., and Romero, P. (1997) Analysis of MAGE-3-specific cytolytic T lymphocytes in human leukocyte antigen-A2 melanoma patients. *Cancer Res.*, **57**, 735–741.

Valmori, D., Fonteneau, J.F., Lizana, C.M., Gervois, N., Lienard, D., Rimoldi, D., Jongeneel, V., Jotereau, F., Cerottini, J.C., and Romero, P. (1998) Enhanced generation of specific tumor-reactive CTL *in vitro* by selected Melan-A/MART-1 immunodominant peptide analogues. *J. Immunol.*, **160**, 1750–1758.

Van den Eynde, B., Peeters, O., De Backer, O., Gaugler, B., Lucas, S., and Boon, T. (1995) A new family of genes coding for an antigen recognized by autologous cytolytic T lymphocytes on a human melanoma. *J. Exp. Med.*, **182**, 689–698.

Van den Eynde, B., and van der Bruggen, P. (1997) T cell defined tumor antigens. *Curr. Op. Immunol.*, **9**, 684–693.

van der Bruggen, P., Traversari, C., Chomez, P., Lurquin, C., De Plaen, E., Van den Eynde, B., Knuth, A., and Boon, T. (1991) A gene encoding an antigen recognized by cytolytic T lymphocytes on a human melanoma. *Science*, **254**, 1643–1647.

van der Bruggen, P., Bastin, J., Gajewski, T., Coulie, P.G., Boel, P., De Smet, C., Traversari, C., Townsend, A., and Boon, T. (1994a) A peptide encoded by human gene MAGE-3 and presented by HLA-A2 induces cytolytic T lymphocytes that recognize tumor cells expressing MAGE-3. *Eur. J. Immunol.*, **24**, 3038–3043.

van der Bruggen, P., Szikora, J.P., Boel, P., Wildmann, C., Somville, M., Sensi, M., and Boon, T. (1994b) Autologous cytolytic T lymphocytes recognize a MAGE-1 nonapeptide on melanomas expressing HLA-Cw*1601. *Eur. J. Immunol.*, **24**, 2134–2140.

van der Burg, S.H., Visseren, M.J.W., Brandt, R.M.P., Kast, W.M., and Melief, C.J.M. (1996) Immunogenicity of peptides bound to MHC class I molecules depends on the MHC-peptide complex stability. *J. Immunol.*, **156**, 3308–3314.

Vierboom, M.P., Nijman, H.W., Offringa, R., van der Voort, E.I., van Hall, T., van den Broek, L., Fleuren, G.J., Kenemans, P., Kast, W.M., and Melief, C.J. (1997) Tumor eradication by wild-type p53-specific cytotoxic T lymphocytes. *J. Exp. Med.*, **186**, 695–704.

Visseren, M.J., van der Burg, S.H., van der Voort, E.I., Brandt, R.M., Schrier, P.I., van der Bruggen, P., Boon, T., Melief, C.J., and Kast, W.M. (1997) Identification of HLA-A*0201-restricted CTL epitopes encoded by the tumor-specific MAGE-2 gene product. *Int. J. Cancer*, **73**, 125–130.

Vissers, J.L., De Vries, I.J., Schreurs, M.W., Engelen, L.P., Oosterwijk, E., Figdor, C.G., Adema, G.J. (1999) The renal cell carcinoma-associated antigen G250 encodes a human leukocyte antigen (HLA)-A2.1-restricted epitope recognized by cytotoxic T lymphocytes. *Cancer Res.*, **59**, 5554–5559.

Vonderheide, R.H., Hahn, W.C., Schultze, J.L., and Nadler, L.M. (1999) The telomerase catalytic subunit is a widely expressed tumor-associated antigen recognized by cytotoxic T lymphocytes. *Immunity*, **10**, 673–679.

Wang, R.-F., Robbins, P.F., Kawakami, Y., Kang, X.-Q., and Rosenberg, S.A. (1995) Identification of a gene encoding a melanoma tumor antigen recognized by HLA-A31-restricted tumor-infiltrating lymphocytes. *J. Exp. Med.*, **181**, 799–804.

Wang, R.-F., Appella, E., Kawakami, Y., Kang, X., and Rosenberg, S.A. (1996a) Identification of TRP-2 as a human tumor antigen recognized by cytotoxic T lymphocytes. *J. Exp. Med.*, **184**, 2207–2216.

Wang, R.-F., Parkhurst, M.R., Kawakami, Y., Robbins, P.F., and Rosenberg, S.A. (1996b) Utilization of an alternative open reading frame of a normal gene in generating a novel human cancer antigen. *J. Exp. Med.*, **183**, 1131–1140.

Wang, R.-F., Johnston, S.L., Southwood, S., Sette, A., and Rosenberg, S.A. (1998a) Recognition of an antigenic peptide derived from tyrosinase-related protein-2 by CTL in the context of HLA-A31 and -A33. *J. Immunol.*, **160**, 890–897.

Wang, R.-F., Johnston, S.L., Zeng, G., Topalian, S.L., Schwartzentruber, D.J., and Rosenberg, S.A. (1998b) A breast and melanoma-shared tumor antigen: T cell responses to antigenic peptides translated from different open reading frames. *J. Immunol.*, **161**, 3596–3606.

Wang, R.-F., Wang, X., Atwood, A.C., Topalian, S.L., and Rosenberg, S.A. (1999a) Cloning genes encoding MHC class II-restricted antigens: mutated CDC27 as a tumor antigen. *Science*, **284**, 1351–1354.

Wang, R.-F., Wang, X., and Rosenberg, S.A. (1999b) Identification of a novel major histocompatibility complex class II-restricted tumor antigen resulting from a chromosomal rearrangement recognized by CD4+ T cells. *J. Exp. Med.*, **189**, 1659–1667.

Wölfel, T., Van Pel, A., Brichard, V., Schneider, J., Seliger, B., Meyer zum Buschenfelde, K.H., and Boon, T. (1994) Two tyrosinase nonapeptides recognized on HLA-A2 melanomas by autologous cytolytic T lymphocytes. *Eur. J. Immunol.*, **24**, 759–764.

Wölfel, T., Hauer, M., Schneider, J., Serrano, M., Wölfel, C., Klehmann-Hieb, E., De Plaen, E., Hankeln, T., Meyer Zum Buschenfelde, K.-H., and Beach, D. (1995) A p16INK4a-insensitive CDK4 mutant targeted by cytolytic T lymphocytes in a human melanoma. *Science*, **269**, 1281–1284.

Yang, D., Nakao, M., Shichijo, S., Sasatomi, T., Takasu, H., Matsumoto, H., Mori, K., Hayashi, A., Yamana, H., Shirouzu, K., and Itoh, K. (1999) Identification of a gene coding for a protein possessing shared tumor epitopes capable of inducing HLA-A24-restricted cytotoxic T lymphocytes in cancer patients. *Cancer Res.*, **59**, 4056–4063.

Yee, C., Gilbert, M.J., Riddell, S.R., Brichard, V.G., Fefer, A., Thompson, J.A., Boon, T., and Greenberg, P.D. (1996) Isolation of tyrosinase-specific CD8+ and CD4+ T cell clones from the peripheral blood of melanoma patients following *in vitro* stimulation with recombinant vaccinia virus. *J. Immunol.*, **157**, 4079–4086.

Yewdell, J.W., and Bennink, J.R. (1992) Cell biology of antigen processing and presentation to major histocompatability complex class I molecule-restricted T lymphocytes. *Adv. Immunol.*, **52**, 1–123.

Zaks, T.Z., and Rosenberg, S.A. (1998) Immunization with a peptide epitope (p369-377) from HER-2/neu leads to peptide specific cytotoxic T lymphocytes which fail to recognize HER-2/neu+ tumors. *Cancer Res.*, **58**, 4902–4908.

Zorn, E., and Hercend, T. (1999) A natural cytotoxic T cell response in a spontaneously regressing human melanoma targets a neoantigen resulting from a somatic point mutation. *Eur. J. Immunol.*, **29**, 592–601.

2 Processing and Presentation of Antigen for the Activation of Lymphocytes to Tumor Cells

Suzanne Ostrand-Rosenberg, Beth A. Pulaski and Vicky Gunther

ABBREVIATIONS

Ii	Class II-associated invariant chain
APC	Antigen-presenting cells
β2m	Beta 2 microglobulin
BcR	Antigen-specific receptor of B lymphocytes
CTL	Cytotoxic T lymphocytes
DC	Dendritic cells
ER	Endoplasmatic reticulum
FDC	Follicular dendritic cells
GM-CSF	Granulocyte-monocyte colony-stimulating-factor
HSP	Heat shock proteins
IFN-γ	Interferon gamma
IL-...	Interleukin-2, -4, -10, -12
MHC	Major histocompatibility complex
MIIC	Major histocompatibility complex class II compartment
NK	Natural killer
NKT	Natural killer T cells
PBMC	Peripheral blood mononuclear cells
TAP1, TAP2	Transporter associated with antigen processing -1, -2
TcR	Antigen-specific receptor of T lymphocytes
T_h	T helper
TNF-α	Tumor necrosis factor alpha

Processing and presentation of tumor antigen

1. **Antigens are processed by specialized antigen-presenting cells (APC) (e.g. dendritic cells, monocytes, B-cells) through endogenous or exogenous pathways which are preferentially used to present peptides to class I and class II MHC molecules, respectively.**
2. **Tumor antigenic proteins are processed and mounted on tumor cell membrane as peptides within the groove of MHC molecules.**
3. **Tumor cells are poor APC since, even when expressing adequate amounts of MHC/peptide complexes, they lack co-stimulatory molecules and cannot activate T cells.**
4. **Tumor cells can become effective APC upon transfection with genes encoding class II MHC and co-stimulatory molecules (e.g. B7-1).**
5. **Cross-priming through host dendritic cells is the most likely mechanism of tumor antigen presentation *in vivo*.**
6. **The MHC encoded class I-like (class Ib) MHC non-polymorphic molecules present peptides and may be involved in surveillance against pathogens and tumor cells.**
7. **Other molecules, homologue to MHC (e.g. CD1), are expressed on APC and can present bacterial or tumor cell glycoplipids antigens. Such glycolipids can induce an antitumor immunity even *in vivo*.**

ANTIGEN PROCESSING AND PRESENTATION ARE CRITICAL COMPONENTS OF LYMPHOCYTE ACTIVATION AND TARGETING

Harnessing the immune response to reject autologous tumor involves at least two processes: 1) activation of tumor-specific lymphocytes and 2) targeting of the activated lymphocytes to tumor cells. For lymphocytes to be successfully activated they must interact via their antigen-specific receptor (TcR for T lymphocytes; BcR for B lymphocytes) with their cognate antigen and receive additional co-stimulatory signals. This process is called antigen presentation and usually professional APC provide both the antigen signal and the co-stimulatory signal. Although the BcR of B lymphocytes can respond to intact antigen, the TcR of T lymphocytes only responds to small fragments of antigen. APC must therefore break down macromolecular antigens into smaller fragments for presentation to T lymphocytes. This process of degradation is called antigen processing and occurs in APC. Because the antigen-specific receptor of T cells only recognizes antigenic fragments bound to specialized antigen-presenting molecules encoded by the MHC, degraded antigen must associate with the antigen presentation molecules encoded by the APC's MHC (e.g. MHC class I, class II, or CD1 molecules) for presentation to T lymphocytes. Because $CD4^+$ T_h lymphocytes are required for both T and B lymphocyte responses, appropriate processing and presentation of antigen is central to both T and B immune responses, and critical for the generation of effective antitumor immunity.

Once lymphocytes are specifically activated to tumor antigens, they must destroy or inhibit the growth of tumor cells for successful antitumor immunity. Recognition of target cells by activated lymphocytes also occurs by lymphocyte receptor binding to antigen. The same antigen-specific receptors are used in the target phase of the immune response as during the activation phase. Therefore, antigen processing is not required for B cell (antibody) targeting, but is essential for T cell targeting. To be targeted by activated T cells, tumor cells, therefore, must present fragmented tumor antigen/MHC complexes at their cell surface.

Antigen presentation, therefore, encompasses a series of events in APC, beginning with the uptake of antigen, followed by processing of antigen, expression of antigen with/without antigen presentation molecules, and co-expression of co-stimulatory molecules. A schematic diagram of these events during the activation of CD8$^+$ and CD4$^+$ T cells is shown in Figure 2.1. A critical step in this activation scheme is the uptake of antigen by

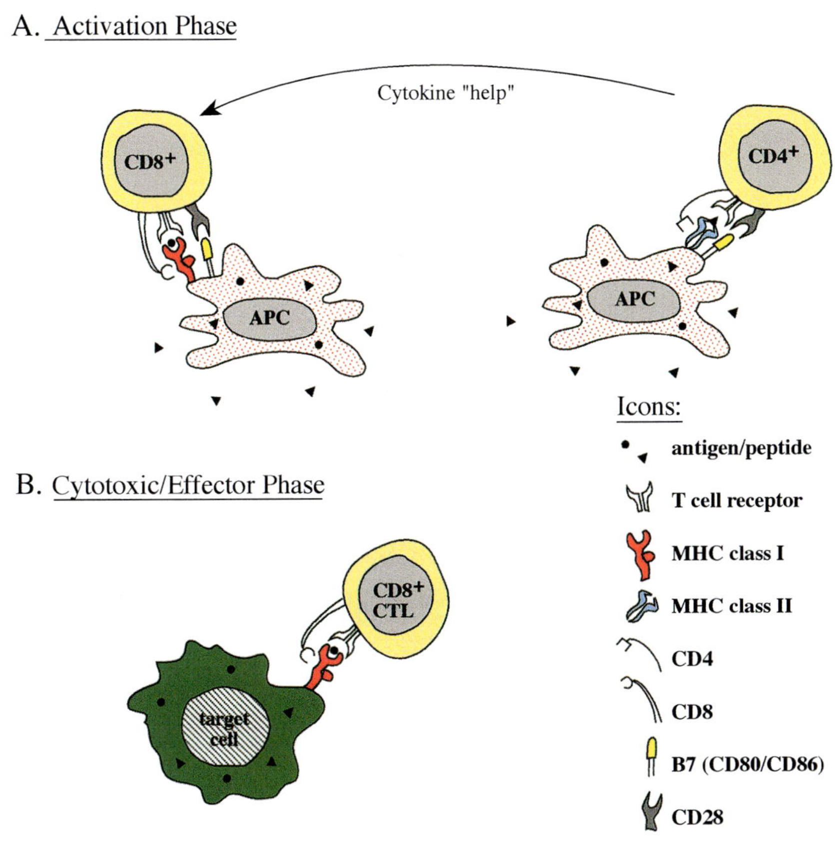

Figure 2.1 Overview of antigen processing and presentation during the activation of CD4$^+$ and CD8$^+$ T lymphocytes. (A) During the activation phase, professional APC pinocytose exogenous antigen, process it into peptides, and re-present it bound to their MHC class II molecules along with a CD80 and/or CD86 co-stimulatory signal to the TcR and CD28 receptors, respectively, of CD4$^+$ T cells. Concomitant with CD4$^+$ T cell activation, CD8$^+$ T cells are being activated by APC presenting processed antigen bound to MHC class I molecules along with co-stimulatory signals. If the activated CD4$^+$ T cell provides "help" in the form of cytokines to the CD8$^+$ T cells, the latter cell will become optimally activated and gain cytotoxic activity. (B) During the cytotoxic or effector phase, the CD8$^+$ cytotoxic T cell recognizes processed antigen bound to MHC class I molecules of the target (tumor) cell and destroys the target.

APC. In conventional immune responses with soluble antigens, antigen is either carried in soluble form or pinocytosed by APC and carried via the lymphatic system to the draining lymph nodes where it is presented to lymphocytes. However, if tumor antigens are not secreted by tumor cells, or if tumor cells do not release cellular debris containing tumor antigens, this conventional route may not be accessible. Various alternative pathways have been suggested, including lymphocyte migration to the tumor site and tumor cell migration to the draining lymph nodes. It has also been suggested that poor antitumor immunity in tumor-bearing patients is due to an inability of tumor antigens to be picked up by professional APC and brought to the draining lymph nodes.

Generation of effective antitumor immunity is critically dependent on optimal presentation of tumor antigens to T and B lymphocytes. Many of the current experimental immunotherapy methods focused on stimulating antitumor immunity are strategies aimed at improving presentation of tumor antigens. To fully appreciate these strategies an understanding of antigen processing and presentation is necessary. The remainder of this chapter, therefore, will address the principle aspects of antigen processing and presentation, including antigen uptake and processing by APC, presentation of antigen by APC, the molecules encoded by the MHC that bind and present antigen, and the various types of professional APC. Since some of these pathways are currently being exploited to improve antitumor immunity in experimental animals and clinical trials, we will also discuss some of the approaches that have been devised to enhance presentation of tumor antigens.

ANTIGEN PROCESSING AND PRESENTATION

T lymphocytes only recognize and respond to peptide fragments of antigen bound to proteins encoded by the MHC. Antigen to be presented to T lymphocytes, therefore, must be ''processed'' within the APC into peptides before it can be presented to T cells. APC use two major intracellular pathways for antigen processing. One pathway is used for antigen synthesized within the APC (endogenously synthesized antigen), while antigen synthesized by another cell and taken up by the APC is handled via a different pathway (exogenously synthesized antigen).

ENDOGENOUS PATHWAY OF ANTIGEN PROCESSING AND PRESENTATION

Virtually all proteins are encoded by APC traffic via the endogenous antigen processing pathway. These molecules include self proteins, plus proteins produced by viruses, bacteria, and other intracellular parasites. In the endogenous or cytosolic pathway, molecules in the cytosol destined for degradation are tagged in the cytoplasm with a small protein called *ubiquitin*. Ubiquinated proteins are then degraded within the proteosome, a cytosolic organelle containing a variety of proteolytic enzymes. Following breakdown of the protein, the peptides are transported via TAP from the cytosol into the ER. Peptide transport is ATP dependent and affinity of peptide for the TAP1 and TAP2 proteins is highest for those peptides of 8–13 amino acids in length. Simultaneous with peptide transport, MHC class I molecules, which have been synthesized within the rough ER, are structurally stabilized by binding to the chaperone calnexin and β2m. This stabilization occurs in parallel to peptide transport. Within the ER, the class I/β2m/ calnexin complex binds to the TAP proteins, facilitating peptide transfer to the antigen binding cleft of class I (see the section on ''Antigen presentation molecules'' for a description of the peptide/class I binding process). Peptide binding to class I stabilizes the class I/β2m complex, thus releasing calnexin, and the class I/β2m/peptide complex then travels via the Golgi complex to the cell surface. Figure 2.2 shows a schematic diagram of the endogenous antigen presentation pathway. Because almost all endogenously encoded proteins are degraded by the proteosome at some point in their existence, the endogenous pathway enables presentation of essentially all proteins synthesized by the APC (York and Rock, 1996). Therefore, tumor cells, like virtually all other cells, can potentially present at their cell surface any fragmented self-peptide bound to MHC class I molecules.

EXOGENOUS PATHWAY OF ANTIGEN PROCESSING AND PRESENTATION

In contrast to the endogenous pathway, the exogenous pathway presents antigens synthesized outside of the APC (see the right-hand side of Figure 2.2 for a schematic diagram of the endogenous pathway). Antigens synthesized external to APC are phagocytosed or pinocytosed by APC (see ''Dendritic Cell'' section for a description of these processes) and travel through a series of endosomal compartments where they are degraded by resident proteases. Successive compartments have decreasing pH, ranging from a pH of 6.0–6.5 in the early endosomal compartments to a pH of 4.5–5.0 in lysosomes. By the time antigen reaches the so-called MHC class II compartment, or MIIC, it has been degraded into peptides of approximately 13–18 amino acids in length.

Class II molecules preferentially present exogenously synthesized antigen because they travel via an intracellular pathway that intersects with the endosomal pathway taken by phagocytosed or pinocytosed antigen. Synthesis of class II molecules is coordinately regulated with synthesis of the class II-associated proteins invariant (Ii) chain and HLA-DM. In the ER the Ii chain binds to the peptide binding groove of newly synthesized MHC class II molecules thereby blocking the binding of other endogenously synthesized peptides present in the ER. From the ER the MHC class II/Ii complex travels to an endosomal compartment in the cytoplasm, guided by a homing sequence contained in the Ii chain. Due to the low pH within the endosome, the Ii chain degrades and ultimately dissociates from the class II molecule, leaving the peptide binding groove accessible to peptides in the endosome. Binding of peptide to available class II molecules in the endosome is facilitated by another molecule encoded within the MHC, the HLA-DM protein. Once loaded with endocytosed peptide, the class II/peptide complex exits the endosomal compartment and is inserted into the plasma membrane (Lanzavecchia, 1996; Watts, 1997). The end result of this process is that MHC class II molecules typically present antigens of the APC's extracellular environment that are phagocytosed or pinocytosed by the APC.

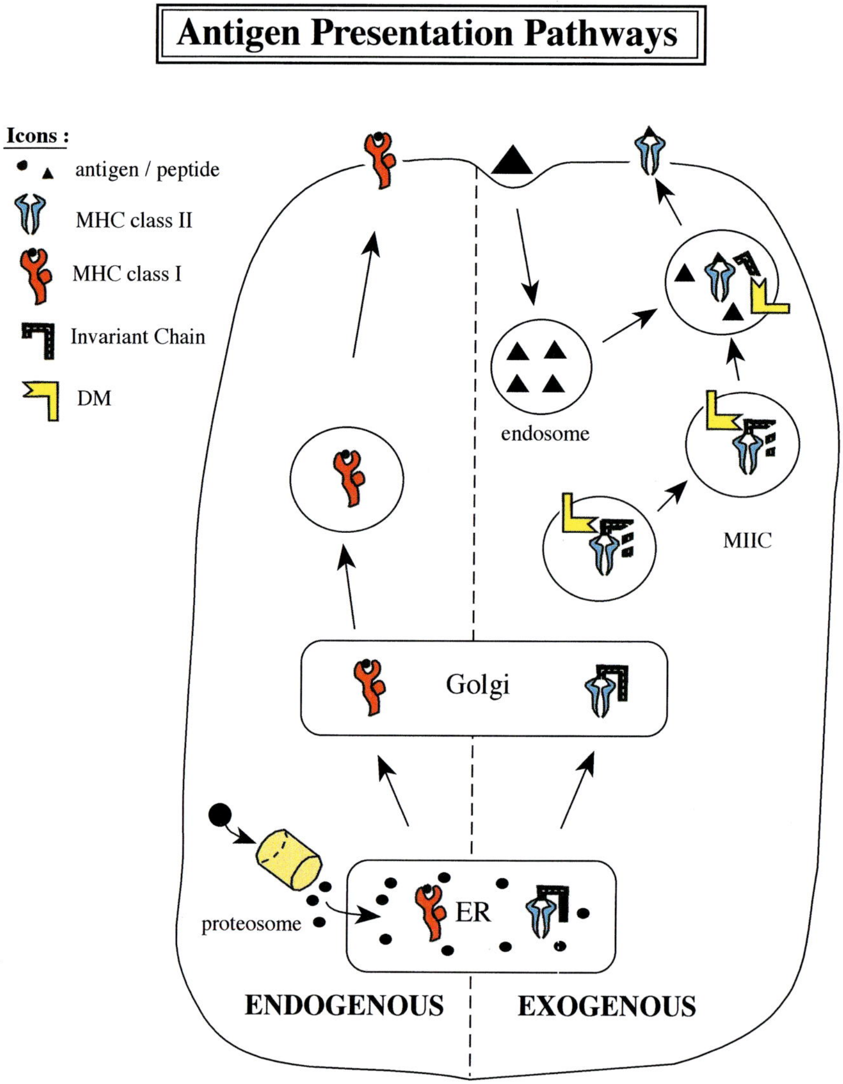

Figure 2.2 Prototypic antigen presentation pathways for endogenously and exogenously synthesized antigens. *Endogenous pathway* (left side of figure): Cytosolic antigen is degraded in the proteosome and transported via TAP-1 and TAP-2 into the ER. Newly synthesized MHC class I molecules then bind the peptides and transport them via the Golgi to the cell surface where the MHC class I/peptide complex is inserted into the plasma membrane. *Exogenous pathway* (right side of figure): Newly synthesized MHC class II molecules associate with the coordinately regulated Invariant chain in the ER and traffic via the Golgi to an endosomal compartment. As the endosomal compartment becomes more acidic the invariant chain is partially degraded and dissociated from the class II molecule, leaving CLIP associated with the binding region. Meanwhile, exogenously synthesized antigen is taken up into the endosomal compartment and degraded into peptides. The MHC class II and peptide compartments then fuse, giving rise to the MIIC. In the MIIC HLA-DM displaces CLIP and facilitates binding of the exogenous peptides to the binding cleft of class II. The MHC class II/peptide complex then traffics to the cell surface and is inserted into the plasma membrane.

In most cases, MHC class I molecules present peptides generated via the endocytic pathway, and MHC class II molecules present peptides generated via the exocytic pathway. However, these pathways are not exclusive and endogenously synthesized antigen can be presented by MHC class II molecules, and exogenously synthesized antigen can be presented by MHC class I molecules. As discussed in more detail later in this chapter, MHC class I molecules can access the endocytic route and thereby present exogenous antigen in B cells (Ke and Kapp, 1996), macrophages (Pfeifer *et al.*, 1993), and DC (Bohm *et al.*, 1995; Bachman *et al.*, 1996; Shen *et al.*, 1997). The antigen trafficking routes, therefore, are not absolute.

ANTIGEN PRESENTATION MOLECULES

Different types of lymphocytes ''see'' antigenic fragments in the context of different antigen presentation molecules. These molecules include the classical class I and class II molecules of the MHC, the non-classical MHC-encoded molecules Qa, Tla, and CD1, and the HSP. Although MHC class I, class II, and CD1 molecules have very distinct amino acid sequences, they share many structural motifs. Likewise, they all have unique antigen binding regions, but they share many antigen binding characteristics. In the next 3 sections these antigen presentation molecules will be discussed. Some of the shared and unique features of these molecules are listed in Table 2.1.

MHC CLASS I MOLECULES PREFERENTIALLY PRESENT ENDOGENOUSLY SYNTHESIZED PEPTIDE ANTIGENS TO CD8$^+$ T CELLS

MHC class I molecules are integral membrane glycoproteins expressed by virtually all nucleated cells and are the molecules that present antigen to $\alpha\beta^+$ CD8$^+$ T lymphocytes.

TABLE 2.1
Binding motifs of CD1 and MHC class I and class II molecules

Features	MHC Class I	MHC Class II	CD1
Peptide-binding domain	$\alpha 1/\alpha 2$	$\alpha 1/\beta 1$	$\alpha 1/\alpha 2$
Nature of cleft	Closed	Open	Closed
Bound peptides	8–10 amino acids	13–23 amino acids	lipids or glycolipids
Peptide composition	– anchor residues found on ends – typically residues are (eg. G, P, Y, L, I, V)	– anchor residues distributed along peptide – typically residues are hydrophobic and aromatic – 30% peptides contain multiple prolines	– hydrophylic head group – 2 aliphatic tails
Position of bound peptide	Structure is secured at the ends and arches away from cleft	Structure held at a constant elevation above cleft	Structure held within the hydrophobic groove by the tails to expose the polar head group outside cleft

The class I molecules were originally defined as the antigens that govern graft rejection, and hence are sometimes referred to as transplantation antigens. In humans there are 3 loci within the MHC or HLA (human leucocyte antigen) complex that encode class I molecules: the HLA-A, HLA-B, and HLA-C loci. All three loci are extremely polymorphic with approximately 40–120 alleles at each locus. Since the class I alleles are co-dominant, each individual may express as many as 6 different HLA class I molecules, resulting in extensive heterogeneity within the population (see Figure 2.3 for a genetic map of the human MHC region).

Each class I molecule consists of a polymorphic heavy chain polypeptide that is non-covalently associated with an invariant molecule called β2m. Each heavy chain consists of 3 extracellular domains (α1, α2, and α3), a hydrophobic transmembrane region that anchors the class I molecule into the plasma membrane, and a cytoplasmic domain that extends into the cytoplasm. Each protein domain is encoded by a corresponding exon within a class I gene (see Figure 2.4 for a schematic diagram of class I molecules).

Landmark X-ray crystallography studies demonstrated that peptide binds to the class I molecule at a cleft that is formed by the interaction of the α1 and α2 domains of the heavy chain (Bjorkman *et al.*, 1988a; Bjorkman *et al.*, 1988b). Since most normal nucleated cells express MHC class I molecules, most cells display self antigens that potentially facilitate recognition by CD8$^+$ T cells and are potential targets for CD8$^+$ cytotoxic T cells.

Peptide binding to class I molecules is governed by the size and configuration of the peptide binding groove, which in turn is determined by the amino acid sequence of the α1 and α2 domains. Typically, bound peptides are 8–11 amino acids in length, and have specific amino acid anchor residues at defined positions. The specific anchor residues and their location are different for HLA-A vs. HLA-B vs. HLA-C molecules and for the different alleles within each locus. For example, HLA-A2 0201 has the peptide binding motif of leucine at position 2 and valine or leucine at position 9, while HLA-B7 0702 has the peptide binding motif of proline at position 2 and a hydrophobic or aromatic residue at

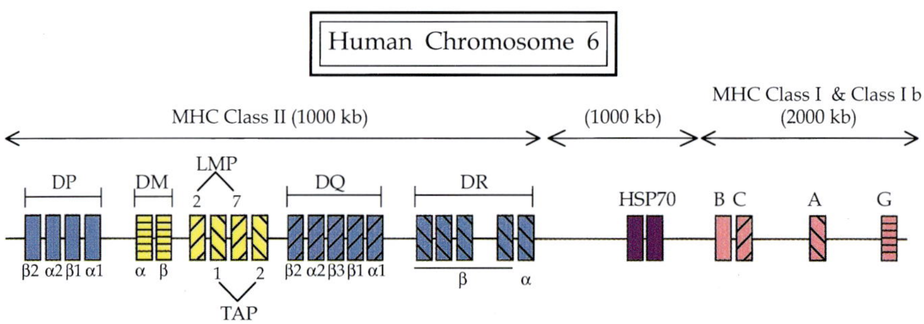

Figure 2.3 Genomic map of HLA antigens found on human chromosome 6 in the Major Histocompatibility Complex. MHC class II and class I/class Ib are shaded in blue and red, respectively. Other molecules important for antigen presentation are also found within the MHC class II region and include HLA-DM, LMP 2 and 7, and TAP1 and TAP2, which are shaded in yellow. The genes encoding the chaperone protein HSP70 (purple) are found in the region between the MHC class II and class I loci. Map is not drawn to scale.

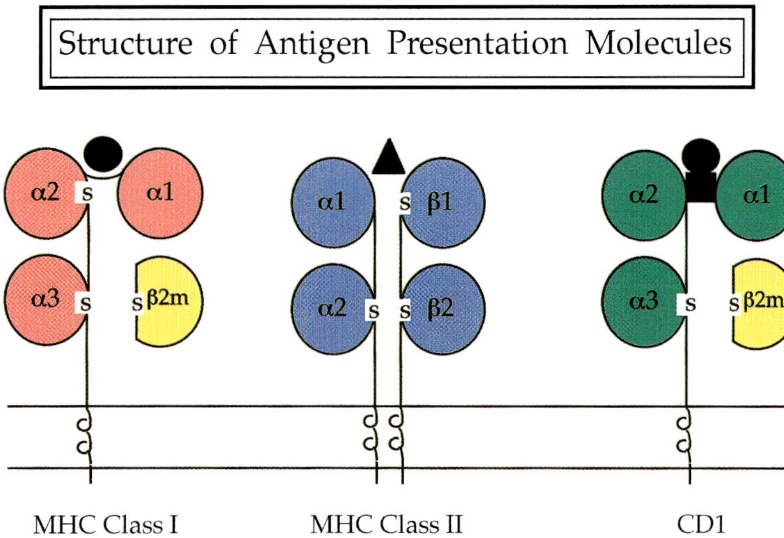

Figure 2.4 Schematic diagrams of the MHC class I, MHC class II, and CD1 molecules showing the different domains and antigen binding clefts for each structure. MHC class I and CD1 both require non-covalent binding of *β*2microglobulin for expression at the cell surface.

position 9. Because of the extensive genetic heterogeneity of class I molecules in the population, different individuals may present different repertoires of class I-restricted antigenic peptides.

As discussed elsewhere in this monograph, various MHC class I-binding tumor peptides have been identified from a variety of tumor types, including malignant melanoma, prostate cancer, mammary carcinoma, colon carcinoma, and renal carcinoma, as well as other tumor types (Ostrand-Rosenberg *et al.*, 1998). All of these antigens and the peptides derived from them are synthesized by tumor cells, and can potentially bind to MHC class I molecules for presentation. Although MHC genotype may limit the quality and quantity of tumor peptides presented by a given individual, theoretically, all MHC class I positive tumor cells should present tumor peptides that can be recognized by $CD8^+$ T lymphocytes. As a result, MHC class I^+ tumors should be targets for $CD8^+$ tumor-specific CTL.

Unfortunately, 15–20% of human tumors do not express a full complement of MHC class I molecules or are completely deficient in MHC class I expression (Garrido *et al.*, 1993). As a result, these cells present a reduced repertoire of tumor peptides, or if totally class I deficient, do not present any peptides to $CD8^+$ T cells. Such tumor cells are poor targets for lysis by $CD8^+$ CTL. Although NK cells can lyse class I-deficient targets (Hoglund *et al.*, 1997) (see also Chapter 3), T lymphocytes are the only cytotoxic effector cells that provide long-term immunological memory. Long-term T cell-mediated immune surveillance against class I-deficient tumors, therefore, may be difficult to achieve and in some cases may not be feasible.

MHC CLASS II MOLECULES PREFERENTIALLY PRESENT EXOGENOUSLY SYNTHESIZED PEPTIDE ANTIGENS

MHC class II molecules are also integral membrane proteins and are the antigen presentation elements that present peptide antigen to $\alpha\beta^+$ $CD4^+$ T_h lymphocytes. Unlike MHC class I molecules, class II molecules are only expressed by professional APC, such as DC, B lymphocytes, Langerhans cells, and macrophages. There are 3 defined class II loci in the human: HLA-DR, HLA-DQ, and HLA-DP. Each MHC class II molecule is a heterodimer of an α and β chain encoded by corresponding genes (see Figure 2.3 for a genetic map including the class II MHC region). With the exception of the HLA-DRα, -DPα, and -DQα loci, the class II loci are extremely polymorphic with approximately 10–125 alleles at each β chain locus. As for the class I alleles, the class II alleles are co-dominant, so that a fully heterozygous individual may express up to 6 different class II molecules.

The α and β chains of class II molecules are non-covalently associated and form a complex including two extracellular domains (the $\alpha1$ and $\alpha2$ domains of the α chain and the $\beta1$ and $\beta2$ domains of the β chain). Each chain also includes a hydrophobic transmembrane region that anchors the class II molecule into the plasma membrane, and a short cytoplasmic domain consistig of the carboxyl termini of the α and β polypeptide chains. Figure 2.4 shows a schematic diagram of an MHC class II molecule.

X-ray crystallography studies of class II molecules demonstrate that class II molecules have a similar overall structure to class I. Antigenic peptide is bound within a cleft formed by the $\alpha1$ and $\beta1$ domains (Brown *et al.*, 1993), however, class II molecules preferentially bind longer peptides than class I (13–21 amino acids vs. 8–11 amino acids for class I), and the anchor residues and binding motifs are less precise for class II molecules as compared to class I molecules.

Although most nucleated cells present class I-restricted peptide antigens, presentation of class II-restricted peptide antigen is much more limited since only specialized professional APC synthesize MHC class II molecules and because antigen must be available for uptake by professional APC. Since activated $CD4^+$ T cells provide help to both $CD8^+$ and B lymphocytes, effective presentation of antigen in the context of MHC class II molecules is critical for generating optimal cellular and antibody-mediated immunity.

In terms of antitumor immunity, adequate activation of $CD4^+$ tumor-specific T cells is dependent on the availability of tumor antigens for uptake by professional APC. It has been proposed that the absence of tumor-specific $CD4^+$ T cells in tumor-bearing patients, especially during early stages of disease, may be limiting, resulting in inadequate activation of $CD4^+$ T_h cells (Ostrand-Rosenberg, 1994; Armstrong *et al.*, 1998b). Various remedies for this deficiency have been proposed and tested, and are discussed later in this chapter.

THE ROLE OF THE MHC-ENCODED CLASS I-LIKE (MHC CLASS IB) MOLECULES IS UNKNOWN

In addition to the already described class I antigens (class Ia), MHC regions of all vertebrates encode non-polymorphic, non-classical class Ib antigens (Shawar *et al.*, 1994; Stroynowski and Forman, 1995; Colonna *et al.*, 1997; O'Callaghan and Bell, 1998). The diversity and structural characteristics of peptides bound to these class Ib molecules are variable. For example, human HLA-G molecules, expressed on class Ia-negative trophoblast, and murine Qa-2 molecules, distributed on a wide variety of tissues, bind large repertoires of peptides similar to ligands of conventional class I molecules (Lee *et al.*, 1995; Tabaczewski *et al.*, 1998). In contrast, ubiquitously expressed HLA-E and its murine homolog Qa-1 bind restricted sets of peptides derived from the leader peptides of selected HLA or H-2 antigens (Aldrich *et al.*, 1994; O'Callaghan *et al.*, 1998). HLA-E has recently been demonstrated to function as a recognition target for inhibitory and activating CD94/NKG2 A, B, C NK cell receptors (Borrego *et al.*, 1998; Braud *et al.*, 1998; Lee *et al.*, 1998), raising a possibility that this class Ib antigen functions in pathogen/tumor immunosurveillance. Similar properties have been postulated for HLA-G (Colonna *et al.*, 1997; Perez-Villar *et al.*, 1997). A recent work demonstrates that NK cells infiltrating the decidua, but not those in the blood, preferentially up-regulate expression of their inhibitory NK receptors that bind to HLA-G that is predominantly expressed by fetal extravillous trophoblasts, thus suggesting that such NK are turned off to allow survival of the fetus (Ponte *et al.*, 1999). Since HLA-G expression has also been reported in human tumor samples, this molecule could contribute to the escape of tumors from immune-mediated destruction (Paul *et al.*, 1999). However, the physiological antigen presentation role of these class Ib molecules is at present only a conjecture. Interestingly, an indirect method for raising alloreactive responses against class Ib Qa-1 molecules has recently been reported to induce immunity against tumor cells expressing Qa-1 (Griffiths *et al.*, 1998). This approach may be explored in the future to develop novel antitumor vaccines independent of MHC polymorphism.

CD1 MOLECULES PRESENT LIPID ANTIGENS

In contrast to the MHC-encoded antigen presentation molecules, CD1 molecules present lipid and glycolipid antigens rather than peptides to T lymphocytes. Although they only share approximately 30% sequence homology with the MHC encoded molecules, they have a striking structural homology to MHC class I molecules having a similar domain structure and association with β2m (see Figure 2.4 for a schematic diagram of CD1) (Zeng *et al.*, 1997).

In humans there are five CD1 genes that map closely together on chromosome 1 and encode antigen presentation elements that have been divided into 2 groups (Melian *et al.*, 1996; Porcelli *et al.*, 1996). Group 1 molecules include CD1a, CD1b, and CD1c. These nonpolymorphic molecules are expressed on many professional APC including DC, some B lymphocytes, and activated monocytes. Extensive studies of the CD1b molecule indicate it presents bacterial lipid antigens such as lipoarabinomannan and phospatidylinositol-mannan glycolipids from *Mycobacterium leporae* and mycolic acid from *Mycobacterium tuberculosis* (Melian *et al.*, 1996). The high hydrophobicity of the α1 and α2 domains and the shape of the antigen binding groove as determined by X-ray crystallography are also consistent with the binding of lipids and glycolipids rather than peptides (Porcelli *et al.*, 1996; Zeng *et al.*, 1997). It is of interest that CD1b can also present self-glycolipids to T cells (Shamshiev *et al.*, 1999).

It is unclear if the group 1 CD1 molecules present intact or partially degraded antigens, although internalization and re-expression of the presented antigen is apparently required since reagents that prevent endosomal acidification interfere with antigen presentation (Porcelli *et al.*, 1996). In fact, presentation of peptide antigens by mouse CD1 requires endosomal localization and protein antigen processing (Tangri *et al.*, 1998). In contrast to peptide antigen presentation, presentation of lipids does not require transport from the cytosol to the ER because TAP-deficient cells efficiently present CD1b-restricted epitopes. Unexpectedly, CD1b trafficks via the MHC class II intracellular pathway to the MIIC, suggesting that antigen loading of CD1b occurs in the same compartment as class II, although HLA-DM, which is required for class II loading, is not obviously involved in CD1b loading (Porcelli *et al.*, 1996; Sugita *et al.*, 1996).

In contrast to the group 1 molecules, the group 2 CD1 molecules, CD1d1 and CD1d2, are expressed predominantly in the intestine. Also unlike group 1 molecules, CD1d1 molecules present peptides, although because of the hydrophobic nature of the peptide binding groove, it is possible that CD1d1 molecules may also bind and present hydrophobic non-peptide fragments. The structural basis for such antigen specificity and CD1 restriction has begun to be worked out (Grant *et al.*, 1999). Group 2 molecules may also present diverse antigens because T cell hybridomas restricted by CD1d with assorted T cell receptors have been isolated (Porcelli, 1995; Melian *et al.*, 1996).

The most direct evidence that CD1, specifically CD1d, plays a role in presentation of antigens relevant to tumors, comes from experiments using IL-12 to up-regulate antitumor immunity (see also Chapter 3). According to these studies, a population of effector cells called ''NKT'' cells that are NK1.1$^+$ (a marker of NK cells) and express Vα14-containing T cell receptor recognize glycosylceramide antigens restricted by CD1d. When tumor-bearing mice are treated with IL-12 there is significant tumor regression and/or extension of survival time which is dependent on the induction of NKT cells (Cui *et al.*, 1997; Kawano *et al.*, 1997). Moreover, DC pulsed with α-galactosylceramide and given to tumor-bearing mice were able to eradicate liver metastases (Toura *et al.*, 1999). CD1 molecules, therefore, may be important molecules for presentation of tumor antigens for the generation of effective antitumor immunity, particularly for tumors that express high levels of lipid and carbohydrate antigens.

HEAT SHOCK PROTEINS ARE CARRIERS FOR A WIDE REPERTOIRE OF PEPTIDES

Heat shock molecules are members of a family of proteins that are induced in virtually all cell types following exposure to excessive heat. They constitute the most abundant family of proteins within the cytosol and ER of most cells. There are several classes of HSP. Each class is defined by size (e.g. HSP 60. 70, 90 and 96 which are 60 KD, 70 KD, 90 KD, and 96 KD, respectively) and is non-polymorphic. Despite their lack of genetic heterogeneity each HSP class binds a wide repertoire of different peptides; however, the mechanism and specificity of peptide-binding remain unknown.

Although HSP do not directly present antigen to lymphocytes, they play an important role in intracellular trafficking of class I-restricted peptides. During antigen processing and presentation, self peptides in the cytosol must travel into the ER so they can encounter and be bound by MHC class I molecules (see Figure 2.2). Current hypotheses speculate that HSP function as chaperones for the peptides and guide them into the ER where the peptides are transferred to MHC class I molecules (Srivastava *et al.*, 1994; Srivastava *et al.*, 1998). This hypothesis predicts that HSP isolated from tumor cells are associated with immunogenic tumor peptides. Indeed, immunization of tumor-bearing mice with tumor-derived HSP/peptide complexes results in antitumor immunity and tumor regression (Suto and Srivastava, 1995). Presumably, during the latter immunization process, the HSP/peptide complex is taken up by professional APC and the peptide is re-presented in the context of host-derived MHC class I molecules via cross-priming (Srivastava *et al.*, 1994).

In addition to their putative role as intracellular chaperones for class I-restricted peptides, HSP may also present tumor peptides to NK cells (Multhoff *et al.*, 1997). Whether HSP present antigen in a fashion similar to that of class I and class II molecules is unclear, and a better understanding of the structural constraints of NK cell recognition may clarify the role of HSP in antigen presentation. HSP, therefore, may function as antigen presentation elements and intracellular transport and delivery agents for peptides, and may be exploited as carriers for tumor peptides for antitumor vaccination and immunotherapy.

ANTIGEN PRESENTATION BY PROFESSIONAL ANTIGEN PRESENTING CELLS

Several cell types within the body are highly specialized to function as APC. These so-called professional APC include DC, macrophages, B lymphocytes, and related cells. Professional APC must scavenge antigen from their surroundings, and subsequently present the antigen along with "second signals" to T and/or B cells. If the process is successfully completed, the T and/or B cells will be "activated." The various professional APC share many common features for antigen processing and presentation. They also have unique features that distinguish their antigen processing and presentation phenotypes.

DENDRITIC CELLS

DC are probably the most efficient APC in the body. Although the first DC, Langerhans cells of the skin, were identified over 20 years ago (Steinman, 1978), their function as potent APC has only recently been appreciated. These recent studies have led to an explosion of subsequent work aimed at using DC as immunization and vaccination agents particularly for inducing antitumor immunity. It was also recently shown that DC may be considered as a link between the two branches of the immune system, the innate immunity, a primitive immunity triggered by a variety of pathogens, and adaptive immunity which is based on specific recognition of antigens (see below). In fact, a very immature form of DC was described that can produce high amounts of interferon-α thus functioning as first barrier in protecting our body from intruders (Siegal *et al.*, 1999).

Antigen Uptake by Dendritic Cells

DC are potent APC for a variety of reasons. They reside in virtually all tissue types and hence are available for antigen uptake at all strategic locations where antigen may be found. They reside in body tissues in their immature form where they are specialized to take up and process antigen into peptides. DC take up antigen by three independent methods: 1) via the fluid phase by macropinocytosis (Sallusto *et al.*, 1995; Lanzavecchia, 1996); 2) via receptor mediated endocytosis using the FcγRII, FcϵR1, mannose receptor (Manca *et al.*, 1991; Stahl, 1992), and possibly additional plasma membrane receptors; or 3) via phagocytosis (Inaba *et al.*, 1993; Lanzavecchia, 1996). Exogenous antigen concentrations as low as 10^{-10} M are efficiently taken up by DC via macropinocytosis, and antigen internalization via the Fc receptors is also highly sensitive (Sallusto and Lanzavecchia, 1994). Since macropinocytosis by DC and Fc receptor expression is constitutive, DC are constantly sampling their environment. Their high efficiency at concentrating antigen, their widespread distribution in the body, and their constant activity, therefore, enable DC to continually and comprehensively present antigen even when antigen is present at very low concentrations in the surrounding locale.

Dendritic Cells Maturation and Migration

Immature DC in the periphery are specialized and focused on antigen uptake. Once antigen enters an immature DC, it resides in the endocytic route and is digested into small peptides by resident degradative enzymes. Within the same endocytic system in the MIIC, high levels of MHC class II molecules reside, along with the accessory molecule, HLA-DM, that facilitates peptide loading (see section on ''Exogenous pathway of antigen processing and presentation''). Within the MIIC, peptide fragments bind to class II molecules, and the complexes travel to the cell surface where they are stably expressed for many days (Pierre *et al.*, 1997). Once DC begin the process of class II/peptide association, the cells mature, becoming less efficient at internalizing antigen, and begin their transition to cells specialized to present antigen.

DC are potent APC and highly efficient activators of T lymphocytes for several reasons: 1) they have a 10–100 fold higher level of expression of MHC/peptide complexes relative to other APC (Inaba *et al.*, 1997); 2) they synthesize large amounts of IL-12, a cytokine that enhances B, T, and NK cell activity; 3) they express high levels of costimulatory and adhesion molecules, such as CD86, that enhance T cell activation (Inaba *et al.*, 1994); 4) mature DC are resistant to the immunosuppressive effects of IL-10 so this inhibitory cytokine which is frequently expressed *in vivo* does not interfere with DC-mediated T cell activation.

Differentiation of DC from an antigen uptake to an antigen presentation mode is accompanied by morphological and functional changes. As class II/peptide complexes traffic to the plasma membrane, the MIIC loses its degradative activity and is unable to generate additional antigenic peptides (Banchereau and Steinman, 1998). The cells also lose some of the markers that characterize them as immature cells, and take on expression of markers that characterize them as mature DC (Table 2.2 lists some of the markers expressed by mature DC). Although the function of some of these markers is

TABLE 2.2
Markers expressed by antigen-presenting cells

Intestazione	Marker	Alternate Name	DC	Macrophage	B Cell
T cell markers	CD3	TcR	no	no	no
	CD4	T4; HIV receptor	yes[a]	yes	no
DC markers	CD83	HB15			
	CD120a	p55; TNFR1	yes[b]	yes	yes
Adhesion molecules	CD58	LFA-3	yes[b]	yes	yes
	CD54	ICAM-1	yes[b]	yes	yes
Co-stimulatory molecules	CD80	B7.1; BB1	yes[b]	yes[d]	yes[e]
	CD86	B7.2; B70	yes[b]	yes[d]	yes[e]
	CD40	Bp50	yes[b]	yes	yes
	CD25	IL2Rα	yes	yes[d]	yes[e]
Homing receptors	CD11c	Axb2; CR4, p150	yes	yes	yes[lo]
Antigen presentation molecules	MHC class I		yes	yes	yes
	MHC class II		yes[c]	yes[d]	yes
	CD1a	R4	yes		
Other markers	CD14	LPS receptor	no	yes	
	CD19		no		yes[f]
	CD16	FcRIIIA/FcRIIIB	no	yes	
	CD13	APN; EC3.4.11.2	yes	yes	
	DEC-205		yes		
	CD115	c-fms; CSF-1R; M	no	yes	
	CD68	gp110; macrosialin	yes	yes	yes[lo]

[a] Some DC isolates express CD4
[b] Expressed at higher levels on mature DC
[c] Expressed on the cell surface of mature DC at high levels; expresed intracellularly on immature DC
[d] Expressed on activated macrophages
[e] Expressed on activated B cells
[f] Not expressed on plasma cells

unclear, other markers are definitely associated with the changing functions of mature vs. immature DC. For example, in immature DC, MHC class II molecules are largely intracellular, while in mature DC intracellular MHC class II levels are very low and plasma membrane expression is high. This change in class II location reflects the migration of MHC class II/peptide complexes from the MIIC to the cell surface and coincides with the increase in antigen presentation. Expression of the co-stimulatory molecules CD80, CD86, and CD40 also increases dramatically with maturation as DC become specialized to present antigen and activate T cells. Likewise, as DC mature they down-regulate their capacity to micropinocytose, and their antigen receptors (FcγRII and mannose receptor) decrease. This final DC maturation process is dependent on exposure to inflammatory cytokines like TNF-α and IL-1 but other stimuli can also be effective (LPS or CD40L). More recently, it has been found that double-stranded RNA treatment of DC results not only in increased antigen presentation and T cell stimulation but in resistance of DC to cytopathic effect of viruses (Cella *et al.*, 1999) (see also the section on ''*In vitro* generation of DC'').

Concomitant with the switch to an antigen presentation phenotype, mature DC gain the ability to migrate from peripheral tissue spaces to lymphoid organs such as the regional lymph nodes and spleen. The ability to migrate to lymph nodes is essential for optimum antigen presentation because T and/or B lymphocytes are concentrated in the lymph nodes and are activated there.

Dendritic Cell-Mediated Activation of B Cells and T cells within The Lymph Nodes

Two types of DC are present in the blood, CD11c^{+} and CD11c^{-}. Both types enter the lymph nodes via the afferent lymphatics and high endothelial venules. It is hypothesized that all DC migrate through T cell dependent areas of the nodes where they mature and have been named interdigitating cells by electron microscopists. The CD11c^{-} DC, also called follicular DC (FDC), migrate to the B-cell dependent germinal centers where they bind antigen/antibody complexes via their Fc and complement receptors. The FDC then present this non-denatured, intact antigen to B lymphocytes which in turn proliferate and undergo somatic hypermutation in their immunoglobulin genes. Following initial activation, the B cells wait for a subsequent antigen signal from the FDC. Delivery of this second signal results in B cell uptake of the presented intact antigen, and subsequent processing and presentation of the processed antigen to T cells. Activation of T cells via this route, therefore, involves antigen presentation of intact antigen by FDC → B cells, and subsequent presentation of the same antigen in a processed form from B cells → T cells (Banchereau and Steinman, 1998).

The second type of DC is CD11c^{+} and is also found in the germinal centers of lymph nodes. In contrast to the CD11c^{-} DC, the CD11c^{+} cells probably carry antigen with them into the lymph node. They are much more potent activators of T cells than of B cells of the germinal centers, and may be the DC that activate T memory lymphocytes (Grouard *et al.*, 1996; Banchereau and Steinman, 1998). Figure 2.5 shows the pathway of lymphocyte activation by CD11c^{+} DC.

The turnover of DC probably occurs within lymph nodes since afferent lymph contains abundant DC, while efferent lymph is deficient for DC. Once DC are charged with antigen, therefore, their raison d'être is to migrate to the lymph node and activate T and B lymphocytes. Once this activation occurs, the useful life of the DC is over and they apoptose.

Of note is recently discovered antitumor activity of CD11c^{+} DC which is mediated by TRAIL (TNF-related apoptosis-inducing ligand). This molecule is a member of the TNF family that induces apoptosis in a variety of cancers. CD11c^{+} DC exposed to IFN-γ or -α acquire expression of TRAIL and the ability to kill TRAIL-sensitive neoplastic cells thus suggesting an innate antitumor role of CD11c^{+} DC (Fauger *et al.*, 1999). Moreover, DC have the capacity to trigger, in addition to T or B cells (adaptive immunity), also NK cells (innate immunity) both *in vitro* and *in vivo* as shown by the ability of Flt3 ligand to expand DC which, in turn, promote NK cell-dependent antitumor destruction (Fernandez *et al.*, 1999).

Cross-Priming or Indirect Antigen Presentation for Activating T Lymphocytes

As discussed earlier, MHC class I molecules typically present endogenously synthesized antigens, while MHC class II molecules usually present exogenously synthesized antigens. However, these pathways are not absolute, and DC and other

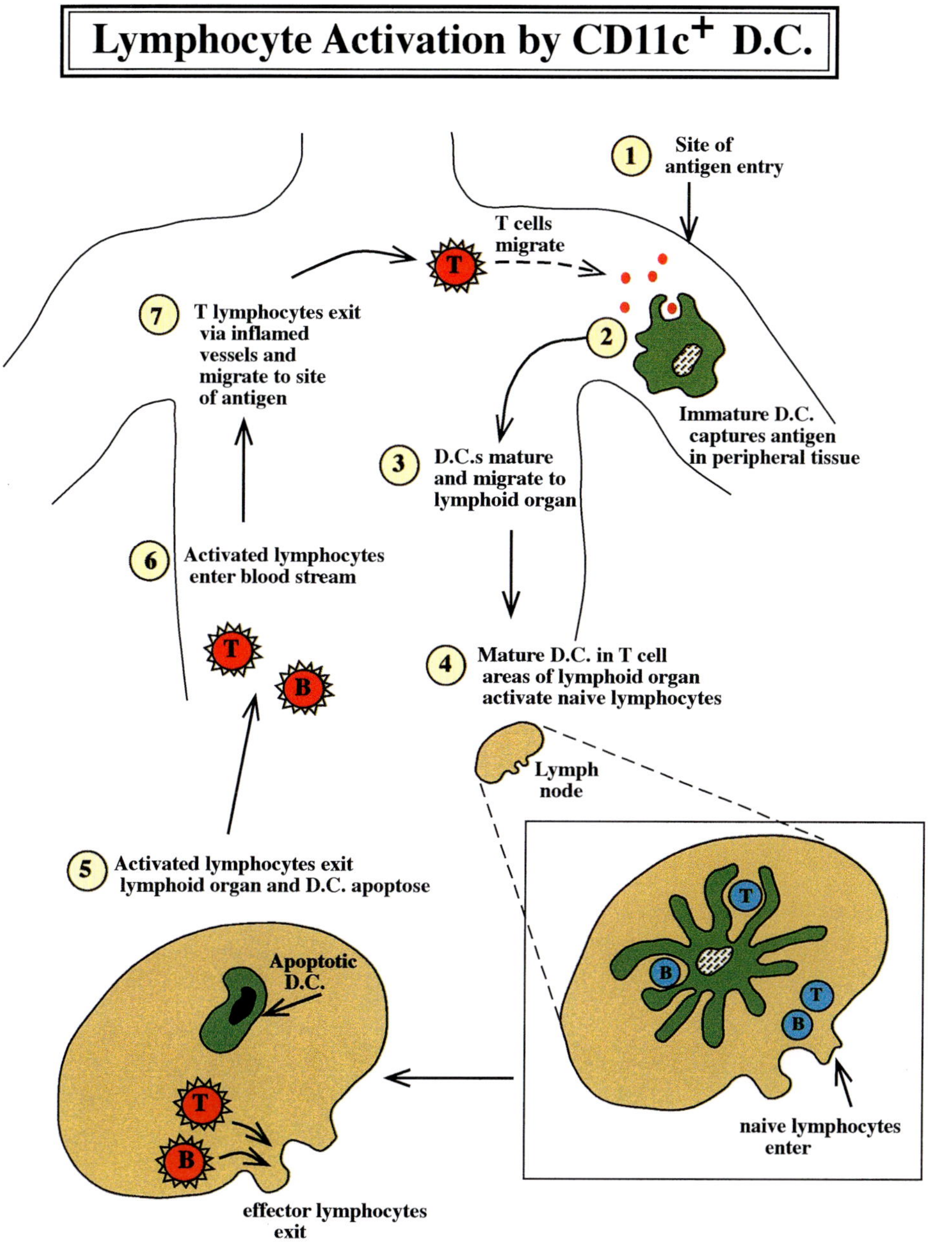

Figure 2.5 Lymphocyte activation and trafficking pathway in response to antigen presentation by CD11c$^+$ dendritic cells. Antigen enters the host and is trapped in the periphery by immature DC which then migrate to lymph nodes and mature. Mature DC then present processed antigen to naive T cells in the lymph nodes. Following activation the DC apoptose and the T cells exit the lymph nodes, enter the blood, and migrate to the site of antigen.

professional APC can present exogenously synthesized antigen bound to MHC class I molecules (Harding, 1996). Presentation of exogenous antigen by MHC class I molecules allows for cross-priming or indirect antigen presentation (Bevan, 1976). As shown in Figure 2.6, in a direct antigen presentation scheme, the cell synthesizing the antigen directly presents processed peptide to responding $CD4^+$ and/or $CD8^+$ T lymphocytes. In contrast, in indirect antigen presentation or cross-priming, antigens are released from the synthesizing cell, taken-up by professional APC, and processed and presented to T cells. Because most MHC class 1^+ cells that are not professional APC do not express co-stimulatory molecules (e.g. CD80, CD86), they are unable to deliver both the antigen-specific signal and the co-stimulatory molecule signal necessary for T cell activation. Therefore, most $CD8^+$ T cell activation probably occurs via cross-priming when endogenously synthesized antigen is taken-up and processed by professional APC and presented along with a co-stimulatory signal to the responding $CD8^+$ T cells. Indeed, activation of tumor-specific $CD8^+$ T lymphocytes has been shown to occur via cross-priming (Huang *et al.*, 1994).

Although the phenomenon of cross-priming for activation of $CD8^+$ T cells is well accepted, the mechanism by which it occurs is not known, and four possible explanations have been proposed (Lanzavecchia, 1996):

1. Partially degraded antigen in the endosomal pathway can leak from an endosome and diffuse into the cytosolic compartment. The resulting degraded antigen may then be further degraded in the proteosome and transported into the ER where it binds to newly synthesized MHC class I molecules (Moore *et al.*, 1988).
2. Phagocytosed antigen could be transferred intact into the cytosolic compartment where it is denatured in the proteosome and transferred into the ER (Pfeifer *et al.*, 1993).
3. Direct peptide exchange of endosomal peptide for class I bound peptide could occur either at the cell surface, or in phagolysosomes when class I molecules are recycled.
4. Capture of HSP-96 and its associated bound peptides by DC and their transport to the ER where the bound peptides are released and available for subsequent binding to MHC class I molecules.

Regardless of the mechanism of class I-restricted presentation of soluble antigen, DC are potent activators of class I-restricted $CD8^+$ CTL, and this capability should be exploited when using DC as anti-tumor vaccines.

Generating Dendritic Cells In Vitro for Immunization/Vaccination Therapies

Although tumor antigens have been defined and demonstrated to be immunogenic, most tumor-bearing patients do not mount effective antitumor immunity. Numerous mechanistic explanations for the lack of an antitumor response have been proposed and many of these are discussed elsewhere in this volume. As research focuses on DC as central regulatory cells in initiating immune responses, insufficiencies in these cells have also been proposed for the absence of significant antitumor immunity (Banchereau and Steinman, 1998). For example, studies with colon and basal-cell carcinomas indicate that the infiltrating DC do not express the co-stimulatory molecules CD80 and/or CD86 (Chaux *et al.*, 1996), so these

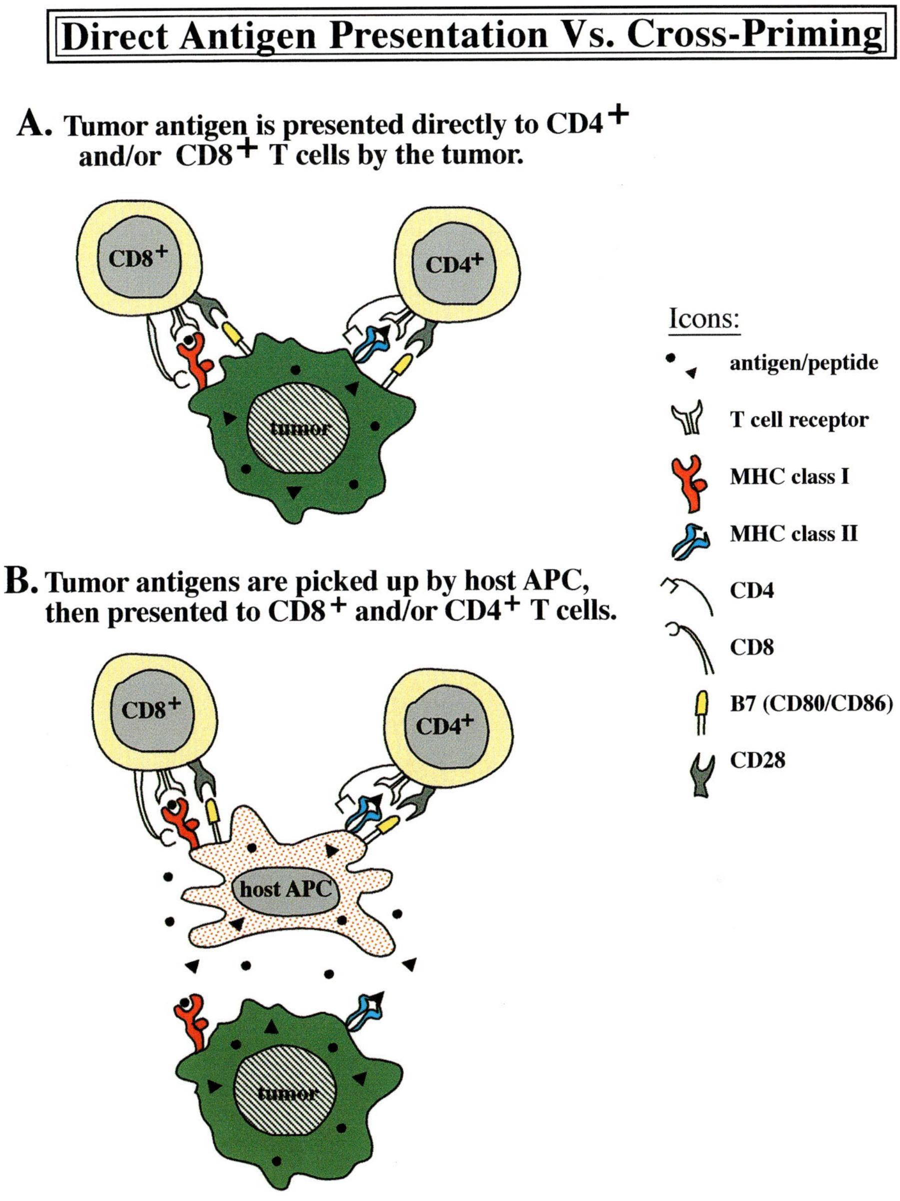

Figure 2.6 Direct antigen presentation vs. cross-priming (indirect antigen presentation) for activation of $CD4^+$ and $CD8^+$ T cells. (A) In the direct antigen presentation model, the antigen-presenting cell (either a professional or non-professional APC) directly presents a processed, endogenously synthesized antigen bound to an MHC molecule, plus a co-stimulatory signal to the responding $CD4^+$ and/or $CD8^+$ T cells. (B) In cross-priming, antigen is released by the cell synthesizing the antigen and is taken up by a professional antigen-presenting cell. The professional APC then processes the antigen and presents it in the context of an MHC class II or class II molecule to responding $CD4^+$ and/or $CD8^+$ T cells, respectively.

DC would be incapable of activating T cells. DC activity in the tumor setting may also be compromised because of soluble molecules produced by tumors. For example, many tumors secrete IL-10, TGF-β, and/or VEGF and these molecules are very effective in reducing DC function and maturation. If the DC secrete high levels of IL-12, however, the immunosuppressive effects of IL-10 can be reversed.

Given the hypothesis that antitumor immunity is suppressed because of inadequate DC function and maturation, investigators working in both experimental animal and subsequently clinical settings have used *ex vivo* matured DC carrying tumor antigens as immunotherapeutic agents. Enough studies have been completed to date in animal systems to indicate that DC loaded with tumor antigens are a promising immunotherapeutic strategy, being able to generate both a prophylactic and a therapeutic response (Mayordomo *et al.*, 1995). Obviously the viability of this strategy is dually dependent on the availability of autologous DC and the ability to successfully load the DC with appropriate tumor antigen (see Ostrand-Rosenberg *et al.*, 1999).

DC can be generated *in vitro* from CD34$^+$ or CD14$^+$ blood, bone marrow, or splenic precursors. The cell yield, however, is low and improved techniques will be necessary to generate sufficient DC for clinical immunotherapy protocols. Although different types of DC have been described, and may be functionally distinguished in the future, at present there are two basic approaches for generating human DC. As shown in Figure 2.7, CD 34$^+$ bone marrow or cord blood precursor cells are cultured *in vitro* for 7–10 days in the presence of GM-CSF and TNF-α. If peripheral blood is the source of the CD34$^+$ precursors, the patients must first be administered G-CSF systemically to increase the level of precursors (Caux *et al.*, 1992; Siena *et al.*, 1995; Strunk *et al.*, 1996). For CD14$^+$ precursors, cells are cultured *in vitro* in GM-CSF and IL-4 (Bender *et al.* 1996; Romani *et al.*, 1996).

Once generated, DC must be tested to ascertain their identity and efficacy for antigen presentation. Typically, cells are phenotyped for the markers characteristic of mature DC (see Table 2.2 and Figure 2.7), particularly HLA-DR and CD86. Functional efficacy is also tested by their ability to stimulate allogeneic PBMC in a mixed lymphocyte reaction (MLR). Cytokine secretion may also be assessed, particularly IL-12.

Based on these findings several clinical studies are ongoing which make use of *in vitro* generated DC to vaccinate cancer patients. DC can be pulsed with known tumor peptide (e.g. tyrosinase, gp100 or Melan-A/MART-1 in melanoma), with tumor lysates or transfected with viral vector containing genes encoding tumor antigens. Preliminary results of such trials are encouraging (Nestle *et al.*, 1998; Murphy *et al.*, 1999; Thurner *et al.*, 1999), though several problems have still to be solved (see also Chapter 5).

MACROPHAGES/MONOCYTES

Macrophages make up a heterogeneous family of cells. In addition to their APC activity, macrophages have many other functions, including their role in inflammation, non-specific and innate immunity, their secretion of cytokines, and phagocytosis of apoptotic and dead cells. Like DC, macrophages can be very effective APC for activating naive T cells; however, their APC activity is highly dependent on their activation. A principal function of macrophages is to phagocytose and destroy invasive microorganisms in a non-specific

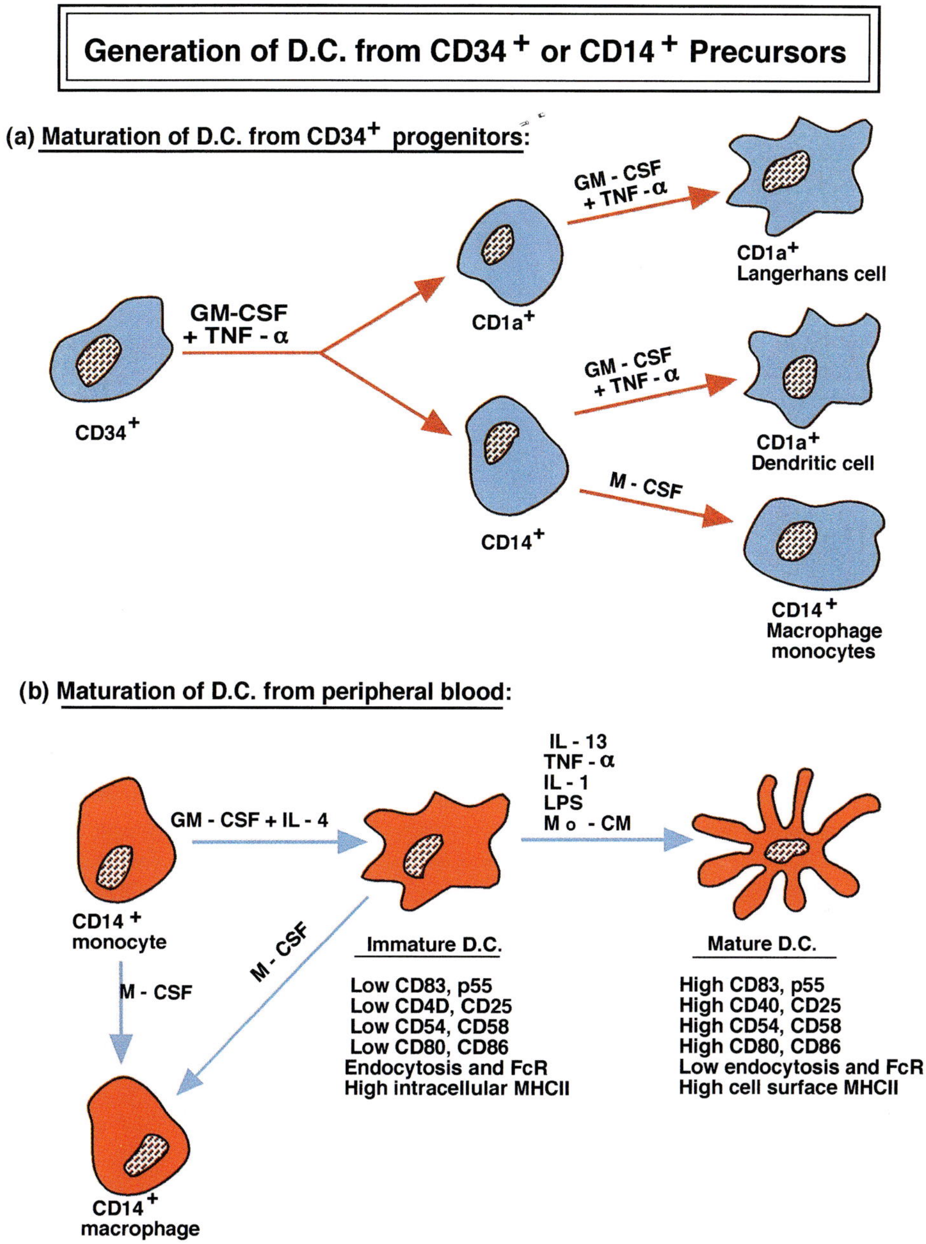

Figure 2.7 Generation and maturation of dendritic cells. DC can be generated from either CD34$^+$ progenitors from the bone marrow or peripheral blood, or from CD14$^+$ monocytes from peripheral blood. Markers of immature vs. mature CD and cytokines that drive maturation are shown.

fashion, and it is during this process that macrophages become activated. Resting macrophages have very low levels of MHC class II and co-stimulatory molecules and hence are unable to effectively present antigen to lymphocytes. Activated macrophages share many antigen presentation properties with DC. Indeed, prior to the appreciation of DC as a distinct cell population, many papers describing antigen presentation used macrophages and DC interchangeably.

Inflammatory and immune stimulators trigger monocyte migration from the bone marrow and blood to tissues. In response to various stimuli in the tissues, principally IFN-γ, the monocytes differentiate into activated macrophages. Activated macrophages display a variety of activities, one of which is the ability to present antigen to lymphocytes. Uptake of antigen by activated macrophages is facilitated by the cell surface expression of receptors that bind antigen. These receptors include the macrophage scavenger receptor (MSR) that mediates endocytosis of lipoproteins; CD14, a receptor for lipopolysaccharide binding protein; sialoadhesin, a lectin that binds sialic acid containing molecules; and probably other as yet uncharacterized receptors. Expression of these receptors enables macrophages to be highly efficient cells for taking up antigenic material from the environment (Gordon *et al.*, 1995).

As shown in Table 2.2, DC and macrophages share some common markers; however, they also display certain distinct markers. Some of the macrophage markers are indicative of macrophages' highly phagocytic phenotype which is due to the high levels of proteolytic phagosomes in their cytoplasm (Allen and Aderem, 1996). Macrophages are more efficient at phagocytozing microbial material than DC and are, therefore, thought to be more important for presentation of microbial antigens. However, macrophages can collaborate with DC by transferring antigenic material (Nair *et al.*, 1995), so that DC are also capable of presenting microbial antigens (Reimann and Kaufmann, 1997).

The variety of cell surface receptors expressed by activated macrophages, combined with potent phagocytic capability, enable macrophages to efficiently take up and process exogenous antigen. These activities combined with high cell surface expression of MHC class II and co-stimulatory molecules make macrophages potent APC for exogenous antigen.

B LYMPHOCYTES

Unlike DC and macrophages, B lymphocytes express a clonally distinct antigen-specific plasma membrane receptor (BcR). This receptor makes B cells unique among APC because it enables them to specifically bind and subsequently internalize soluble protein. This ability distinguishes them from other professional APC, and enables them to serve a strategic role in presentation of exogenous, soluble antigen to T cells. Indeed, optimal T cell responses to soluble antigen are usually obtained using B cells rather than DC or macrophages as the APC. Unlike DC and macrophages, B cells are not phagocytic and hence are unable to internalize and present particulate microbial or tumor material.

B lymphocytes constitutively express high levels of MHC class II molecules and process exogenously ingested antigen via the endocytic route. However, like macrophages, they do not constitutively express co-stimulatory molecules unless they are activated. Activation, resulting in the up-regulation of CD80 and CD86, occurs when B cells contact antigen, microorganisms or bacterial extracts. In addition, B cell encoded CD40 can signal the induction of CD80 and CD86 when bound by CD40 ligand which is expressed on activated T cells. As a result, B cells are potent APC for naive T cells, provided they are induced to express CD80 and CD86. Since non-activated B lymphocytes may present soluble antigen without delivering a co-stimulatory signal, B lymphocytes may also serve a role in tolerance induction.

Soluble antigen is not present at high concentrations during bacterial and viral infections, and hence antigen presentation by B lymphocytes may not be a major route of naive T cell activation during infections. However, immunization and vaccination strategies against tumors using soluble tumor antigens and/or peptides may depend on B cells as APC.

The phenotypes and relative antigen presentation activity of B lymphocytes, macrophages, and DC are summarized in Tables 2.2 and 2.3.

NON-PROFESSIONAL ANTIGEN PRESENTATION BY TUMOR CELLS

Many current immunotherapy strategies involve immunization with defined tumor antigens or tumor peptides. For many tumors, tumor antigens or tumor peptides have not been identified, and for those tumor antigens/peptides identified, it is not clear which, if any, are suitable targets for immunotherapy. Given these uncertainties, alternative approaches for immunotherapy have been developed which do not depend on a precise identification of an immunogenic peptide. These alternative approaches use gene transfer techniques to introduce antigen presentation molecules into tumor cells to generate cell-based antitumor vaccines. This strategy is based on two assumptions: 1) tumor cells constitutively express their tumor antigens, so identification of particular antigens is not necessary and immunization with the tumor cells should present any and all relevant tumor peptides; 2) provided tumor cells express the critical molecules important for antigen presentation and T cell activation, they should function as APC for their tumor peptides and directly activate T lymphocytes (Ostrand-Rosenberg, 1994). Genetically modified

TABLE 2.3
Comparison of the antigen presentation activity of dendritic cells, macrophages, and B lymphocytes

Characteristic	Dendritic cells[a]	Macrophages		B Lymphocytes	
		Resting	Activated	Resting	Activated
Requirements for activation	None	LPS or IFN-γ		Antigen	
MHC class I expression	High	High	High	High	High
MHC class II expression	High	Very low	high	High	High
Co-stimulatory molecules	Constitutive CD80, CD86	None	Inducible for CD80, CD86[b]	None	Inducible for CD80, CD86[b]
T cells activated	Naive, effector, memory	None	Naive, effector, memory	Effector, memory[c]	Naive, effector, memory

[a] Dendritic cells are the only professional APC that constitutively are efficient APC. Macrophages and B lymphocytes must be activated to be efficient APC.

[b] Macrophages and B lymphocytes up-regulate CD80 and CD86 expression with antigen presentation.

[c] Co-stimulation is not required for activation of effector or memory T lymphocytes.

tumor cells have been designed as cell-based antitumor vaccines for the activation of both $CD8^+$ and $CD4^+$ T lymphocytes.

ACTIVATION OF $CD8^+$ T LYMPHOCYTES

As discussed earlier, activation of T cells requires two signals: an antigen-specific signal consisting of an MHC/peptide complex, followed by a co-stimulatory signal such as CD80 or CD86. Approximately 85% of tumors constitutively express MHC class I molecules and, therefore, theoretically can present tumor peptides to $CD8^+$ T cells. However, since most tumor cells do not constitutively express co-stimulatory molecules or synthesize IL-2, $CD8^+$ T cells may actually be anergized, rather than activated when they encounter MHC class I^+ tumor cells (Figure 2.8). To overcome this potential problem, class I^+ tumor cells have been transfected with cytokine genes and/or co-stimulatory genes under the assumption that the genetically modified tumor cells will directly present antigen to $CD8^+$T cells (see Figure 2.7A for a schematic representation of direct antigen presentation by tumor cells). A wide variety of cytokine genes (e.g. IL-2, GM-CSF, IL10) has been utilized in this approach. In animal models some of the vaccines provide protection against future tumor challenge, or mediate regression of small established tumors (reviewed by Blankenstein *et al.*, 1996). Some of these vaccines have been tested in phase I clinical trials; however, patients in these trials have had very advanced disease and responses have been modest (see http://cancernet.nci.nih.gov for listing of cancer clinical trials). It is the hope that more dramatic antitumor responses will be seen when these vaccines are tested in patients with smaller tumor loads and who have a more robust immune response, since high tumor load is frequently associated with immunosuppression (Ostrand-Rosenberg *et al.*, 1998).

Similar results have been found with tumor cells modified by gene transfection to express the co-stimulatory molecules CD80 or CD86 (reviewed in Blankenstein *et al.*, 1996). As for the cytokine transfected tumor cells, the assumption is that the transfectants directly present antigen to $CD8^+$ T cells. Immunization of mice with CD80/CD86 transfected tumor cells, in some cases, also provides protection against subsequent challenge with wild-type tumors, and in more limited mouse experiments, the transfectants sometimes mediate regression of small, established tumors.

Interestingly, studies designed to test if the genetically modified vaccines are APC have given contradictory results. Early studies using GM-CSF transfected mouse tumor cells showed that direct antigen presentation by the tumor cells to $CD8^+$ T cells did not occur. Instead, tumor antigen was picked up by professional APC and presented to $CD8^+$ T cells by cross-priming (see Figure 2.7B for a diagram of cross-priming or indirect antigen presentation) (Huang *et al.*, 1994). Similar experiments using CD80-transfected mouse tumor cells showed that direct antigen presentation occurred (Cayeux *et al.*, 1997), while for other tumors cross-priming predominated (Huang *et al.*, 1996).

ACTIVATION OF $CD4^+$ T LYMPHOCYTES

Concurrent with the experiments targeting the activation of $CD8^+$ T cells, cell-based tumor vaccines have also been designed to directly activate $CD4^+$ T lymphocytes. Since most

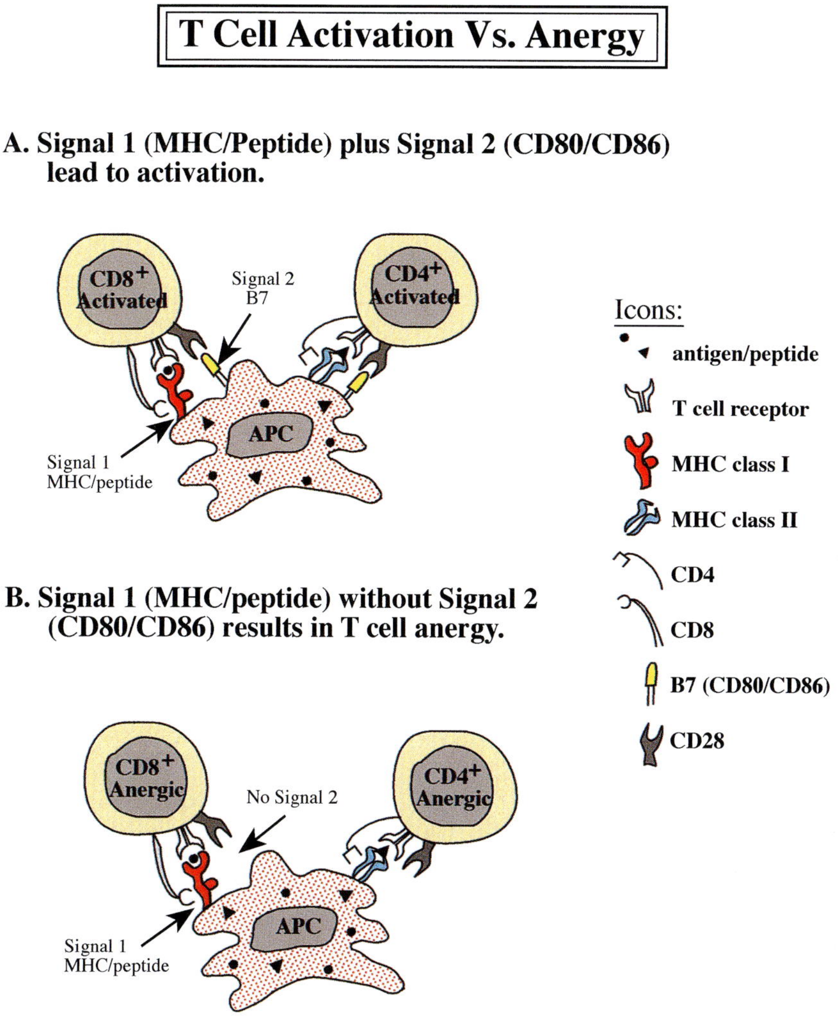

Figure 2.8 T lymphocytes can be either activated or anergized following exposure to antigen. (A) T cell activation requires the delivery of two signals from the antigen presenting cell to the responding CD4$^+$ and/or CD8$^+$ T cell. The first signal is the antigen-specific signal delivered by peptide bound to the MHC class I or class II molecule for CD4$^+$ or CD8$^+$ T cells, respectively. The second signal is the binding of CD80 and/or CD86 on the APC to its cognate receptor, CD28, on the responding CD4$^+$ and/or CD8$^+$ T cell. (B) T cell anergy occurs if the antigen-specific signal is delivered without the co-stimulatory signal.

tumor cells do not constitutively express MHC class II molecules they cannot deliver an antigen-specific signal to CD4$^+$ T cells which recognize antigen in the context of class II molecules. To enable class II-restricted presentation, tumor cells were transfected with syngeneic MHC class II genes plus the co-stimulatory molecule CD80 or CD86 (Baskar *et al.*, 1993; Ostrand-Rosenberg *et al.*, 1996). Immunization of mice with these transfectants induced immunity to subsequent challenge with wild-type tumors. The transfectants were also effective immunotherapeutic agents for the treatment of mice with established primary, solid sarcomas and metastatic breast carcinoma (Baskar *et al.*, 1995; Pulaski and Ostrand-Rosenberg, 1998).

Professional APC usually present exogenously synthesized antigen bound to MHC class II molecules because the co-expression of class II and invariant chain targets class II complexes to the endosome where they bind processed, exogenously synthesized antigens (see section on ''Endogenous pathway of antigen presentation''). The class II-transfected tumor cells, however, are designed to present endogenously synthesized tumor encoded antigens/peptides because the tumor cells do not co-express invariant chain. *In vitro* antigen presentation experiments confirmed the hypothesis that tumor cells expressing class II plus Ii preferentially present exogenous antigen, while cells expressing class II without Ii preferentially present endogenous antigen. Furthermore, only the class $II^{+}Ii^{-}$ tumor cells were effective vaccines (Armstrong *et al.*, 1997). Since tumor cells that constitutively express MHC class II co-express Ii, tumors that are normally class II^{+} are not more immunogenic than class II^{-} tumors.

In contrast to activation of CD8-targeted vaccines, the class II transfectants directly present antigen to $CD4^{+}$ T cells *in vivo* (Armstrong *et al.*, 1998a). The reason for the dichotomy between presentation to $CD4^{+}$ vs. $CD8^{+}$ T cells is unclear (reviewed in Armstrong *et al.*, 1998b). Despite the controversy, however, genetically modified tumor vaccines can be effective preventative and immunotherapeutic agents, and their continued development is warranted.

CONCLUSIONS

Antigen processing and presentation occupies a critical cross-roads in lymphocyte activation. Without adequate antigen processing and/or presentation lymphocytes may not be activated and without concomitant costimulation, lymphocytes may be anergized rather than activated. Rapid progress has been made in identifying processing and presentation pathways that favor optimal lymphocyte activation, elucidating the relevant antigen presentation elements, and characterizing and preparatively isolating potent APC. These and other advances in gene transfer techniques provide many potential novel approaches for enhancing immunity to tumor antigens and for harnessing the immune response against cancer.

ACKNOWLEDGMENTS

The authors appreciate the informative comments of Dr. Iwona Stroynowski during preparation of the manuscript. Original studies from the authors' lab were supported by NIH RO1 CA52527, US Army DAMD 17-94-J-4323, and US Army DAMD 17-1-7152.

REFERENCES

Aldrich, C., DeCloux, A., Woods, A., Cotter, R., Soloski, M., and Forman, J. (1994) Identification of a TAP-dependent leader peptide recognized by alloreactive T cells specific for a class Ib antigen. *Cell*, **79**, 649–658.

Allen, L., and Aderem, A. (1996) Mechanims of phagocytosis. *Curr. Op. Immunol.*, **8**, 36–40.

Armstrong, T., Clements, V., Martin, B., Ting, J.P.-Y., and Ostrand-Rosenberg, S. (1997) Major histocompatibility complex class II-transfected tumor cells present endogenous antigen and are potent inducers of tumor-specific immunity. *Proc. Natl. Acad. Sci. USA*, **120**, 123–128.

Armstrong, T., Clements, V., and Ostrand-Rosenberg, S. (1998a) MHC class II-transfected tumor cells directly present antigen to tumor-specific $CD4^+$ T lymphocytes. *J. Immunol.*, **160**, 661–666.

Armstrong, T., Pulaski, B., and Ostrand-Rosenberg, S. (1998b) Tumor antigen presentation: changing the rules. *Cancer Immunol. Immunother.*, **46**, 70–74.

Bachman, M., Lutz, M., Layton, G., Harris, S., Fehr, T., Rescigno, M., and Ricciardi-Castagnoli, P. (1996) Dendritic cells process exogenous viral proteins and virus-like particles for class I presentation to $CD8^+$ cytotoxic T lymphocytes. *Eur. J. Immunol.*, **26**, 2595–2600.

Banchereau, J., and Steinman, R. (1998) Dendritic cells and the control of immunity. *Nature*, **392**, 245–252.

Baskar, S., Ostrand-Rosenberg, S., Nabavi, N., Nadler, L.M., Freeman, G. J., and Glimcher, L.H. (1993) Constitutive expression of B7 restores immunogenicity of tumor cells expressing truncated major histocompatibility complex class II molecules. *Proc. Natl. Acad. Sci. USA*, **90**, 5687–5690.

Baskar, S., Glimcher L., Nabavi N., Jones R. T., and Ostrand-Rosenberg S. (1995) Major histocompatibility complex class $II^+B7\text{-}1^+$ tumor cells are potent vaccines for stimulating tumor rejection in tumor-bearing mice. *J. Exp. Med.*, **181**, 619–629.

Behar, S.M., Podrebarac, T.A., Roy, C.J., Wang, C.R., and Brenner, M.B. (1999) Diverse TCRs recognize murine CD1. *J. Immunol.*, **162**, 161–167.

Bender, A., Sapp, M., Schuler, G., Steinman, R., and Bhardwaj, N. (1996) Improved methods for the geneation of dendritic cells from nonproliferating progenitors in human blood. *J. Immunol. Methods*, **196**, 121–135.

Bevan, M. (1976) Cross-priming for a secondary cytototxic response to minor H antigens with H-2 congenic cells which do not cross-react in the cytotoxic assay. *J. Exp. Med.*, **143**, 1283–1288.

Bjorkman, P., Saper, M., Samraoui, B., Bennett, W., Strominger, J., and Wiley, D. (1988a) Structure of the human class I histocompatibility antigen, HLA-A2. *Nature*, **329**, 506–512.

Bjorkman, P., Saper, M., Samraoui, B., Bennett, W., Strominger, J., and Wiley, D. (1988b) The foreign antigen binding site and T cell recognition regions of class I histocompatibility antigens. *Nature*, **329**, 512–518.

Blankenstein, T., Cayeux, S., and Qin, Z. (1996) Genetic approaches to cancer immunotherapy. *Rev. Phys. Biochem. Pharm.*, **129**, 1–49.

Bohm, W.S., Elbe, R.A., Melber, K., Diminsky, D., Kraal, G., Van Rooijen, N., Barenholz, Y., and Reimann, J. (1995) Exogenous hepatitis B surface antigen particles processed by dendritic cells or macrophages prime murine MHC class I-restricted cytotoxic T lymphocytes *in vivo*. *J. Immunol.*, **155**, 3313–3321.

Borrego, F., Ulbrecht, M., Weiss, E., Coligan, J., and Brooks, A. (1998) Recognition of uman histocompatibilityleukocyte antigen (HLA)-E complexed with HLA class I signal sequence-derived peptides by CD94/NKG2 confers progection from natural killer cell-mediated lysis. *J. Exp. Med.*, **187**, 813–818.

Braud, V., Allan, D., O'Callaghan, C., Soderstrom, K., D'Andrea, A., Ogg, G.S., Lazetic, S., Young, N., Bell, J., Phillips, J., Lanier, L., and McMichael, A. (1998) HLA-E binds to natural killer cell receptors CD94/ NKG2A, B, and C. *Nature*, **391**, 795–799.

Brown, J., Jardetzky, T., Gorga, J., Stern, L., Urban, R., Strominger, J., and Wiley, D. (1993) Three-dimensional structure of the human class II histocompatibility antigen HLA-DR1. *Nature*, **364**, 33–39.

Caux, C., Dezutter-Dambuyant, C., Schmitt, D., and Banchereau, J. (1992) GM-CSF and TNF-alpha cooperate in the generation od dendritic Langerhans cells. *Nature*, **360**, 258–261.

Cayeux, S., Richter, G., Noffz, G., Dorken, B., and Blankenstein, T. (1997) Influence of gene-modified (IL-7, IL-4, and B7) tumor cell vaccines on tumor antigen presentation. *J. Immunol.*, **158**, 2834–2841.

Cella, M., Salio, M., Sakakibara, Y., Langen, H., Julkunen, I., and Lanzavecchia, A. (1999) Maturation, activation and protection of dendritic cells induced by double-stranded RNA. *J. Exp. Med.*, **189**, 821–829.

Chaux, P., Moutet, M., Faivre, J., Martin, F., and Martin, M. (1996) Inflammatory cells infiltating human colorectal carcinomas express HLA class II but not B7-1 and B7-2 costimulatory moleculs forT-cell activation. *Lab. Invest.*, **74**, 975–983.

Colonna, M., Navarro, F., Bellon, T., Llano, M., Garcia, P., Samaridis, J., Angman, L., Cella, M., and Lopez-Botet, M. (1997) A common inhibitory receptor for Major Histocompatibility Complex Class I molecules on human lymphoid and myelomonocytic cells. *J. Exp. Med.*, **186**, 1809–1818.

Cui, J., Shin, T., Kawano, T., Sato, H., Kondo, E., Toura, I., Kaneko, Y., Koseki, H., Kanno, M., and Taniguchi, M. (1997) Requirement for V alpha 14 NKT cells in IL-12-mediated rejection of tumors. *Science*, **278**, 1623–1626.

Fauger, N.A., Maliszewski, C.R., Schooley, K., and Griffith, T.S. (1999) Human dendritic cells mediate cellular apoptosis via tumor necrosis factor-related apoptosis-inducing ligand (TRAIL). *J. Exp. Med.*, **190**, 1155–1164.

Fernandez, N.C., Lozier, A., Flament, C., Ricciardi-Castagnoli, P., Bellet, D., Suter, M., Perricaudet, M., Tursz, T., Maraskovsky, E., and Zitvogel, L. (1999) Dendritic cells directly trigger NK cell functions: cross-talk relevant in innate anti-tumor immune responses *in vivo*. *Nature Med.*, **5**, 405–411.

Garrido, F., Cabrera, T., Concha, A., Glew, S., Ruiz-Cabello, F., and Stern, P. (1993) Natural history of HLA expression during tumour development. *Immunol. Today*, **14**, 491–499.

Gordon, S., Clarke, S., Greaves, D., and Doyle, A. (1995) Molecular immunobiology of macrophages: recent progress. *Curr. Op. Immunol.*, **7**, 24–33.

Grant, E.P., Degano, M., Rosat, J.-P., Stenger, S., Modlin, R.L., Wilson, I.A., Porcelli, S.A., and Brenner, M.B. (1999) Molecular recognition of lipid antigens by T cell receptors. *J. Exp. Med.*, **189**, 195–205.

Griffiths, E., Ong, H., Soloski, M., Bachmann, M., Ohashi, P., and Speiser, D. (1998) Tumor defense by murine cytotoxic T cells specific for peptide bound to nonclassical MHC class I. *Cancer Res.*, **58**, 4682–4687.

Grouard, G., Durand, I., Filgueira, L., Banchereau, J., and Liu, Y. (1996) Dendritic cells capable of stimulating T cells in germinal centres. *Nature*, **384**, 364–367.

Harding, C. (1996) Class I MHC presentation of exogenous antigens. *J. Clin. Immunol.*, **16**, 90–96.

Hoglund, P., Sundback, J., Olsson-Alheim, M., Johansson, M., Salcedo, M., Ohlen, C., Ljunggren, H., Sentman, C., and Karre, K. (1997) Host MHC class I gene control of NK-cell specificity in the mouse. *Immunol. Rev.*, **155**, 11–28.

Huang, A., Golumbek, P., Ahmadzadeh, M., Jaffee, E., Pardoll, D., and Levitsky, H. (1994) Role of bone marrow-derived cells in presenting MHC class I-restricted tumor antigens. *Science*, **264**, 961–965.

Huang, A., Bruce, A., Pardoll, D., and Levitsky, H. (1996) Does B7-1 expression confer antigen-presenting cell capacity to tumors *in vivo*? *J. Exp. Med.*, **183**, 769–776.

Inaba, K., Inaba, M., Naito, M., and Steinman, R. (1993) Dendritic cell progenitors phagocytose particulates, including bacillus Calmette-Guerin organisms, and sensitize mice to mycobacterial antigens *in vivo*. *J. Exp. Med.*, **178**, 479–488.

Inaba, K., Witmer-Pack, M., Inaba, M., Hathcock, S., Sakuta, H., Azuma, M., Yagita, H., Okumura, K., Linsley, P., Ikehara, S., Muramatsu, S., Hodes, R., and Steinman, R. (1994) The tissue distribution of the B7-2 costimulator in mice: abundant expression on dendritic cells in situ and during maturation *in vitro*. *J. Exp. Med.*, **180**, 1849–1860.

Inaba, K., Pack, M., Inaba, M., Sakuta, H., Isdell, F., and Steinman, R. (1997) High levels of a major histocompatibility complex II-self peptide complex on dendritic cells from lymph node. *J. Exp. Med.*, **186**, 665–672.

Kawano, T., Cui, J., Koezuka, Y., Toura, I., Kaneko, Y., Motoki, K., Ueno, H., Nakagawa, R., Sata, H., Kondo, E., Koseki, H., and Taniguchi, M. (1997) CD1d-restricted and TCR-mediated activation of V alpha 14 NKT cells by glycosylceramides. *Science*, **278**, 1626–1629.

Ke, Y., and Kapp, J. (1996) Exogenous antigens gain access to the major histocompatiblity complex class I processing pathway in B cells by receptor-mediated uptake. *J. Exp. Med.*, **184**, 1179–1184.

Lanzavecchia, A. (1996) Mechanisms of antigen uptake for presentation. *Curr. Op. Immunol.*, **8**, 348–354.

Lee, N., Malacko, A., Ishitani, A., Chen, M., Bajorath, J., Marquardt, H., and Geraghty D. (1995) The membrane bound and soluble forms of HLA-G bind identical sets of endogenous peptides but differ with respect to TAP-association. *Immunity*, **3**, 591–600.

Lee, N., Llano, M., Carretero, M., Ishitani, A., Navarro, F., Lopez-Botet, M., and Geraghty, D. (1998) HLA-E is a major ligand for the natural killer inhibitory receptor CD94/NKG2A. *Proc. Natl. Acad. Sci. USA*, **95**, 4791–4794.

Manca, F., Fenoglio, D., Li-Pira, G., Kunkl, A., and Celada, F. (1991) Effect of antigen/antibody ratio on macrophage uptake, processing, and presentation to T cells of antigen complexed with polyclonal antibodies. *J. Exp. Med.*, **173**, 37–48.

Mayordomo, J.I., Zorina, T., Storkus, W.J., Zitvogel, L., Celluzzi, C., Falo, I.D., Melief, C.J., Ildstad, S.T., Martin Kast, W., Deleo, A. B., and Lotze, M.T. (1995) Bone marrow-derived dendritic cells pulsed with synthetic tumour peptides elicit protective and therapeutic antitumour immunity. *Nature Med.*, **1**, 1297–1302.

Melian, A., Beckman, E., Porcelli, S., and Brenner, M. (1996) Antigen presentation by CD1 and MHC-encoded class I-like molecules. *Curr. Op. Immunol.*, **8**, 82–88.

Moore, M., Carbone, F., and Bevan, M. (1988) Introduction of soluble protein into the class I pathway of antigen processing and presentation. *Cell*, **54**, 777–785.

Multhoff, G., Botzler, C., Jennen, L., Schmidt, J., Ellwart, J., and Issels, R. (1997) Heat shock protein 72 on tumor cells. *J. Immunol.*, **158**, 4341–4350.

Murphy, J.P., Tjoa, B.A., Simmons, S.J., Jarisch, J., Bowes, V.A., Ragde, H., Rogers, M., Elgamal, A., Kenny, G.M., Cobb, O.E., Ireton, R.C., Troychak, M.J., Salgaller, M.L., and Boynton, A.L. (1999) Infusion of dendritic cells pulsed with HLA-A2-specific prostate-specific membrane antigen peptides: a phase II prostate cancer vaccine trial involving patients with hormone-refractory metastatic disease. *Prostate*, **38**, 73–78.

Nair, S., Buiting, A., Rouse, R., Van Rooijen, N., Huang, L., and Rouse, B. (1995) Role of macrophages and dendritic cells in primary cytotoxic T lymphocyte responses. *Int. Immunol.*, **4**, 679–688.

Nestle, F. O., Alijagic, S., Gilliet, M., Sun, Y., Grabbe, S., Dummer, R., Burg, G., and Schadendorf, D. (1998) Vaccination of melanoma patients with peptide- or tumor lysate-pulsed dendritic cells. *Nature Med.*, **4**, 328–332.

O'Callaghan, C., and Bell, J. (1998) Structure and function of the human MHC class Ib molecules HLA-E, HLA-F, HLA-G. *Immunol. Rev.*, **163**, 129–138.

O'Callaghan, C.A., Tormo, J., Willcox, B., Braud, V., Jokobsen, B., Stuart, D., McMichael, M., Bell, J., and Jones, E. (1998) Structural features impose tight peptide binding specificity in the nonclassical MHC molecule HLA–E. *Mol. Cell.*, **1**, 531–541.

Ostrand-Rosenberg, S. (1994) Tumor immunotherapy: the tumor cell as an antigen-presenting cell. *Curr. Op. Immunol.*, **6**, 722–727.

Ostrand-Rosenberg, S., Baskar, S., Patterson, N., and Clements, V. (1996) Expression of MHC class II and B7-1 and B7-2 costimulatory molecules accompanies tumor rejection and reduces the metastatic potential of tumor cells. *Tissue Antigens*, **47**, 414–421.

Ostrand-Rosenberg, S., Gunther, V., Armstrong, T., Pulaski, B., Pipeling, M., and Clements, V. (1998) Immunologic targets for the gene therapy of cancer. In *Gene Therapy of Cancer*, eds. E. Lattime, S. Gerson, in press. San Diego, Academic Press.

Ostrand-Rosenberg, S., Pulaski, B.A., Clemente, V.K., Qi, L., Pipeling, M.R., and Hanyok, L.A. (1999) Cell-based vaccines for the stimulation of immunity to metastatic cancers. *Immunol. Rev.*, **170**, 101–114.

Paul, P., Cabestré, F., Le Gal, F.-A., Khalil-Daher, I., Le Danff, C., Schmid, M., Mercier, S., Avril, M.-F., Guillet, J.-G., and Carosella, E. D. (1999) Heterogeneity of HLA-G gene transcription and protein expression in malignant melanoma biopsies. *Cancer Res.*, **59**, 1954–1960.

Perez-Villar, J., Melero, I., Navarro, F., Carretero, M., Bellon, T., Llano, M., Colonna, M., Geraghty, D., and Lopez-Botet, M. (1997) The CD94/NKG2-A inhibitor receptor complex is involved in natural killer cell-mediated recognition of cells expressing HLA-G1. *J. Immunol.*, **158**, 5736–5743.

Pfeifer, J., Wick, M., Roberts, R., Findlay, K., Normark, S., and Harding, C. (1993) Phagocytic processing of bacterial antigens for class I MHC presentation to T cells. *Nature*, **361**, 359–362.

Pierre, P., Turley, S., Gatti, E., Hull, M., Meltzer, J., Mirza, A., Inaba, K., Steinman, R., and Mellman, I. (1997) Developmental regulation of MHC class II transport in mouse dendritic cells. *Nature*, **388**, 787–792.

Ponte, M., Cantoni, C., Biassoni, R., Tradori-Cappai, A., Bentivoglio, G., Vitale, C., Bertone, S., Moretta, A., Moretta, L., and Mingari, M.C. (1999) Inhibitory receptors sensing HLA-G1 molecules in pregnancy: decidua-associated natural killer cells express LIR-1 and CD94/NKG2A and acquire p49, an HAL-G1-specific receptor. *Proc. Natl. Acad. Sci. USA*, **96**, 5674–5679.

Porcelli, S. (1995) The CD1 family: a third lineage of antigen presentation molecules. *Adv. Immunol.*, **59**, 1–97.

Porcelli, S., Morita, C., and Modlin, R. (1996) T-cell recognition of non-peptide antigens. *Curr. Op. Immunol.*, **8**, 510–516.

Pulaski, B., and Ostrand-Rosenberg, S. (1998) Reduction of established spontaneous mammary carcinoma metastases following immunotherapy with MHC class II and B7.1 cell-based tumor vaccines. *Cancer Res.*, **58**, 1486–1493.

Reimann, J., and Kaufmann, S. (1997) Alternative antigen processing pathways in anti-infective immunity. *Curr. Op. Immunol.*, **9**, 462–469.

Romani, N., Reider, D., Heuer, M., Ebner, S., Eibl, B., Niederweiser, D., and Schuler, G. (1996) Generation of mature dendritic cells from human blood: an improved method with special regard to clinical applicability. *J. Immunol. Methods*, **196**, 137–151.

Sallusto, F., and Lanzavecchia, A. (1994) Efficient presentation of soluble antigen by cultured human dendritic cells is maintained by GM-CSF plus IL-4 and downregulated by TNF alpha. *J. Exp. Med.*, **179**, 1109–1118.

Sallusto, F., Cella, M., Danieli, C., and Lanzavecchia, A. (1995) Dendritic cells use macropinocytosis and the mannose receptor to concentrate macromolecules in the MHC class II compartment: downregulation by cytokines and bacterial products. *J. Exp. Med.*, **182**, 389–400.

Shamshiev, A., Donda, A., Carena, I., Mori, L., Kappos, L., and De Libero, G. (1999) Self glycolipids as T-cell autoantigens. *Eur. J. Immunol.*, **29**, 1667– 1675.

Shawar, S., Vyas, J., Rodgers, J., and Rich, R. (1994) Antigen presentation by major histocompatibility complex class Ib molecules. *Annu. Rev. Immunol.*, **12**, 839–880.

Shen, Z., Reznikoff, G., Dranoff, G., and Rock, K. (1997) Cloned dendritic cells can present exogenous antigens on both MHC class I and class II molecules. *J. Immunol.*, **158**, 2723–2730.

Siegal., F.P., Kadowaki, N., Shodell, M., Fitzgerald-Bocarsly, P.A., Shah, K., Ho, S., Antonenko, S., and Liu, Y.J. (1999) The nature of the principal type 1 interferon-producing cells in human blood. *Science*, **284**, 1835–1837.

Siena, S., Di Nicola, M., Bregni, M., Mortarini R., Anichini, A., Lombardi, L., Ravagnani, F., Parmiani G., and Gianni, M. (1995) Massive *ex vivo* generation of functional dendritic cells from mobilized CD34+ blood progenitors for anticancer therapy. *Exp. Hematol.*, **23**, 1463–1471.

Srivastava, P., Udono, H., Blachere, N., and Li, Z. (1994) Heat shock proteins transfer peptides during antigen processing and CTL priming. *Immunogenetics*, **39**, 93–98.

Srivastava, P., Menoret, A., Basu, S., Binder, R., and McQuade, K. (1998) Heat shock proteins come of age: primitive functions acquire new roles in an adaptive world. *Immunity*, **8**, 657–665.

Stahl, P. (1992) The mannose receptor and other macrophage lectins. *Curr. Op. Immunol.*, **4**, 49–52.

Steinman, R. (1978) Lymphoid dendritic cells are potent stimulators of the primary mixed leukocyte reaction in mice. *Proc. Natl. Acad. Sci. USA*, **75**, 5132– 5136.

Stroynowski, I., and Forman, J. (1995) Novel molecules related to MHC antigens. *Curr. Op. Immunol.*, **7**, 97–102.

Strunk, D., Rappersberger, K., Egger, C., Strobl, H., Kromer, E., Elbe, A., Maurer, D., and Stingl, G. (1996) Generations of human dendritic cells-Langerhans cells from circulating CD34+ hematopoietic progenitor cells. *Blood*, **87**, 1292–1302.

Sugita, M., Jackman, R., Van Donselaar, E., Behaar, S., Rogers, R., Peters, P., Brenner, M., and Porcelli, S. (1996) Cytoplasmic tail-dependent localization of CD1b antigen-presenting molecules to MIICs. *Science*, **273**, 349–352.

Suto, R., and Srivastava, P. (1995) A mechanism for the specific immunogenicity of heat shock protein-chaperoned peptides. *Science*, **269**, 1585–1588.

Tabaczewski, P., Chiang, E., Henson, M., and Stroynowski, I. (1998) Alternative peptide binding motifs of Qa-2 class Ib molecules define rules for binding of self and nonself peptides. *J. Immunol.*, **152**, 2771–2781.

Tangri, S., Brossay, L., Burdin, N., Lee, D.J., Corr, M., and Kronenberg, M. (1998) Presentation of peptide antigens by mouse CD1 requires endosomal localization and protein antigen processing. *Proc. Natl. Acad. Sci. USA*, **95**, 14314–14319.

Thurner, B., Haendle, I., Röder, C., Dieckmann, D., Keikavoussi, P., Jonuleit, H., Bender, A., Maczek, C., Schreiner, D., von den Driesch, P., Bröcker, E.B., Steinman, R.A., Enk, A., Käompgen, E., and Schuler, G. (1999) Vaccination with MAGE-3A.1 peptide-pulsed mature, monocyte-derived dendritic cells expands specific cytotoxic T cells and induces regression of some metastases in advanced stage IV melanoma. *J. Exp. Med.*, **190**, 1669–1678.

Toura, I., Kawano, T., Akutsu, Y., Nakayama, T., Ochiai, T., and Taniguchi, M. (1999) Cutting edge: inhibition of experimental tumor metastasis byd endritic cells pulsed with α-galactosylceramide. *J. Immunol.*, **163**, 2387–2391.

Watts, C. (1997) Capture and processing of exogenous antigens for presentation on MHC molecules. *Annu. Rev. Immunol.*, **15**, 821–850.

York, I., and Rock, K. (1996) Antigen processing and presentation by the class I major histocompatibility complex. *Annu. Rev. Immunol.*, **14**, 369–396.

Zeng, Z., Castano, A., Segelke, B., Stura, E., Peterson, P., and Wilson, I. (1997) Crystal structure of mouse CD1: an MHC-like fold with a large hydrophobic binding groove. *Science*, **277**, 339–345.

3 Cellular Recognition of Tumors by T and NK Cells

Andrea Anichini and Roberta Mortarini

ABBREVIATIONS

APC	Antigen-presenting cells
CML	Chronic myelogenous leukemia
CTL	Cytotoxic T lymphocytes
CTLp	Cytotoxic T lymphocytes precursor
DC	Dendritic cells
DTH	Delayed type hypersensitivity
GM-CSF	Granulocyte-monocyte colony-stimulating-factor
HEVs	High endothelial venules
HLA	Human leukocyte antigen
IFN-γ	Interferon gamma
IL-...	Interleukin-2, -4, -5, -6, -7, -10, -12, -13, -15
LAK	Lymphokine activated killer
NK	Natural killer
PCR	Polymerase chain reaction
TCR	Antigen-specific receptor of T lymphocytes
TH	T helper
TNF-α	Tumor necrosis factor alpha
TSTA	Tumor-specific transplantation antigens

Cellular immune response to tumors

1. **Tumor antigens can be recognized by patients' T cells in MHC-restricted fashion.**
2. **Recognition occurs *in vivo* when tumor cells are admixed with autologous lymphocytes; these cultures result in expansion of tumor-specific T cells (CD4$^+$ and/or CD8$^+$).**
3. **T cell expansion is often oligoclonal, suggesting a preferential recognition of given tumor antigen peptide by lymphocytes with a specific receptor.**
4. **T cells infiltrate primary tumors and their presence is associated with a better prognosis.**
5. **However, T cells infiltrate metastatic lesions less frequently and are often anergic, i.e. unable to destroy tumor cells *in vivo*.**
6. **Tumor antigen-specific T cells can be identified by the use of tetramers in a bulk population of CD8$^+$ lymphocytes.**
7. **NK cells recognize those tumor cells that, due to lack or down-regulation of HLA, cannot be seen by T cells. In fact, HLA deliver inhibitory signal to NK cells which express killer inhibitory receptors (KIR) with some degree of specificity for different HLA alleles.**
8. **A new population of lymphocytes has recently been described, the NKT cells, which can recognize target cells bearing non-proteic, glycolipid antigens presented by non-classical MHC (e.g. CD1). These NKT cells can destroy neoplastic cells and are activated, both *in vivo* and *in vitro*, by some glycoplipids.**
9. **Lymphocytes circulate through the body and traffic through normal and neoplastic tissues. This property is dependent on expression of tissue-specific homing molecules. These molecules are heterogeneous and their expression is the result of activation with cognate ligands.**
10. **Memory, antigen-activated T cells express a profile of homing molecules different from that of naive, unstimulated T cells. This reflects their different ability to circulate between lymphoid tissues and other tissues.**

BASIS FOR T CELL RECOGNITION OF TUMORS

The evidence for the existence of tumor-specific antigens leading to tumor rejection was obtained almost 50 years ago (Prehn and Main, 1957). At that time it was shown that chemically induced, transplanted mouse tumors can be rejected if the recipient mice have been previously rendered ''immune'' to the same tumor by a single round of tumor growth and surgical excision. Rejection of neoplastic cells was tumor-specific, since no protection against subsequent tumor growth could be achieved by transplanting normal tissues or tumor cells different from those used for challenge. Although the initial experiments performed by Foley, Prehn and the Kleins in the 1950s and 1960s formally established the existence of TSTA, it took more than 35 years of research in molecular biology, immunology, and genetics to understand the molecular nature of tumor antigens. This achievement, obtained for the first time by T. Boon and his group, first in mouse and then in human tumors at the beginning of the 1990s (see Boon *et al.*, 1994), represented the final success of a long chain of discoveries that contributed to the shaping of modern immunology. The discovery of the MHC restriction in 1974 by Zinkernagel and Doherty, the elucidation of the crystal structure of HLA molecules in 1987 by P. Bjorkmann, and the understanding of the genetic basis for the expression and function of TCRs by M. Davis in 1984 are just a few of the seminal findings that opened the way to deciphering the molecular nature of antigens recognized by T cells, including tumor antigens. We now know that tumor antigens recognized by T cells are short peptides bound to MHC class I or II molecules. The MHC–peptide complex is the ''antigenic epitope'' recognized by the specific receptor for antigen (TCR) expressed by each T cell. The rules dictating how a T cell will recognize the peptide antigen for which it possesses a specific TCR are universal; therefore, at the structural level T cell recognition of a tumor antigen is no different from recognition of viral antigens on an infected cell (see Figure 3.1). The elucidation of the structure of the TCR has revealed a clonally distributed heterodimer made up of two chains (α and β) bound by a disulphide link. Each of the two TCR chains is transcribed from families of gene segments coding for the variable (V), joining (J) and constant (C) regions. The β chain contains an additional D region. Somatic rearrangement, taking place during T cell differentatiation within the thymus, joins together different VDJ segments that are then linked by splicing to the constant region transcripts. The region of the TCR coded for by the V, J and D regions represents the most important segment for interaction with the ligand (the MHC–peptide complex) and is named CDR3 (complementarity determining region 3, Figure 3.1). The unique sequences in the CDR3 region contribute to defining the ligand specificity of the TCR. By taking advantage of these unique sequences, it is even possible to identify and quantitate *in vivo* (in lesions) or *in vitro* (in T cell lines selected for tumor recognition) tumor-specific T cells.

ROLE OF T CELLS IN ANTITUMOR RESPONSES

Understanding the molecular nature of tumor antigens has required several decades of research. Similarly, the recognition of the role of T cells in antitumor responses against both experimental and human tumors has taken more than 20 years, with experiments beginning in the 1950s (see Kedar and Weiss, 1983). At that time, and during the following decades, attempts to control tumor growth were carried out by transfer of lymphoid cells, isolated from immunized donors, to tumor-bearing hosts. In some instances T cell-deficient tumor-bearing hosts were used that showed the need for T cells to mediate tumor rejection. In 1955 Mitchinson first reported that transfer of lymph node cells from mice that had rejected a tumor graft could confer accelerated tumor rejection to the recipients. Subsequent experiments, published during the 1960s and 1970s, showed that large numbers of immune cells (at least 10^8) were needed, that such cells had to survive for some days in the host tissues, and that removal of suppressor cells in treated animals, or combination with chemotherapy, could increase the antitumor activity. Antitumor activity was measured as the reduction in the number of pulmonary

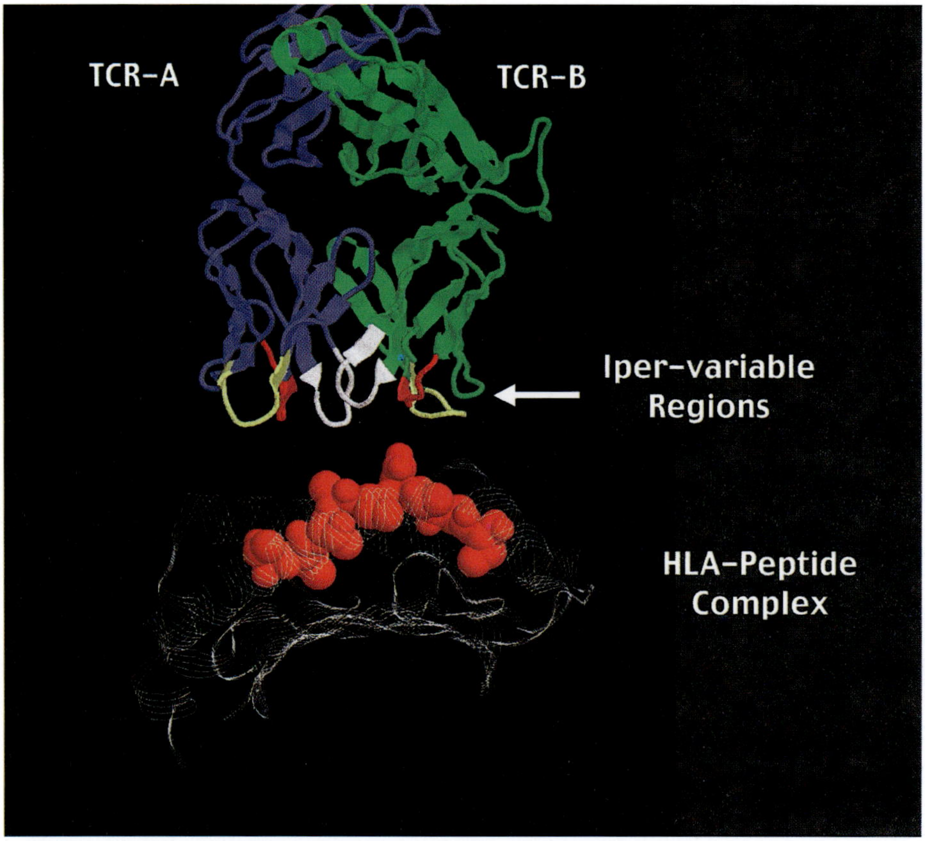

Figure 3.1 Interaction of TCR with peptide–MHC complex. The figure shows a TCR (TCRA and TCRB chains in green and blue respectively) while interacting with an MHC–peptide complex (peptide, shown in red, bound to an HLA molecule, shown in white). Only the $\alpha1$ and $\alpha2$ domains of the HLA molecule are represented, while both the $\alpha3$ domain and $\beta2$ microglobulin were omitted. The peptide, originating from intra-cellular degradation of proteins, fits a binding groove formed by the tridimensional folding of $\alpha1$ and $\alpha2$ MHC domains. Secondary pockets existing in the floor of the groove in the MHC molecules dictate the rules of peptide binding. These rules define the specificity of peptide binding to MHC and allow only a subset of peptides with defined residues in critical positions to bind a particular MHC allele. At the level of the peptide-binding groove, the main difference in structure between MHC class I and II molecules is that the groove of MHC class II molecules is open at one end, thus allowing binding of peptides longer (18–23 aminoacids) than those (8–10 aminoacids) that bind the closed groove of MHC class I molecules. TCR specificity is determined by the aminoacids that establish contact with the MHC–peptide surface. Information from crystal structures of TCR–MHC–peptide complexes suggests a common orientation of different TCR in the interaction with the same MHC–peptide complex. According to this model, both the hypervariable regions of the TCR (shown in white and corresponding to CDR3 segments) as well as variable regions (shown in yellow and red and corresponding to CDR1 and CDR2 segments) participate in establishing contacts with various portions of the MHC–peptide surface. To achieve this, the TCR binds the MHC–peptide complex in a conserved diagonal manner with respect to the long axis of the MHC–peptide surface (the axis parallel to the peptide). This conserved geometry in binding of the TCR is believed to have significance for allowing the formation of supramolecular assemblies needed to initiate TCR signaling. Furthermore, one model put forward by C. Janeway suggests that the conserved geometry in the binding of different TCR to the same MHC–peptide complex originates from the positive selection process, occurring in the thymus. At that time the whole TCR repertoire is shaped by interaction of many different TCR with a limited set of different self-MHC–self-peptide complexes expressed by thymic cortical epithelial cells.

metastases and, sometimes, even as the cure of a fraction of the tumor-bearing animals. However, it was only in the early 1980s that adoptive transfer of tumor-specific T cells firmly established the role of both CD4$^+$ and CD8$^+$ tumor-specific T cells in the rejection of tumor grafts of high or low immunogenicity (Greenberg, 1991; Kedar and Klein, 1992). One of the most successful models, described by Philip Greenberg and colleagues (chemoimmunotherapy of FBL-3 erythroleukemia), showed that adoptive transfer of tumor-specific CD4$^+$ or CD8$^+$ T cells, in association with cyclophosphamide, could cure a significant fraction of mice bearing a disseminated tumor (Greenberg, 1991). The same FBL-3 system has provided the framework to prove the role both of MHC-class II-restricted T cells with a helper phenotype (CD4$^+$) and of MHC-class I-restricted T cells with a cytolytic phenotype (CD8$^+$) in the therapy of experimental tumors. The general model that emerged from those studies was one based on a cooperation between the two main T cell subsets. In that model CD4$^+$ T cells are important in the generation of the immune response through the production of cytokines. The CD4$^+$-derived cytokines eventually induce proliferation and differentiation of tumor-specific CD8$^+$ T cells to cytolytic effectors. This scenario has now been substantially revised, although not rejected, by including professional APC in the picture. Two key findings, both dealing with the function of APC in their interaction with T cells, have produced a new model of the early phases of T cell mediated immune responses, including response to tumor antigens. The first finding is the recent discovery of the role of CD40–CD40L interaction as a main pathway through which CD4$^+$ T cells provide "help" by inducing DC maturation to a state that enables APCs to prime naive CD8$^+$ T cells (Schoenberger *et al.*, 1998). The second key discovery is the recognition that DC act as a temporal bridge between CD4$^+$ and CD8$^+$ antigen-specific T cells (Ridge *et al.*, 1998) (see also Chapter 2).

CD4$^+$ T LYMPHOCYTES AND CANCER

At the time Greenberg and colleagues published their results with the FBL-3 model it was also shown that, in appropriate experimental conditions, cure of tumor-bearing animals could be achieved by a transfer of tumor-specific CD4$^+$ non-cytolytic T cells, unable to interact directly with MHC-class II tumor cells. These initial results indicated that tumor destruction does not necessarily require direct lysis by cytolytic lymphocytes and that CD4$^+$ T cells are important players in establishing protective antitumor immunity. Further experiments by several investigators, beginning in 1990, indicated that, in some but not all models, gene-modified tumor cells (e.g. those transfected with genes coding for cytokines, for MHC class II antigens or for co-stimulatory molecules such as B7-1) or direct administration of cytokines to tumor-bearing animals could activate effective antitumor immune responses mediated by CD4$^+$ T cells (Arca *et al.*, 1996; Pardoll and Topalian, 1998). For example, regional, peri-lymphatic administration of cytokines as IL-4 could inhibit tumor growth in models of poorly immunogenic or non-immunogenic tumors by a CD4-dependent mechanism. These models also provided evidence for the induction of immunological memory against tumor re-challenge. Similar results were obtained with different cytokines.

DIRECT VS. INDIRECT ANTIGEN PRESENTATION IN CD4$^+$-MEDIATED IMMUNE RESPONSE

The initial experiments, while establishing the role of CD4$^+$ T cells in blocking tumor growth and providing immunological memory, did not address the issue of direct (by the tumor cells) rather than indirect (by specialized class II host-derived cells) antigen presentation. This question had been raised by results obtained in the FBL-3 model, since at that time the role of DC in priming immune responses was not recognized. However, the results obtained by Greenberg and colleagues had a relevant implication, namely that generation of tumor-specific MHC class II-restricted CD4$^+$ T cells, directed against a class-II-negative tumor, could not take place unless a phase of ''antigen presentation'', through MHC class II$^+$ specialized cells, was involved. The idea that antigen from a given cell type could be transferred to a different cell type and only then be seen by T cells in an immunogenic form leading to T cell priming had been suggested more than 20 years ago. In fact, in 1976 Bevan showed priming of CTL response to minor histocompatibility antigens using cells mismatched for the MHC: he termed this phenomenon ''cross-priming'' (Bevan, 1976). We now know that this indirect antigen presentation is accomplished when tumor cells release antigens that are processed and presented by professional APC such as DC (see also Chapter 2). Direct evidence for a mechanism based on cross-priming to induce antitumor immunity was obtained in 1994 by Huang and co-workers by showing that bone marrow derived cells, and not the vaccinating tumor, function as APC for tumor antigen presentation *in vivo* (Huang *et al.*, 1994). The recognition of the role of professional APC in priming antitumor responses has also enabled different investigators to show that splenic DC or epidermal Langerhans cells can be used *in vitro* to generate antitumor CD4$^+$ T cells from vaccinated mice. In these models it was demonstrated that CD4$^+$ T cells from immunized mice will proliferate in an MHC class II-restricted fashion in the presence of DC that have been allowed to process tumor antigens from tumor lysates. These models represent the experimental basis that underlies the recent attempts to vaccinate patients with autologous DC loaded with tumor antigens. More recently, several models have provided further support to the role of CD4$^+$ in antitumor responses. Both CD4 depletion experiments as well as use of CD4 knock-out mice have been used to show abrogation of antitumor immunity induced by either tumor cells or recombinant viral vaccines or recombinant bacterial vaccines (Pardoll and Topalian, 1998; Toes *et al.*, 1999).

Cross-priming, as a mechanism to induce CD4-mediated antitumor immunity, is not the only priming mechanism. Several models have recently shown that direct antigen presentation by tumors engineered to express class II antigens can occur and activate a CD4$^+$ immune response. Even though the ''normal'' route for class II antigen presentation is based on processing of exogenously synthesized antigen, nevertheless, the attempt to perform immunotherapy with MHC class II$^+$ tumor cells is based on the assumption that the tumor cells themselves can present endogenously synthesized tumor peptides in the context of MHC class II molecules to activate CD4$^+$ tumor-specific T cells. Recent results obtained by Ostrand-Rosenberg and colleagues (see also Chapter 2 in this volume) have shown that MHC class II-transfected tumor cells can directly present tumor antigens to CD4$^+$ T cells and thus induce potent antitumor immunity (see Armstrong *et al.*, 1998). It is, however, to be pointed out that in the human system (for example in melanoma) expression of HLA class II antigens on tumor cells is sometimes constitutive. Unfortunately, this does not appear to lead to efficient activation of an effective antitumor response, at least in a large fraction of patients.

WHY THE HELPER ARM OF THE IMMUNE RESPONSE TO TUMORS MAY BE DEFECTIVE

In contrast to data emerging from experimental models, the evidence for a role of $CD4^+$ T cells in immunity to human tumors is, to say the least, disappointing. One of the possible explanations for the failure of the human immune system to control tumor growth is that the helper arm of the response is defective. IL-2, released by activated $CD4^+$ T cells, is a critical component for the recruitment of $CD8^+$ T cells and absence of this cytokine is a frequent finding in tissue sections of human tumors even when infiltrated by $CD4^+$ T cells. Indirect evidence in support of a defective release of IL-2 as the mechanism to explain failure to reject tumor grafts came in 1990 by experiments carried out by Fearon and colleagues. These authors showed that a poorly immunogenic mouse tumor, modified to release IL-2, could be rejected, thus ''bypassing'' the helper arm of the immune response, although in that system no immunological memory could be established (Fearon *et al.*, 1990). An alternative mechanism, leading to a defective helper arm of the response, is tumor-specific $CD4^+$ T cell tolerance. This may occur when tumor-associated antigens are also expressed by some normal cells, a condition supported by the finding that human melanoma may express several $CD4^+$ T cell epitopes coded for by a cell lineage-specific gene (tyrosinase) expressed as such not only in melanoma but also in normal melanocytes (see class II HLA-restricted antigens in Chapter 1).

The condition of tumor-associated antigens shared with normal cells has been replicated in mouse models to test the consequences on immune response. In one mouse model (the FBL-3 leukemia) the Friend mouse leukemia virus *env* gene product is recognized by $CD4^+$ T cells on the tumor. Transgenic mice, where the *env* gene was also expressed on some normal lymphoid cells, could not be vaccinated against the *env* protein, as these mice showed an immune response against tumor re-challenge (Hu *et al.*, 1993). Interestingly, tumor rejection could be achieved by adoptive transfer of *env*-specific $CD4^+$ T cells from non-transgenic mice to the transgenic ones. However, in the adoptive transfer setting, no immune response against the normal lymphoid cells expressing low levels of *env* gene was observed. Taken together these results prove that tolerance to tumor-associated antigens can develop when the same epitopes are also expressed on normal cells. However, the adoptive transfer of tumor-specific T cells from non-tolerant mice suggests that *ex vivo* generated antitumor $CD4^+$ T cells might be used in adoptive immunotherapy in patients with a tolerant arm of the immune system. More recently, in a model system based on transfer of TCR-transgenic T cells with specificity for a model tumor antigen, Staveley-O'Carrol and colleagues showed that progressive and antigen-specific $CD4^+$ anergy developed in tumor-bearing mice (Staveley-O'Carroll *et al.*, 1998). The transgenic T cells isolated from tumor-bearing animals did not respond to antigen-pulsed APC. Interestingly, in this model the tumor was MHC class II^+ and $B7^+$, suggesting that anergy induction can be the end result even when the tumor is apparently equipped as a functional APC. In other words, direct antigen presentation (through tumor MHC class II) and T cell co-stimulation (through tumor B7) do not necessarily induce T cell activation but, rather, may result in tolerization. Another mechanism that can block an effective $CD4^+$-mediated antitumor response has been recently described by Blankenstein and colleagues (Qin *et al.*, 1998). These authors have taken into consideration the fact that different APC (such as B cells, macrophages and DC) can compete for antigen and have shown, using B cell deficient mice, that the presence of B cells (as APC for $CD4^+$ T cell priming) in the priming phase of the antitumor response diverts the $CD4^+$ T cell response from a TH1-type (resulting in help for CTL-mediated tumor immunity) to a TH2-type non-protective humoral response (see also Chapter 4). These results have led the authors to suggest that the frequent observation of tumor-reactive antibodies in cancer patients may indeed reflect a non-protective TH2-type humoral response resulting from $CD4^+$ T cell priming by B cells as APC for tumor-associated antigens.

BOTH TH1 AND TH2 $CD4^+$ T CELLS CAN COOPERATE IN ANTITUMOR RESPONSES

The role of antitumor $CD4^+$ T cells in inducing protective tumor immunity is not only that of providing help for CTL induction. Results obtained by the end of the last decade had clearly indicated that a major mechanism of the antitumor effect of $CD4^+$ T cells is the production of cytokines leading to the activation and recruitment of other effector cells such as macrophages (Figure 3.2). The discovery that $CD4^+$ T cells can be classified into two functionally polarized subsets (TH1 and TH2), depending on the cytokines they produce, has prompted an evaluation of how these two subsets may contribute to antitumor response. TH1 T cells produce IFNγ, TNF-α and IL-2, and play a major role in cell-mediated immunity (through the activation of CTL, NK cells and macrophages) and in promoting delayed-type hypersensitivity reactions. TH2 T cells produce IL-4, IL-5, IL-10 and IL-13, and play a role in antibody responses and eosinophil activation (see Romagnani, 1997). Cytokines not only affect cell types regulated by $CD4^+$ T cells but are also involved in inducing the differentiation of naive $CD4^+$ T cells along the TH1 or the TH2 pathway. Thus, IL-4 and IL-6 are responsible for TH2 differentiation, while IL-12 and IFN promote TH1 differentiation.

On the basis of the different immunological functions regulated by the two $CD4^+$ subsets, it was suggested by Clerici and co-workers (Clerici *et al.*, 1996) that conditions that promote TH2 development may inhibit cell-mediated immunity to tumors through release of cytokines (such as IL-10) that down-regulate TH1 differentiation. On the contrary, cytokines as IL-12 may favour cell-mediated immunity to tumors by inducing TH1 cells and by activating the cytolytic activity of NK and CTL. According to these authors, TH2-type responses might even provide an explanation for the phenomenon of tumor enhancement (enhanced tumor growth by transfer of antiserum specific for the tumor), described at the beginning of the twentieth century by Flexner and Jobling (1907). Tumor enhancement had been initially attributed to antibodies covering immunologically relevant sites on tumor cells but, according to the hypothesis put forward by Clerici and co-workers, it might reflect a skewing of immune response towards a non-protective, antibody-dominated TH2-type response. Experimental models of adoptive transfer of tumor-specific TH2 T cells have indeed shown enhanced production of pulmonary metastases in mice bearing implants of low metastatic B16F1

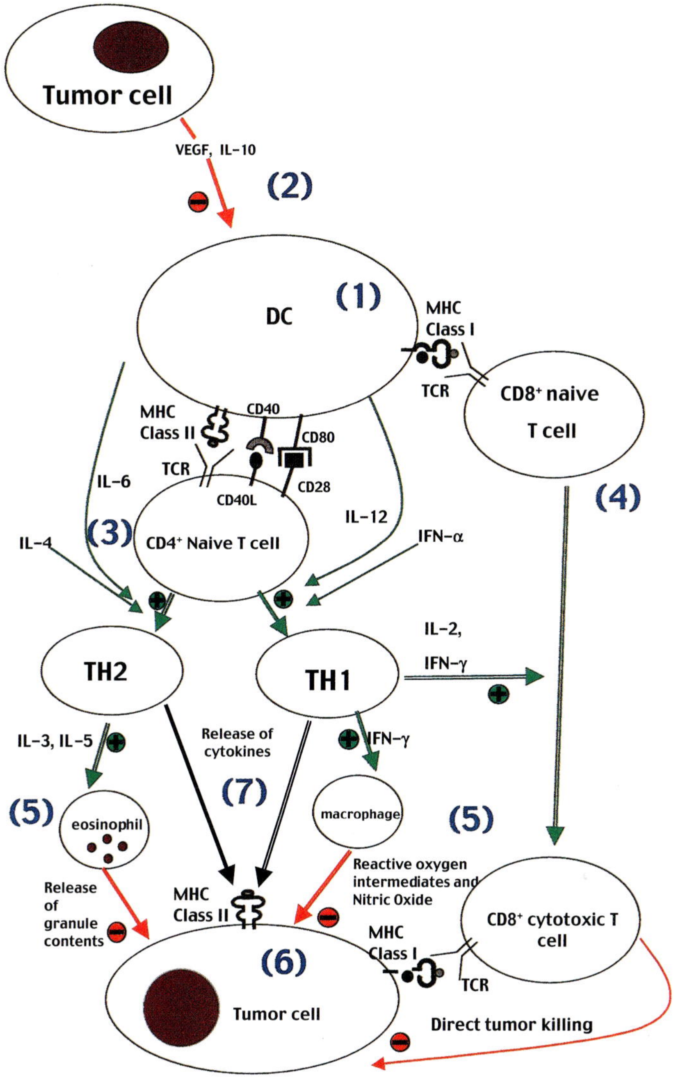

Figure 3.2 Cytokine pathways in antitumor response. Tumor antigens are presented by DCs (1) to CD4$^+$ T cells; such recognition promotes activation of DCs (via CD40L–CD40 and CD86–CD80 interactions) to release IL-12 that plays a central role in differentiation of naive CD4$^+$ T cells to TH1 cells (3). Activated DCs can prime antigen-specific CD8$^+$ T cells (4) that, through cytokines released by TH1 CD4$^+$ T cells, can proliferate and differentiate to CTL effectors able to directly mediate lysis of antigen$^+$ tumor cells. Alternatively, under the influence of different cytokines (IL-6, IL-4) naive CD4$^+$ T cells can differentiate to TH2 cells. TH1 and TH2 T cells can both contribute to antitumor responses by directly recognizing MHC class II$^+$, antigen$^+$ tumors (6) and releasing cytokines, or indirectly by activating other effectors such as eosinophils and macrophages (5). Note that tumor cells can release factors that negatively affect the maturation and/or antigen-presenting function of DCs (1). Pathways leading to activation of other cell types are marked by green arrows and a ''plus'' symbol, while inhibitory pathways or those associated with antitumor effects are marked by red arrows or a red ''minus'' sign. Note that a number of additional cytokines, not shown here, are produced by either CD4$^+$ or CD8$^+$ T cells and may contribute to antitumor response. For example, CD4$^+$ TH2 cells release IL-10 which, in some models, has been shown to promote antitumor responses rather than inhibiting them as initially thought.

melanoma (Kobayashi *et al.*, 1998), thus supporting a detrimental role of TH2 T cells in antitumor immunity. Furthermore, in the same model, injection of antibody to IL-4 (an important TH2 cytokine) in mice receiving TH2 T cells resulted in inhibition of pulmonary metastases, confirming that blocking of TH2 responses could restore a protective immunity against tumor growth.

This view that TH2-derived cytokines and TH2-type responses are detrimental to protective tumor immunity has now been challenged by additional reports indicating that, in mouse models, IL-10 (an important TH2-derived cytokine) has anti-metastatic activity (dependent on the function of NK cells) and antitumor activity (dependent on T cells) (Kundu *et al.*, 1996). Recent studies in mouse models have shown that both TH1 and TH2 $CD4^+$ T cells can activate additional effector pathways, independent from CTLs, and that these pathways may cooperate in tumor destruction. For example, tumor-specific TH1 T cells can activate macrophages to release reactive oxygen intermediates and nitric oxide, while TH2 T cells can recruit and activate eosinophils to release their granule contents. In these models, both macrophages and eosinophils can mediate the antitumor responses independently from CTLs. In a recent study using tumor cells engineered to release GM-CSF, Hung and colleagues have indeed shown that after vaccination with cytokine-releasing tumor both TH2 and TH1 $CD4^+$ T cells are induced which orchestrate the antitumor immune response (Hung *et al.*, 1998).

$CD4^+$ T LYMPHOCYTES AND HUMAN CANCER

In the human system, although tumor-specific $CD4^+$ T cells have not been shown to control tumor growth, several *in vitro* studies have demonstrated reactivity of $CD4^+$ T cells to autologous tumor cells from melanoma, lymphoma, colon cancer, breast cancer and sarcoma patients (see Pardoll and Topalian, 1998). During 1999, several shared and unique human tumor antigens that elicit an *in vitro* CD4+ T cell response were identified (see Toes *et al.*, 1999, and Chapter 1), though a role for $CD4^+$ in controlling human tumor growth *in vivo* is yet to be proved. The isolation of tumor-reactive $CD4^+$ T cells recognizing the idiotypic Ig sequence of the autologous B cell lymphoma, or the junctional sequence of *bcr-abl* fusion protein in CML, or even mutated p21 *ras* sequences in pancreatic cancer has been also accomplished by using synthetic peptide to generate CD4 T cells *in vitro*.

Apart from all mechanisms of tumor escape (see Chapter 6), it is quite possible that most human tumors do not activate a $CD4^+$ helper response simply because the immune response needs an ''inflammatory milieu'' to be triggered and this condition may not occur during tumor growth. This inflammatory reaction can be induced by the release of cytokines in experimental models with cytokine-transduced tumors (see Musiani *et al.*, 1997) but, apparently, it does not take place during development of tumors in patients. According to the ''danger model'' proposed by P. Matzinger, the goal of the immune system is not that of distinguishing self from non-self, but that of activating a response against tissue distress, a condition that might be triggered by inflammatory reactions (Fuchs and Matzinger, 1996). Thus, without an inflammatory milieu, cancer may not appear dangerous to the immune system and T cell responses are not activated. This mechanism may provide an explanation for the lack of immunogenicity of human tumors, even when antigens potentially recognized by $CD4^+$ T cells are expressed.

$CD8^+$ T LYMPHOCYTES AND CANCER

By the beginning of the 1990s, it was clear that tumor-specific $CD8^+$ CTL represent an important arm of the antitumor response. In some models, cure of tumor-bearing mice could be achieved by adoptive transfer of $CD8^+$ tumor-specific T cells, without any contribution of the $CD4^+$ T cells subset. However, in contrast to the results obtained with tumor-specific $CD4^+$ T cells, adoptive transfer of tumor-specific $CD8^+$ T cells achieved tumor regression of tumor-bearing mice only when IL-2 was administered for several days, following $CD8^+$ T cell transfer. The requirement for IL-2 in these models was interpreted as an indication that tumor-specific $CD8^+$ T cells needed a $CD4^+$-derived cytokine for survival and proliferation into the tumor-bearing host (Greenberg, 1991). More importantly, these findings indicate that the phase of priming of the immune reponse could be bypassed by the adoptive transfer of antigen-specific $CD8^+$ T cells.

$CD8^+$ T CELLS IN HUMAN CANCER

At the time the mouse models had established a role for $CD8^+$ T cells in antitumor responses, it was also understood, thanks to several studies performed during the 1980s, that antitumor $CD8^+$, HLA class I-restricted CTL could be isolated from cancer patients' lymphocytes after expansion *in vitro* in the presence at autologous tumor cells and IL-2. During the 1990s new molecular techniques were developed (based on PCR in most instances) that have enabled the investigating of whether selective accumulation/expansion of tumor-specific T cells occurs in neoplastic lesions. These techniques allow tumor-specific T cells in tumor tissue to be traced and quantitated and are based on the identification of unique molecular sequences of the TCR expressed by these T cells (usually either variable region or hypervariable region sequences are used for tracing specific T cells). These investigations have clearly shown that at least in some human tumors, an oligoclonal expansion of $CD8^+$ tumor-specific T cells occurs in a proportion of patients (see Sensi and Parmiani, 1995).

More recent data have been obtained by the technique based on staining antigen-specific T cells with fluorescent MHC–peptide tetrameric complexes. T cells expressing a TCR that recognizes the tetramer can be stained and quantified by flow cytometry. This technique has indeed shown that in some melanoma patients a high number of tumor-specific $CD8^+$ T cells with a memory phenotype can be found in metastatic lymph nodes (Romero *et al.*, 1998). These selective clonal expansions are thought to reflect an antigen-driven process leading to proliferation and/or accumulation of antigen-specific $CD8^+$ T cell clones directed to both known and unknown antigens. Additional evidence, obtained in our laboratory by the limiting dilution analysis (LDA) technique, has indicated that tumor-specific $CD8^+$ CTL precursors (CTLp) can be found at high frequency in peripheral blood of some metastatic melanoma patients. Interestingly, when we looked at the type of antigens these CTLp were recognizing in HLA-$A2^+$ patients, we found that most of the immune repertoire was directed to antigens expressed only on the tumor and not shared with normal melanocytes (Anichini *et al.*, 1996). This raised the possibility that tumor-specific antigens, expressed as result of neoplastic transformation, may play an important role in tumor recognition. The role of such antigens may be even more relevant than that of the well-known lineage-specific antigens of melanoma (such as Melan-A/MART-1, gp100, tyrosinase and TRP-2). The recent molecular identification of the first example of the class of "melanoma-specific antigens" (resulting from translation of a retained intron of the TRP-2 gene) provided direct evidence for a mechanism, occurring only in transformed cells of the melanocyte lineage, that may lead to the expression of CTL-defined antigens on melanomas but not on melanocytes nor on other tumors of different histological origin (Lupetti *et al.*, 1998). More recent data indicate that a state of systemic immunity to a single melanoma antigen (such as Melan-A/MART-1) can be found in peripheral blood of some metastatic melanoma patients as an expanded pool of peptide-specific CTL with a memory phenotype (CD45RO$^+$) (Anichini *et al.*, 1999).

Thus, the results of several studies are consistent with immunogenicity of at least some human tumors. The question, however, is whether the evidence for local or systemic immunity to tumor antigens reflects an effective CD8 T lymphocytes response. In fact, all available data do not necessarily imply that infiltrating CD8$^+$ T cells can indeed exert an antitumor activity. On the one hand, activation signals needed to promote the cytolytic function of antigen-specific CD8$^+$ T cells may be missing in the tumor-tissue. On the other hand, antigen-specific CD8$^+$ T cells isolated from tumor-infiltrating lymphocytes have been shown to release a pattern of cytokines (upon tumor recognition) that may in fact suppress immune responses (for example due to the presence of IL-10). Therefore, the simple and attractive hypothesis that infiltrating CD8$^+$ T cells represent evidence of antitumor immune response needs a re-evaluation, since this can be true in some instances but not in all tumors or in all stages of disease.

WHY CD8$^+$-MEDIATED T CELL RESPONSES MAY FAIL TO TAKE PLACE EVEN WHEN TUMORS ARE ANTIGENIC

In spite of the presence of antigens on at least some human tumors, the available evidence suggests that tumor-destructive CTL-mediated immune response does not take place (Anichini *et al.*, 1999). One possibility is that immunogenicity of most human tumors may be impaired or absent. Animal models have been developed to test whether tumor immunogenicity can be improved. To this end many investigators have assessed whether peri-tumoral injection of cytokines or modification of tumor cells by cytokine genes transduction could induce CTL-mediated immune responses even when apparently non-immunogenic tumors were used. Several reports have indeed shown that cytokine-activated tumor rejection occurs, indicating that tumor immunogenicity can be boosted, providing that T cell-defined antigens are expressed on the tumor. These models have also shown that rejection of cytokine-producing tumors can lead to the establishment of immunological memory against poorly or non-immunogenic tumors (see Parmiani *et al.*, 1997). The mechanism underlying this process is activated by the cytokine used to modify the tumor. The initial destruction of tumor cells induces release of tumor antigens that can load host APC and promote priming of tumor-specific T cells. Interestingly, as reported by Forni and colleagues (Musiani *et al.*, 1997), in the TSA mammary adenocarcinoma model (a spontaneous tumor of a BALB/c mouse), in several instances, when the tumor had been modified to release IL-2, IL-7, IL-10, IFN-γ and TNF-α, the main memory response was found to be dependent on CD8$^+$ CTL, confirming the relevance of this subset in antitumor immunity. Thus, an adequate priming of the immune response of tumor-free animals results in long-lasting immunity. This is in agreement with current models indicating that CD8$^+$ T cell memory persists indefinitely in the absence of the priming antigen (Lau *et al.*, 1994). Unfortunately, appropriate priming of the immune response may not occur during tumor growth in patients. Furthermore, in patients with advanced disease, activation of antitumor response (by vaccination with any of the various available approaches such as gene-modified tumor cells or with tumor antigen loaded APC) is usually performed in the presence of a significant tumor burden. This suggests that tumor escape from immune mechanisms as well as tumor-induced immune suppression may significantly hamper the attempts to boost tumor immunogenicity and to establish CD8$^+$ T cell memory (see also Chapter 6).

DIRECT VS. INDIRECT ANTIGEN PRESENTATION IN CD8$^+$-MEDIATED ANTI-TUMOR RESPONSES

A critical point established by mouse models of immunization with gene-modified tumor cells is that activation of CD8$^+$-mediated anti-tumor responses occurs in many instances by cross-priming. This was found to be true when using cytokine-producing tumors as well as when the immunizing tumor has been engineered to express co-stimulatory molecules as B7-1. The model of cross-presentation, through specialized APC for priming of CD8$^+$ CTL responses, is considered important for the induction of immunity towards antigens expressed in peripheral, extra-lymphoid organs (see also Chapter 2). As reviewed recently by Carbone and colleagues (Carbone *et al.*, 1998), naive and resting T cells are thought to recirculate between secondary lymphoid organs through blood and lymphatic vessels and to avoid peripheral tissues. In fact, to penetrate peripheral tissues T cells need to be primed within the lymph nodes that drain peripheral organs. This explains why antigens (such as viral or even tumor antigens) have to be processed by professional APC in the periphery before being presented in an immunogenic form by such APC to naive T cells in lymph nodes. As a consequence, it is necessary to use professional APC, loaded with tumor antigen, in order to prime naive CD8$^+$ T cells. The model of indirect antigen presentation for priming CD8$^+$ T cells has been shown to be true not only in mouse models but even in the human system, where several HLA class I-restricted T cell epitopes recognized by CD8$^+$ CTL have been identified in different tumors. It is well established that human tumor cells, although antigenic in some instances, usually cannot behave as professional APC, due to the lack of important co-stimulatory molecules. For this reason, vaccination approaches should not rely on the use of tumor cells as APC, unless they have been modified by gene transfer, but must use indirect antigen presentation through autologous DCs. Indeed, both *in vitro* data as well as results of *in vivo* vaccination studies indicated that DC loaded with tumor peptides can induce tumor-specific CTL, in the absence of a CD4$^+$ help. Thus, vaccination approaches to cancer therapy can be designed even using only CD8$^+$-recognized antigens as targets for immune intervention. This principle is in agreement with results obtained during the 1980s showing that, in appropriate animal models, tumor rejection can be achieved even by transfer of a single CD8$^+$ CTL clone recognizing a tumor antigen (Greenberg, 1991). This does not exclude the possibility that these approaches may fail in the human system due either to tumor heterogeneity for antigen expression, or to lack of an effective helper arm of the response that may be necessary for maintaining the CTL activity induced by the vaccination procedure. This concern represents the basis for the development of both experimental models and some clinical trials where $CD4^+$-derived cytokines that affect proliferation (IL-2), long-term survival (IL-7) and cytotoxic activity (IL-12) of $CD8^+$ CTL have been included in the immunization scheme or even expressed, by retroviral vectors, in professional APC.

Alternatively, instead of providing CD4-derived cytokines, immunization attempts could be designed in such a way as to directly activate both a $CD4^+$-mediated response and $CD8^+$ CTL. One way of obtaining this result in human cancers is by expressing, into professional APC, the whole genes that code for tumor epitopes recognized by CTL. The hope is that, within the protein sequence coded for by the tumor antigen gene, additional peptides may be expressed by the APC and behave as the target antigens of $CD4^+$ T cells. This indeed has been shown to occur with at least two different melanoma antigens (tyrosinase and Melan-A/MART-1) whose genes, when expressed by viral vectors into DCs, can indeed activate both $CD4^+$ and $CD8^+$ T cells directed against different peptides within the protein sequence of the same antigens (Yee *et al.*, 1996; Perez-Diez *et al.*, 1998).

ROLE OF NATURAL KILLER LYMPHOCYTES

Both in rodents and humans, NK cells are a subset of large granular lymphocytes characterized by absence of CD3 and expression of CD56 and CD16 (Whiteside and Herberman, 1995). The initial interest in the role of NK cells as antitumor effectors derives from the original definition of their *in vitro* function (i.e. the ability to lyse tumor and virus-infected cells but not normal cells in a MHC-unrestricted fashion and without the need for prior sensitization) and from the finding that their cytotoxic activity could be significantly boosted by T cell-derived factors. The observation by Rosenberg's group that culture of peripheral blood lymphocytes with IL-2 could induce MHC-unrestricted cytotoxic cells (LAK) prompted several studies that investigated the potential use of LAK cells against fresh human tumor cells. These studies eventually revealed that LAK cells are mostly activated NK cells endowed with enhanced cytotoxic activity effective even against otherwise NK-resistant targets. The clinical trials conducted during the 1980s, employing LAK cells and IL-2, have indeed shown that it is possible to achieve significant and durable tumor regression, though in a limited fraction of patients, by adoptive transfer of these effectors (Rosenberg *et al.*, 1989). However, these trials were associated with significant toxicity, mainly due to the side effects of high-dose IL-2, and high cost and this therapeutic approach, therefore, has been abandoned.

THE BASIS FOR NK CELL RECOGNITION OF TUMORS

In spite of the limited clinical success in the use of activated NK cells as therapeutic agents, recent evidence on the mechanism of NK cell recognition of targets has renewed interest in this subset for their potential role in antitumor response. This new information has explained observations made in tumor models and with virally infected cells during the past 20 years or so. In 1982 Gorelik and colleagues reported that NK cells could control the metastatic potential of tumor cells (Gorelik *et al.*, 1982) and, more than 10 years ago, it became evident from studies with mouse models that the reduced expression of MHC class

I antigens on target cells correlated with increased susceptibility to NK cell lysis. For example, transfection of MHC antigens on tumors lacking them conferred protection against NK-mediated lysis and could even restore tumorigenicity. A similar relationship between NK cell function and absence of MHC molecules had been documented even in virally infected cells. This evidence led Ljunggren and Karre (1990) to propose the ''missing self'' hypothesis, predicting that NK cells evolved as a defense against cells that may have lost MHC antigens. Loss of MHC molecules may indeed prevent T cell recognition of both virally infected and transformed cells, and it seems reasonable to assume that an alternative immune mechanism (NK cells) has evolved to counteract loss of MHC molecules. Indeed, adenoviruses and herpesviruses, including HSC and HCMV, can induce down-regulation of expression of MHC molecules upon infection (Fruh *et al.*, 1997). The recent observation that several human tumors frequently do not express *in vivo* one or more HLA alleles (Garrido *et al.*, 1997) is consistent with a potential role of NK cells as a defense against tumor growth when MHC-restricted recognition of tumor antigens by either $CD4^+$ or $CD8^+$ T cells is no longer possible. It is, however, to be pointed out that in the human system there is no convincing evidence for an immune surveillance mechanism against tumor growth based on NK cell-mediated recognition of HLA-loss variants. For example, a relationship between the loss of HLA on tumor cells and the presence of infiltrating NK cells in the neoplastic tissue has not been found.

In spite of this uncertainty, the recent elucidation of the molecular basis for NK cell recognition of targets missing HLA molecules has provided new tools to re-evaluate the potential role of this lymphocyte subset in anti-cancer responses. Results obtained by Moretta and colleagues at the beginning of the 1990s have profoundly changed our view of how NK cells interact with targets that may or may not express MHC antigens (Moretta and Moretta, 1997). The early reports indicated that NK cells could lyse MHC-deficient targets, while the same targets became resistant to NK recognition after transfection of certain MHC alleles. Moreover, susceptibility to NK cell-mediated lysis of class I HLA-positive human melanomas was shown to reflect the level of expression of different HLA alleles (Pende *et al.*, 1998). Now we know that this lymphocyte subset expresses receptors for MHC molecules and that these receptors may be inhibitory or non-inhibitory for NK cell functions. Molecular cloning of the genes coding for these receptors has revealed transmembrane receptors of the C-type lectin superfamily expressed as disulfide-bonded heterodimers (the CD94/NKG2 receptors) and an Ig superfamily (the KIR receptors), where each member is characterized by two or three Ig-like domains in the extracellular portions (Figure 3.3) (Lanier, 1998). The available evidence indicates that each NK clone can simultaneously express several receptors of the KIR and CD94/NKG2 type and these receptors can function independently. Thus NK cell function depends on a balance between positive and negative signals deriving from these receptors when they engage a target expressing a defined HLA profile. This evidence may help in deciding which NK subsets may be effective against a tumor that has lost a particular HLA allele.

However, whether the information on structure and function of NK receptors can be translated into effective clinical trials against HLA-loss variants arising in patients during tumor progression remains an open question. As in the field of immunotherapy with T cells, even immune intervention targeted at activating NK cells faces two possible

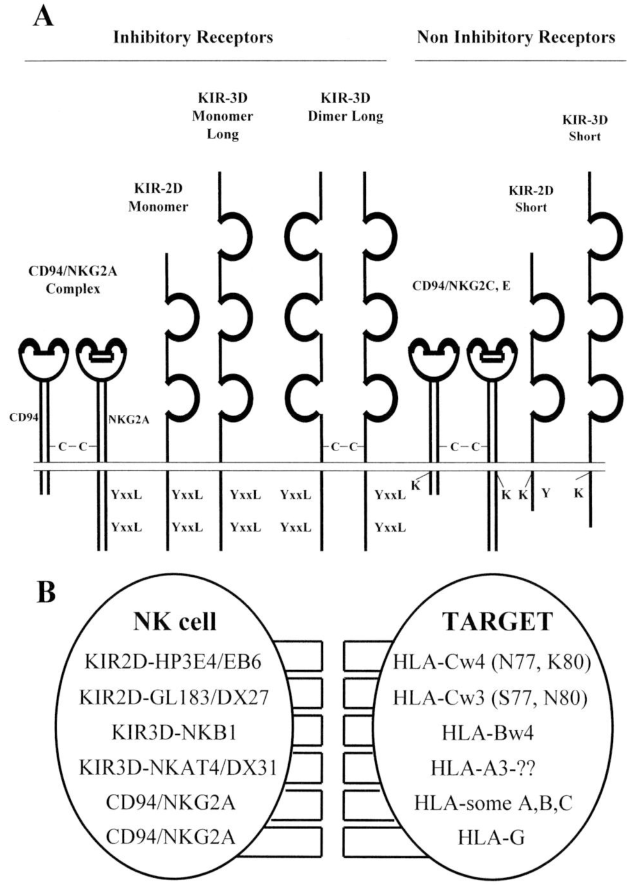

Figure 3.3 Human NK cell receptors for MHC. (**A**) Human NK receptors for MHC belong to two distinct molecular families. The CD94/NKG2A complex belongs to the family of C-type lectins that code for type II glycoproteins expressed as disulfide-linked heterodimers. CD94 is an invariant subunit linked to distinct proteins encoded by the NKG2 gene family (comprising 4 genes: NKG2A, NKG2C, NKG2E and NKG2D/F). CD94 and the four NKG2 genes map to the human ''NK complex'' on chromosome 12p12.3–p13.1. CD94 has essentially no cytoplasmic tails, indicating lack of function in signal transduction. The function of CD94 is thought to be that of a chaperone that allows transport of the NKG2 proteins to the cell surface. The killer inhibitory receptors (KIR) genes code for glycoproteins of the Ig superfamily. The KIR genes are located on chromosome 19q13.4 and about 12 genes are thought to exist. KIR receptors are classified into two subfamilies according to the number of Ig-like domains (two in KIR2D receptors and three in KIR3D receptors). In addition, marked heterogeneity in the cytoplasmic domain of KIR receptors has been described. KIRs with long cytoplasmic tails (such as KIR2DL) contain ''immunoreceptor tyrosine-based inhibition motifs'' (ITIM sequences = I/VxYxxL/V) that mediate the inhibitory function of the receptor. KIRs with short cytoplasmic tails (such as KIR3DS) lack ITIM sequences but have a charged aminoacid residue (K in the figure). KIR2DS and KIR3DS are activating rather than inhibiting receptors for MHC. KIR are expressed as monomers, with the exception of KIR3DL which may be expressed as monomer or as homodimer. (**B**) Examples of ligand–receptor interaction. The CD94/NKG2A heterodimer has promiscuous binding specificity and can recognize several HLA-A, -B, -C and -G ligands. KIR2D molecules recognize mainly HLA-C ligands, but different members of the KIR2D family can discriminate HLA-C alleles on the basis of residues at position 77 (N rather than K as the receptors recognized by mAbs HP3E4 or EB6) and 80 (S rather than N, as receptors recognized by mAbs GL183 or DX27) in the HLA-C heavy chain. KIR3DL (recognized by mAb DX31) is directed to HLA-B allotypes that have the Bw4 motif at residues 77–83 of the HLA-B heavy chain. Note that recognition of polymorphic HLA-B and HLA-C ligands by KIR3D and KIR2D molecules respectively depends even on the nature of peptides bound to the groove of the MHC class I molecule.

alternatives, *ex vivo* selection followed by adoptive transfer or *in vivo* activation. The first approach might focus on selecting the appropriate NK subset expressing the inhibitory MHC receptor directed to HLA alleles lost in the tumor. The second approach could aim at an *in vivo* NK activation by cytokines (such as IFN-γ, IL-2, IL-12, IL-15) known to affect the proliferation, differentiation and function of this subset.

Finally we should point out that inhibitory receptors for MHC have been described even on some T cells, including antitumor CTL (Mingari *et al.*, 1996; Spieser *et al.*, 1999). This has a significant implication for tumor immunology, since a single CTL may express a TCR directed against a tumor antigen in the context of one of the HLA alleles and an inhibitory receptor directed to a different HLA molecule expressed on the same tumor. Under such a condition, T cell activation resulting from TCR-mediated recognition of the tumor antigen would be prevented by the MHC-specific inhibitory receptor. This is a new tumor escape mechanism that has been shown by Coulie and colleagues to occur in a melanoma patient where an HLA-A24-restricted CTL directed to the PRAME antigen (a normal gene overexpressed in melanoma) also expressed the KIR2DL inhibitory receptor and could only recognize a metastatic variant (lacking the HLA-Cw7, the ligand for KIR2DL) but not the parental melanoma (Ikeda *et al.*, 1997). Expression of the MHC inhibitory receptors on antitumor T cells is intriguing and suggests that it may be part of a protective mechanism to prevent autoimmunity against normal non-mutated gene products (Such as the PRAME protein). However, further studies are needed to clarify whether expression of inhibitory receptors for MHC is more frequent on T cells with specificity for self-antigens rather than on T cells directed to epitopes resulting from mutations.

NKT CELLS

A new subset of lymphocytes has recently been described both in mice and in man. These cells express the marker CD161 (NKR-P1) and a restricted TCR that, in humans, encompasses Vα24JαQ predominantly paired with Vβ11 (Exley *et al.*, 1998). These CD4+ NKT cells specifically recognize an (α-galactosylceramide presented by CD1d and, when stimulated, release a large amount of IL-12, IL-4 and IFN-γ; they were previously referred as Th0. Since α-galactosylceramide may be expressed by tumor cells, such effectors may contribute to an antitumor immune response which may synergize with or complement that mediated by T cells. It is of note that, in the mouse system, these NKT cells have been shown to mediate antitumor activity of IL-12 (Cui *et al.*, 1997).

CIRCULATION AND HOMING OF TUMOR-SPECIFIC T AND NK CELLS, AND THE ROLE OF HOMING-ASSOCIATED ADHESION MOLECULES AND OF CHEMOKINES

The development of T cell mediated antitumor response is critically dependent on the ability of lymphocytes to recirculate between blood and secondary lymphoid organs and on their migratory properties through tissues. Both processes, recirculation and migration, are dependent on the interplay between adhesion/homing receptors, chemokines and cytokines. Receptors for cell adhesion and homing receptors are a heterogeneous class of surface molecules and cognate ligands that are expressed on several cell types and enable leukocytes to interact with other cell types, including endothelial cells. These receptors are responsible both for selective recruitment of lymphocyte subsets and for transducing activation signals that contribute to development of effector functions. On the basis of molecular structure these receptors and their cognate ligands belong to at least 5 families, the Ig superfamily (e.g. ICAM-1,4, CD31, VCAM-1, and NCAM), mucins-like vascular addressins (e.g. MAdCAM-1), selectins (e.g. E-, L- and P-selectin), integrins (e.g. LFA-1, Mac-1, $\alpha 4\beta 1$ and $\alpha 4\beta 7$) and fucosylated tetrasaccharides (Such as sialyl Lewis X) (for review and details on expression and receptor-ligand specificity see Carlos and Harlan, 1994). The selective recruitment of leukocyte subsets at sites of inflammation or immune reactions has been described (Carlos and Harlan, 1994) as a combinatorial process whose outcome depends on the adhesion receptor and chemokine/cytokine receptor profile of each leukocyte subset. Thus, distinct lymphocyte subsets (depending on functional differentiation and activation stage) will express a well-defined profile for adhesion receptors and chemokine receptors. This phenotype will contribute to define the homing characteristics of each subset and their response to the milieu of chemokines found in a particular microenvironment. With respect to the homing and migratory patterns of lymphocyte subsets, chemokines and cytokines (produced at sites where immune responses will take place) play at least two major roles, regulation of expression and functional status of adhesion receptors (e.g. integrins expressed on either leukocyte subsets or endothelial cells), and selective chemoattraction.

The interplay between homing receptors and chemokines can be understood by looking at the process that enables naive T cells to reach those areas of lymph nodes that contain professional APCs. In fact, in the priming phase of the immune response, naive T cells need to enter lymph nodes where they can interact with APCs (DC) that will present tumor antigens. To enter lymph nodes, naive T cells leave the blood-stream via HEVs, a specialized endothelium for lymphocyte migration that lines postcapillary venules of lymph nodes and Peyers' patches (Girard and Springer, 1996). At this level, lymphocyte adherence and transendothelial migration are regulated by distinct families of adhesion/homing receptors that promote initial attachment and rolling, then firm adhesion and arrest, and finally migration through endothelial cell junctions. While rolling is mediated by selectins, adhesion and extravasation are mediated by integrins (Carlos and Harlan, 1994). L-selectin (which binds to CD34, GlyCAM-1 and to MAdCAM-1 on endothelial cells) and LFA-1 (an integrin which binds to ICAM-1 on endothelial cells) are the molecules that control lymphocyte interaction with HEVs. In order for T cells to bind to HEVs and to migrate across the endothelial wall, the adhesion receptors (integrins) involved in the process need to be activated to full functional status by a process known as inside-out signaling promoted by chemokines expressed on the surface of endothelial cells or produced in the lymphoid tissue (Sallusto *et al.*, 1999). The process is mediated by chemokines such as SDF-1, SLC and ELC that bind to chemokine receptors CXCR4 and CCR7 expressed at the highest levels on the naive T cells. After trans-endothelial migration, additional chemokines (such as ELC and DC-CK1), released by DCs, drive T cells to lymph node areas containing APCs. After priming, T cells will leave the lymph node through efferent lymph.

In the antitumor responses, the role of L-selectin in migration of naive T cells to lymph node areas where T cell priming occurs has been investigated in a mouse tumor model involving *in vivo* treatment with anti-L selectin monoclonal antibody (Rosato *et al.*, 1996). In mice treated with this monoclonal antibody, the authors found impaired generation of tumor-specific CTL (directed to viral antigens expressed on a Moloney murine sarcoma virus-induced tumor) in the tumor-draining lymph node (where homing of naive CTL precursors depends on L-selectin) but not in the spleen (where T cell localization is independent of L-selectin).

Depending on the combination of cytokines at the time of T cell priming, T cells will be polarized into either type 1 or type 2. This leads to polarization even at the level of the expression of chemokine receptors on TH1 and TH2 T cells, thus predisposing a mechanism for differential migration of these subsets to peripheral sites (see Sallusto *et al.*, 1999) depending on the type of immune response (e.g. type-1 responses as DTH reactions or type-2 responses as allergic reactions) and on the pattern of chemokines produced at sites of immune responses. As result of priming, memory T cells can develop that express a different adhesion/homing and chemokine receptor profile in comparison to naive counterparts. Although the existence of a clear-cut distinction in the homing properties of naive and memory T cells has been questioned (Westermann and Pabst, 1996), nevertheless some differences have been found. For example, memory T cells can migrate into non-lymphoid organs (e.g. skin) where they can mount secondary responses. To achieve this, memory T cells express specific homing receptors that enable them to bind to cognate ligands on endothelial cells expressed in different tissues. One of these receptors, the CLA antigen, enables binding to E-selectin on endothelium of skin venules. Other receptors mediate homing to mucosal lymphoid tissues. One of these receptors, the integrin $\alpha4\beta7$, defines a subset of memory T cells able to home to intestinal sites.

Another difference between naive and memory T cells involves the increased ability of the latter to exhibit rolling under flow on cytokine-activated endothelial cells, a process dependent on T cell interaction with E- and P-selectin as well as on VCAM-1 expressed on endothelial cells (Lichtman *et al.*, 1997). This feature of memory T cells is clearly useful to direct these cells at sites where a secondary response is needed. At these sites inflammation can promote the release of cytokines that will activate the expression of adhesion molecules on endothelial cells and this, in turn, can signal circulating lymphocytes that they have to leave the bloodstream. In this respect, one of the reasons for the failure to mount an effective immune response against tumors, in spite of their immunogenicity, may be the lack of appropriate inflammatory milieu at sites of tumor growth. As documented by several reports, the whole process of T cell priming in the human neoplasms may be functional and lead to the development of a memory T cell pool. However, in the absence of clear "signals" for recruitment, extravasation and activation, even circulating memory T cells with specificity for tumor antigens may never leave the bloodstream in sufficient numbers and home to the neoplastic tissue. Evidence for this mechanism has been obtained in transgenic mice where a transgene (the oncoprotein large T antigen) expressed in β cells leads first to hyperplasia of the islets and then to tumors (Onrust *et al.*, 1996). In hyperplastic β islets the authors found lymphocyte infiltration associated with up-regulation on blood vessels of ligands (GlyCam-1) for lymphocyte homing receptors L-selectin and $\alpha4\beta7$. In contrast, in tumors evolving from β islets no lymphocyte infiltration nor expression of ligands for the lymphocyte homing receptors was found. Thus, the lack of appropriate inflammatory milieu in the tumor tissue may prevent the expression of endothelial cell ligands for homing receptors expressed by T cells.

In spite of this possible limitation, it is known that the migratory activity of lymphocyte subsets, including T cells and NK cells, can be modulated by cytokines such as IL-2, IL-12 and IFN-γ. Thus, there is a rational basis for designing immune intervention approaches aimed at redirecting lymphocyte circulation and migration patterns to sites of neoplastic growth. For example, it is known that IL-2 can increase adhesion of NK cells to mucosal HEVs (Uksila *et al.*, 1997). The process depends on the function of adhesion receptors such as CD34 and α4 integrins whose expression is boosted by IL-2. Furthermore, recent evidence indicates that NK cells can be transiently recruited to the liver by treating mice with IL-2 or IL-12 (Fogler *et al.*, 1998). The two cytokines act by different mechanisms, as IL-12-induced, but not IL-2-induced, hepatic recruitment of NK cells depends on production of IFN-γ. Interestingly, IL-12 can induce recruitment to liver of both NK cells and T cells although with different kinetics (Fogler *et al.*, 1998). However, both NK and T cells migrate to liver after IL-12 treatment, thanks to the function of an important endothelial cell adhesion molecule, VCAM-1 (Fogler *et al.*, 1998). Expression of homing receptors on lymphocyte subsets, depending on differentiation status, can even be exploited to enrich tumor-specific T cells. For example, as a result of activation with tumor antigens, lymphocytes from tumor-draining lymph nodes contain a fraction of tumor-specific $CD4^+$ T cells that can be identified on the basis of low expression of L-selectin (Kagamu and Shu, 1998). These cells, after purification, can mediate significant antitumor effects in adoptive immunotherapy of intracranial growing tumors.

REFERENCES

Anichini, A., Mortarini, R., Maccalli, C., Squarcina, P., Fleischhauer, K., Mascheroni, L., and Parmiani, G. (1996) Cytotoxic T cells directed to tumor antigens not expressed on normal melanocytes dominate the HLA-A2.1-restricted immune repertoire to melanoma. *J. Immunol.*, **156**, 208–217.

Anichini, A., Molla, A., Mortarini, R., Tragni, G., Bersani, I., Di Nicola, M., Gianni, M., Pilotti, S., Dunbar, R., Cerundolo, V., and Parmiani, G. (1999) An expanded peripheral T cell population to a cytotoxic T lymphocyte (CTL)-defined, melanocyte-specific antigen in metastatic melanoma patients impacts on generation of peptide-specific CTL, but does not overcome tumor escape from immune surveillance in metastatic lesions. *J. Exp. Med.*, **190**, 651–668.

Arca, M.J., Mule, J.J., and Chang, A.E. (1996) Genetic approaches to adoptive cellular therapy of malignancy. *Sem. Oncol.*, **23**, 108–117.

Armstrong, T.D., Pulaski, B.A., and Ostrand-Rosenberg, S. (1998) Tumor antigen presentation, changing the rules. *Cancer Immunol. Immunother.*, **46**, 70–74.

Bevan, M.J. (1976) Cross-priming for a secondary cytotoxic response to minor H antigens with H-2 congenic cells which do not cross-react in the cytotoxic assay. *J. Exp. Med.*, **143**, 1283–1288.

Boon, T., Cerottini, J.-C., Van den Eynde, B., van der Bruggen, P., and Van Pel, A. (1994) Tumor antigen recongized by T lymphocytes. *Ann. Rev. Immunol.*, **12**, 337–365.

Carbone, F.R., Kurts, C., Bennet, S.R., Miller, J.F., and Heath, W.R. (1998) Cross-presentation, a general mechanism for CTL immunity and tolerance. *Immunol. Today*, **19**, 368–372.

Carlos, T.M., and Harlan, J.M. (1994) Leukocyte-endothelial adhesion molecules. *Blood*, **84**, 2068–2101.

Clerici, M., Clerici, E., and Shearer, G.M. (1996) The tumor enhancement phenomenon, reinterpretation from a TH1/TH2 perspective. *J. Natl. Cancer Inst. USA*, **88**, 461–462.

Cui, J., Shin, T., Kawano, T., Sato, H., Kondo, E., Toura, I., Kaneko, Y., Kosiki, H., Kanno, M., and Taniguchi, M. (1997). Requirement for Vα14 NKT cells in IL-12-mediated rejection of tumors. *Science*, **278**, 1623–1626.

Exley, M., Porcelli, S., Furman, M., Garcia, J., and Balk, S. (1998) CD161(NKR-P1A) costimulation of CD1d-dependent activation of human T cells expressing invariant V α24JαQ T cell receptor α chains. *J. Exp. Med.* **188**, 867–876.

Fearon, E.R., Pardoll, D.M., Itaya, T., Golumbek, P., Levitsky, H.I., Simons, J.W., Karasuyama, H., Vogelstein, B., and Frost, P. (1990) Interleukin-2 production by tumor cells bypasses T helper function in the generation of an antitumor response. *Cell* **60**, 397–403.

Flexner, S., and Jobling, J.W. (1907) On the promoting influence of heated tumor emulsions on tumor growth. *Proc. Soc. Exp. Biol. Med.*, **4**, 156–169.

Fogler, W.E., Volker, K., Watanabe, M., Wigginton, J.M., Roessler, P., Brunda, M.J., Ortaldo, J.R., and Wiltrout, R.H. (1998) Recruitment of hepatic NK cells by IL-12 is dependent on IFN-gamma and VCAM-1 and is rapidly down-regulated by a mechanism involving T cells and expression of Fas. *J. Immunol.*, **161**, 6014–6021.

Fruh, A., Ahn, K., and Paterson, P.A. (1997) Inhibition of MHC class I antigen presentation by viral proteins. *J. Mol. Med.*, **75**, 18–27.

Fuchs, E.J., and Matzinger, P. (1996) Is cancer dangerous to the immune system? *Sem. Immunol.*, **8**, 271–280.

Garrido, F., Ruiz-Cabello, F., Cabrera, T., Perez-Villar, J.J., Lopez-Botet, M., Duggan-Keen, M., and Stern, P.L. (1997) Implications for immusurveillance of altered HLA class I phenotype in human tumours. *Immunol. Today*, **18**, 89–95.

Girard, J.P., and Springer, T.A. (1996) High endothelial venules (HEVs), specialized endothelium for lymphocyte migration. *Immunol. Today*, **16**, 449–457.

Gorelik, E., Wiltrout, R.H., Okumura, K., Habu, S., and Herberman, R.B. (1982) Role of NK cells in the control of metastatic spread of tumor cells in mice. *Int. J. Cancer*, **30**, 107–112.

Greenberg, P.D. (1991) Adoptive T cell therapy of tumors, mechanisms operative in the recognition and elimination of tumor cells. *Adv. Immunol.*, **49**, 281–355.

Hu, J., Kindsvogel, W., Busby, S., Bailey, M.C., Shi, Y.Y., and Greenberg, P.D. (1993) An evaluation of the potential to use tumor-associated antigens as targets for antitumor T cell therapy using transgenic mice expressing a retroviral tumor antigen in normal lymphoid tissues. *J. Exp. Med.*, **177**, 1681–1690.

Huang, A.Y., Golumbek, P., Ahmadzadeh, M., Jaffee, E., Pardoll, D., and Levitsky, H. (1994) Role of bone marrow-derived cells in presenting MHC class I-restricted tumor antigens. *Science*, **264**, 961–965.

Hung, H.M., Urba, W.J., and Fox, B.A. (1998) Gene-modified tumor vaccine with therapeutic potential shifts tumor-specific T cell response from a type 2 to a type 1 cytokine profile. *J. Immunol.*, **161**, 3033–3041.

Hung, K., Hayashi, R., Lfond-Walker, A., Lowenstein, C., Pardoll, D., and Levitsky, H. (1998) The central role of CD4+ T cells in the antitumor immune response. *J. Exp. Med.*, **188**, 2357–2368.

Ikeda, H., Lethé, B., Lehmann, F., van Baren, N., Baurain, J.F., De Smet, C., Chambost, H., Vitale, M., Moretta, A., Boon, T., and Coulie, P.G. (1997) Characterization of an antigen that is recognized on a melanoma showing partial HLA loss by CTL expressing an NK inhibitory receptor. *Immunity*, **6**, 199–208.

Kagamu, H., and Shu, S. (1998) Purification of L-selectin^{low} cells promotes the generation of highly potent CD4 antitumor effector T lymphocytes. *J. Immunol.*, **160**, 3444–3452.

Kedar, E., and Weiss, D. (1983) The *in vitro* generation of effector lymphocytes and their employment in tumor immunotherapy. *Adv. Cancer Res.*, **38**, 171–287.

Kedar, E., and Klein, E. (1992) Cancer immunotherapy, are the results discouraging? can they be improved? *Adv. Cancer Res.*, **59**, 245–323.

Kobayashi, M., Kobayashi, H., Pollard, R.B., and Suzuki, F. (1998) A pathogenic role of TH2 cells and their cytokine products on the pulmonary metastasis of murine B16 melanoma. *J. Immunol.*, **160**, 5869–5873.

Kundu, N., Beaty, T.L., Jackson, M.J., and Fulton, A.M. (1996) Antimetastatic and antitumor activities of interleukin 10 in a murine model of breast cancer. *J. Natl. Cancer Inst. USA*, **88**, 536–541.

Lanier, L.L. (1998) NK cell receptors. *Annu. Rev. Immunol.*, **16**, 359–393.

Lau, L.L., Jamieson, B.D., Somasundaram, T., and Ahmed, R. (1994) Cytotoxic T cell memory without antigen. *Nature*, **369**, 648–652.

Lichtman, A.H., Ding, H., Henault, L., Vachino, G., Camphausen, R., Cumming, D., and Luscinskas, F.W. (1997) CD45RA-RO+ (memory) but not CD45RA+RO- (naive) T cells roll efficiently on E- and P-selectin and vascular cell adhesion molecule-1 under flow. *J. Immunol.*, **158**, 3640–3650.

Ljunggren, H.G., and Karre, K. (1990) In search of the ''missing self'', MHC molecules and NK cell recognition. *Immunol. Today*, **11**, 237–244.

Lupetti, R., Pisarra, P., Verrecchia, A., Farina, C., Nicolini, G., Anichini, A., Bordignon, C., Sensi, M., Parmiani, G., and Traversari, C. (1998) Translation of a retained intron in tyrosinase-related protein (TRP) 2 mRNA generates a new cytotoxic T lymphocyte (CTL)-defined and shared human melanoma antigen not expressed in normal cells of the melanocytic lineage *J. Exp. Med.*, **188**, 1005–1016.

Moretta, A., and Moretta, L. (1997) HLA class I specific inhibitory receptors. *Curr. Op. Immunol.*, **9**, 694–701.

Musiani, P., Modesti, A., Giovarelli, M., Cavallo, F., Colombo, M., Lollini, P.L., and Forni, G. (1997) Cytokines, tumour-cell death and immunogenicity, a question of choice. *Immunol. Today*, **18**, 32–36.

Onrust, S.V., Hartl, P.M., Rosen, S.D., and Hanahan, D. (1996) Modulation of L-selectin ligand expression during an immune response accompanying tumorigenesis in transgenic mice. *J. Clin. Invest.*, **97**, 54–64.

Pardoll, D.M., and Topalian, S. (1998) The role of CD4+ T cell responses in antitumor immunity. *Curr. Op. Immunol.*, **10**, 588–594.

Parmiani, G., Colombo, M.P., Melani, C., and Arienti, F. (1997) Cytokine gene transduction in the immunotherapy of cancer. *Adv. Pharmacol.*, **40**, 259–307.

Pende, D., Accame, L., Pareti, L., Mazzocchi, A., Moretta, A., Parmiani, G., and Moretta, L. (1998) The susceptibility to natural killer cell-mediated lysis of HLA class I-positive melanomas reflects the expression of insufficient amounts of HLA class I alleles. *Eur. J. Immunol.*, **28**, 2384–2394.

Perez-Diez, A., Butterfield, L.H., Li, L., Chakraborty, N.G., Economou, J.S., and Mukherji, B. (1998) Generation of $CD8^+$ and $CD4^+$ T-cell response to dendritic cells genetically engineered to express the MART-1/Melan-A gene. *Cancer Res.*, **58**, 5305–5309.

Prehn, R.T., and Main, J.M. (1957) Immunity to methylcholanthrene-induced sarcomas. *J. Natl Cancer Inst. USA*, **18**, 768–778.

Qin, Z., Richter, G., Schuler, T., Ibe, S., Cao, X., and Blankenstein, T. (1998) B cells inhibit induction of T cell-dependent tumor immunity. *Nature Med.*, **4**, 627–630.

Ridge, J.P., Di Rosa, F., and Matzinger, P. (1998) A conditioned dendritic cell can be a temporal bridge between a CD4+ T-helper and a T-killer cell. *Nature*, **393**, 474–477.

Romagnani, S. (1997) The TH1/TH2 paradigm. *Immunol. Today*, **18**, 263–266.

Romero, P., Dunbar, P.R., Valmori, D., Pittet, M., Ogg, G.S., Rimoldi, D., Chen, J.L., Liénard, D., Cerottini, J.-C., and Cerundolo, V. (1998) *Ex vivo* staining of metastatic lymph nodes by class I major histocompatibility complex tetramers reveals high numbers of antigen-experienced tumor-specific cytolytic T lymphocytes. *J. Exp. Med.*, **188**, 1641–1650.

Rosato, A., Zambon, A., Macino, B., Mandruzzato, S., Bronte, V., Milan, G., Zanovello, P., and Collavo, D. (1996) Anti-L-selectin monoclonal antibody treatment in mice enhances tumor growth by preventing CTL sensistization in peripheral lymph nodes draining the tumor area. *Int. J. Cancer*, **65**, 847–851.

Rosenberg, S.A., Lotze, M.T., Yang, J.C., Aabersold, P.M., Linehan, W.M., Seipp, C.A., and White, D.E. (1989) Experience with the use of high-dose interleukin-2 in the treatment of 652 cancer patients. *Ann. Surg.*, **210**, 474–485.

Sallusto, F., Lanzavecchia, A., and Mackay, C.R. (1999) Chemokines and chemokine receptors in T-cell priming and TH1/TH2-mediated responses. *Immunol. Today*, **19**, 568–574.

Schoenberger, S.P., Toes, R.E.M., van der Voort, E.I.H., Offringa, R., and Melief, C.J.M. (1998) T-cell help for cytotoxic T lymphocytes is mediated by CD40-CD40L interactions. *Nature*, **393**, 480–483.

Sensi, M., and Parmiani, G. (1995) Analysis of TCR usage in human tumors, a new tool for assessing tumor-specific immune responses. *Immunol. Today*, **16**, 588–595.

Speiser, D.E., Pittet, M.J., Valmori, D., Dunbar, R., Rimoldi, D., Liénard, D., McDonald, H.R., Cerottini, J.-C., Cerundolo, V., and Romero, P. (1999) *In vivo* expression of natural killer cell inhibitory receptors by human melanoma-specific cytolytic T lymphocytes. *J. Exp. Med.*, **190**, 775–782.

Staveley-O'Carroll, K., Sotomayor, E., Montgomery, J., Borrello, I., Hwang, L., Fein, S., Pardoll, D., and Levitsky, H. (1998) Induction of antigen-specific T cell anergy, An early event in the course of tumor progression. *Proc. Natl. Acad. Sci. USA*, **95**, 1178–1183.

Toes, R.E.M, Ossendorp, F., Offringa, R., and Melief, C.J.M. (1999) CD4 T cells and their role in antitumor immune responses. *J. Exp. Med.*, **189**, 7753–756.

Uksila, J., Salmi, M., Butcher, E.C., Tarkkanen, J., and Jalkanen, S. (1997) Function of lymphocyte homing-associated adhesion molecules on human natural killer and lymphokine-activated killer cells. *J. Immunol.*, **158**, 1610–1617.

Westermann, J., and Pabst, R. (1996) How organ-specific is the migration of ''naive'' and ''memory'' T cells? *Immunol. Today*, **17**, 278–282.

Whiteside, T.L., and Herberman, R.B. (1995) The role of natural killer cells in immune surveillance of cancer. *Curr. Op. Immunol.*, **7**, 704–710.

Yee, C., Gilbert, M.J., Riddel, S.R., Brichard, V.G., Fefer, A., Thompson, J.A., Boon, T., and Greenberg, P.D. (1996) Isolation of tyrosinase-specific $CD8^+$ and $CD4^+$ T cell clones from the peripheral blood of melanoma patients following *in vitro* stimulation with recombinant vaccinia virus. *J. Immunol.*, **157**, 4079–4086.

4 Humoral Recognition of Cancer

Philip O. Livingston

ABBREVIATIONS

ADCC	Antibody-dependent cellular cytotoxicity
APL	Acute promyelocytic leukemia
BCG	Bacillus Calmette-Guérin
CT	Computerized tomography
KLH	Keyhole limpet hemocyanin
mAbs	Monoclonal antibodies
NK	Natural killer
SCLC	Small cell lung cancer

Humoral recognition of cancer

1. **B lymphocytes mature in the bone marrow, then migrate to B cell rich areas of lymph nodes, spleen and gastrointestinal tract and recirculate in the blood.**
2. **B cells bind antigens through the antibody molecule (receptor) on the membrane. Such a binding results in a functional change with activation of effector mechanisms and release of antigen-specific antibodies.**
3. **Antibodies may directly affect tumor cells, but usually their antitumor effector mechanism involves activation of complement, opsonization and ADCC.**
4. **Antibodies that recognize cell surface antigens, on malignant and normal tissues were found in a proportion of cancer patients. These antigens have a very different distribution on various malignancies.**
5. **Antigens recognized by antibodies include gangliosides, mucins, the oncoprotein HER-2/neu, etc.**

6. **Vaccines have been made with some glycolipids that were able to elicit antibody responses without evident toxic effect. This suggests that those normal antigens are sequestered from the immune system.**
7. **By using autologous patient's sera, expression cDNA libraries from human tumors were screened. Such an approach (SEREX) allowed the discovery of a large number of antigens some of which were already known to elicit a T-cell response.**
8. **At least with some antigens, the antibody response may correlate with the evolution of antigen-positive tumors.**
9. **Passively administered and vaccine induced antibodies have been shown to correlate with improved disease-free and overall survival.**
10. **Antibodies can be used for imaging tumors for diagnostic purposes. New technology allows the use of $F(ab)_2$, single chain fv; these are molecules smaller than the parental natural antibody and can better penetrate tissues and be more rapidly cleared.**
11. **Molecular technology now allows antibody fragments to be produced in bacteria by lysing the genetically engineered bacteria and detecting antigen-specific F(ab) fragments by immunoassay. Phage display libraries are another approach to this end.**
12. **Several antibodies (often chimerized or humanized) are now used effectively in the clinic, such as herceptin (anti-HER2 neu) in breast cancer, rituximab (anti-B cells) in non-Hodgkin's lymphoma, 3F8 (anti-GD2) in neuroblastoma, and 17-1a (anti-epithelial antigen KSA) in colon cancer patients.**

MECHANISMS FOR B CELL RECOGNITION OF TUMOR ANTIGENS AND FOR EFFECTOR ACTIONS

Unlike T lymphocytes, which recognize processed (partially digested) antigens, antibodies recognize antigens in their natural configuration. For an individual to make antibodies against the full range of pathogens continually encountered, B-lymphocytes expressing a diverse repertoire of immunoglobulins must be generated continually. Each B cell expresses immunoglobulin against a single antigenic epitope, with the immunoglobulin expressed at the cell surface where it acts as a specific receptor for that antigen. The diversity of specificities in different B cells is generated largely by gene rearrangements in new B cells, which continue to be generated throughout life. In their early development, B cells with immunoglobulins against ubiquitous self-antigens are eliminated. This elimination of B cells reactive to autoantigens is not absolute, however, as a broad array of mAbs and serum antibodies against autoantigens have been derived from experimental animals and humans. Peripheral blood B cells consist of these naive and relatively short-lived B cells, long-lived memory B cells resulting from maturation in response to antigenic stimulation, and a small population of B cells expressing germ line specificities, also termed CD5 B cells (Fearon *et al.*, 1997).

B cells are not sessile; after maturation in the bone marrow they migrate through the peripheral blood to B cell rich areas such as follicles of lymph nodes, spleen and gastrointestinal tract and may continue recirculating. If its antigen is encountered in these tissues, the B lymphocyte is detained in the T cell rich areas where, if appropriate T cell help is provided, it may be activated to proliferate. This T cell help does not have to be induced by the same antigen. Chemical conjugation of the original antigen to highly immunogenic bacterial or xenogeneic proteins, or expression of the antigen in bacterial or viral vectors, are widely used approaches to ensuring adequate T cell help in vaccines. The result is antibody-secreting plasma cells and germinal centers where hypermutation in variable genes and class and subclass switching occur. The consequence is plasma cells secreting increasingly higher affinity IgG antibodies. In addition, some B cells which generally recognize non-protein antigens can be stimulated to proliferate in the absence of T-cell help. Class switching, affinity maturation and memory B cells generally do not occur. Low affinity IgM antibodies of shorter duration result.

The immunoglobulin variable region (Fv) determining antibody specificity is located in the Fab and is critical for effective recognition of tumor antigens (Fab and Fc are the immunoglobulin degradation products from papain digestion, in the hinge region). However, the constant region (Fc) where class and subclass are determined is equally critical (see Figure 4.1). Binding of antibody to antigen results in a functional change in the Fc portion and activation of several effector mechanisms. IgM antibodies are synthesized early in the response against protein antigens but at all times in the response to most non-protein antigens and are found mainly in the blood. The IgM pentameric structure is specialized to increase avidity of binding to repeated antigens and to activate complement

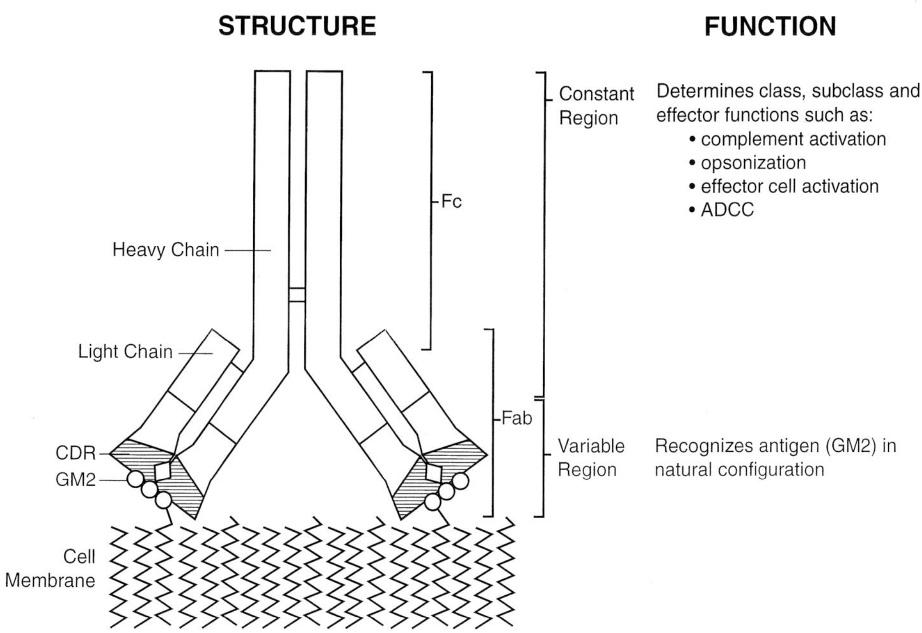

Figure 4.1 Correlation between antibody structure and function shown for GM2 antibody.

efficiently. Complement activation results in opsonization, activation of and uptake by macrophages, monocytes, neutrophils and dendritic cells, as well as membrane attack complex formation and pathogen lysis. IgG antibodies are synthesized later in the response to protein antigens, are usually of higher affinity, and can be found in the extracellular fluid as well as in the blood. IgG1 and IgG3 antibodies in humans are especially effective in activating complement and also in sensitizing of pathogens for killing by NK cells (see Table 4.1).

Opsonization for ingestion and destruction by phagocytes can occur through complement activation, but also occurs directly as a consequence of Fc receptors on phagocytic cells. NK cells are non-T, non-B lymphoid cells. Fc receptors on cell surface bound IgG1 and IgG3 are the primary targets for effector cells mediating ADCC of tumor cells. FcδRI (CD64), FcδRII (CD32), and FcδRIII (CD16) receptors on a range of effector cells, including especially NK cells, but also cells of myeloid lineage, react with these tumor cell bound antibodies, resulting in activation of inherent cytotoxic mechanisms in the effector cells (see Table 4.2).

While in some cases the antibody may have direct effects against tumor cells, for example by inhibiting tumor cell attachment or growth hormone receptors, in general the interaction of the antibody and the tumor cell antigen is without significance unless Fc-mediated secondary effector mechanisms are activated. Of these various effector mechanisms, activation of the complement system, opsonization and ADCC are the most important.

TABLE 4.1
Correlation between antibody Fc isotype and function

Functional activity	*IgM*	*IgG1*	*IgG2*	*IgG3*	*IgG4*
Opsonization	–	+++	–	++	+
Sensitization for NK killing	–	++	–	++	–
Complement activation	++++	++	–	++	–

TABLE 4.2
Features of Fc receptors on accessory cells

Receptor	FcγRI (CD64)	FcγRII (CD32)	FcγRIII (CD16)
Target	IgG1	IgG1	IgG1
Affinity	10^8 m^{-1}	2×10^6 m^{-1}	5×10^5 m^{-1}
Order of affinity	1) IgG1 2) IgG3 = IgG4 3) IgG2	1) IgG1 2) IgG3 = IgG4 3) IgG2	1) IgG1 = IgG3
Cell type	macrophages neutrophils eosinophils	macrophages neutrophils eosinophils platelets Langerhans' cells	macrophages neutrophils eosinophils NK cells Langerhans' cells
Effect of binding	uptake	uptake, granule release	induction of killing (NK cells)

TARGET CANCER ANTIGENS

We have used mAbs to screen for the expression of a large panel of cell surface antigens on malignant and normal tissues by immunohistochemistry (Zhang *et al.* 1997a; Zhang *et al.* 1997b; Zhang *et al.* 1998a). This has been confirmed in the case of ganglioside antigens by extraction of biopsy specimens and immune thin layer chromatography (Hamilton *et al.*, 1993). Since recognition of antigens on living cancer cells by antibodies is largely restricted to the cancer cell surface, the focus is on cell surface antigens. In general, ganglioside antigens and blood group or mucin-related antigens had very different distributions on various malignancies. The antigens strongly expressed on 60% or more of biopsy specimens are listed in Table 4.3. Antigens expressed in fewer than 60% of tumor specimens are not shown, but some, such as HER2/neu which is overexpressed in 30% of breast cancer specimens, may still be suitable targets for immune attack in patients with positive cancers.

Expression of gangliosides on normal tissues was very different from that of the other antigens, but consistent with the expression on tumors. GM2, GD2 and GD3 were all expressed in brain cells, especially GD2 which is also expressed on some peripheral nerves. Unexpectedly, GD2 was expressed on B lymphocytes in the spleen and lymph nodes, and GM2 was expressed at the secretory borders of most epithelial tissues. GD2 and GD3 were also expressed, though at lower levels, in connective tissues of multiple organs and GD3 is known to be expressed on a subset of human T lymphocytes (Merritt *et al.*, 1996). Fucosyl GM1 was expressed only on occasional cells in the islets of Langerhans and in some sensory neurones in the dorsal root ganglia. Polysialic acid was expressed significantly in brain and some bronchial epithelial cells. Globo H, the Lewis antigens, Tn, sialyl Tn, TF, mucins MUC1, 2 and 5AC, KSA, PSMA and CEA were expressed exclusively at the secretory borders of a variety of epithelial tissues and sTn was found on Leydig cells of the testis. Contributing to tumor mucin specificity is the less intense glycosylation of tumor mucins than normal mucins, involving shorter carbohydrate chains. The simplified structures of these antigens in relation to the cancer cell surface lipid bilayer are shown in Figure 4.2. MUC2 and MUC5AC are in parentheses because they have no transmembrane domain and so are not technically cell surface antigens. They are, however, large secreted molecules which tend to surround cancer cells *in vivo*.

TABLE 4.3
Antigens expressed on 50% or more of tumor cells in 60% or more of tumor specimens as detected by immunohistochemistry

Tumor	Antigens (mAb)
Melanoma	GM2, GD2, GD3
Neuroblastoma	GM2, GD2, GD3, Polysialic acid
Sarcoma	GM2, GD2
B cell lymphoma	GM2, GD2
Small cell lung cancer	GM2, Fucosyl GM1, Polysialic Acid, Globo H, Sialyl Le^a, KSA
Breast	GM2, Globo H, TF, MUC1, MUC5AC, KSA, CEA
Prostate	GM2, Tn, sTn, TF, Le^Y, MUC2, KSA, PSMA
Lung	GM2, Globo H, Le^Y, MUC1, KSA, CEA
Colon	GM2, sTn., TF, Sialyl Le^a, Le^Y, MUC2, KSA, CEA
Ovary	GM2, Globo H, sTn, TF, Le^Y, MUCl, KSA
Stomach	GM2, Le^Y, Le^a, Sialyl Le^a, MUC5AC, KSA, CEA

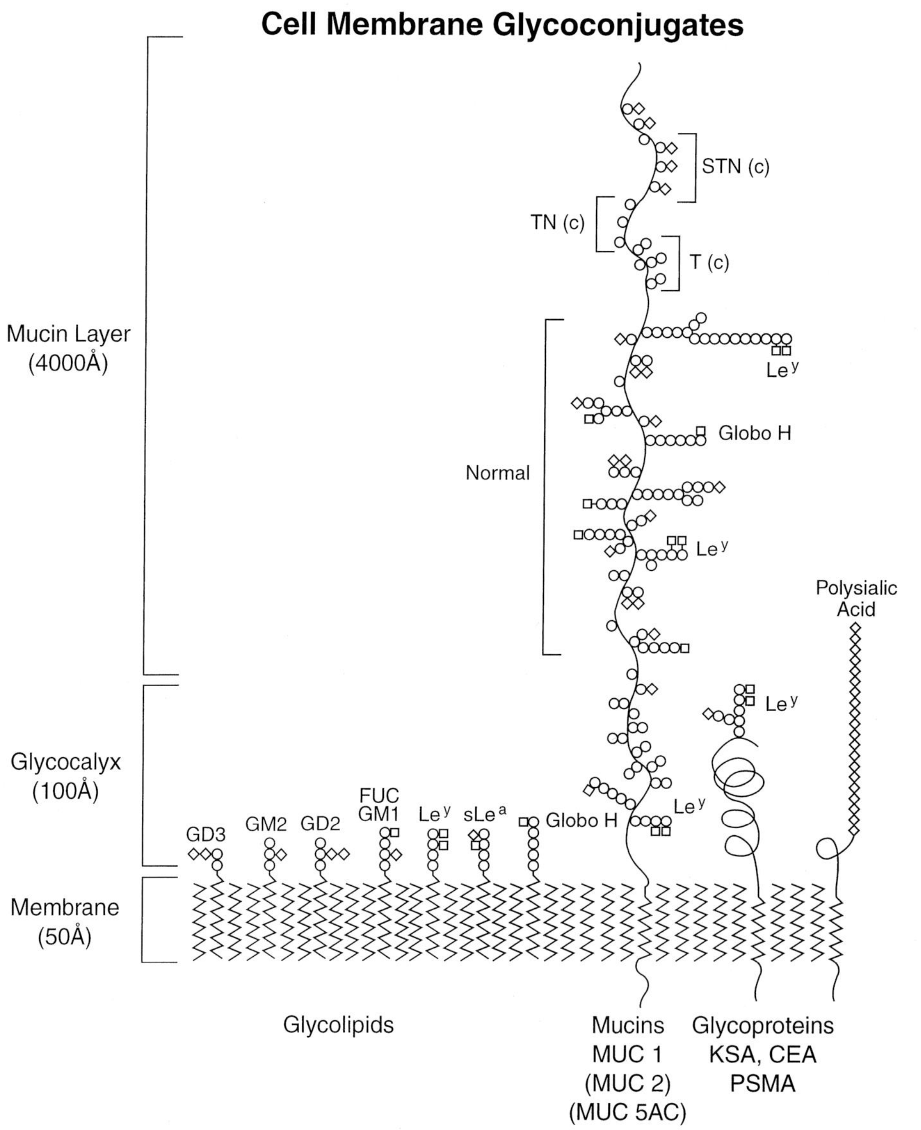

Figure 4.2 Glycolipid and glycoprotein antigens expressed at the cancer cell surface. Symbols: ◇ = sialic acid; □ = fucose; ○ = glucose, galactose, N-acetylgalactosamine or N-acetylglucosamine.

There is now sufficient experience from clinical trials with vaccine-induced antibody responses against GM2, GD2, TF, sTn, MUC1 and KSA antigens, and passive administration of mAbs against GD2, GD3, Le^X, sTn and KSA to draw conclusions about the consequences of antigen distribution on various normal tissues. GM2, GD2 and GD3 exposure on cells in the brain and GM2, sTn, TF, MUC1, KSA and CEA antigen expression in cells at the secretory borders of epithelial tissues induce neither immunological tolerance nor autoimmunity once antibodies are present, suggesting they are sequestered from the immune system. Against this background, GM2, GD3, polysialic acid, T, Tn, sTn, Globo H, sLe^a, MUC1, MUC2, MUC5AC and CEA all appear to be good targets for active immunotherapy with vaccines and passive immunotherapy with mAbs.

The use of GD2, fucosyl GM1 and Le^Y as targets for vaccine therapy may be more problematic. The known expression of Le^X and sialyl Le^X on polymorphonucleocyte, and the granulocytopenia lasting several days after each treatment of patients with mAb FC-2.15 (Capurro *et al.*, 1998) later found to recognize Le^X, may exclude these two carbohydrates as candidates for vaccine construction where long-term maintenance of antibody titers is the goal. In addition, the consequences of antibodies against antigens such as GD2 and fucosyl GM1 expressed on B cells, Islets of Langerhans and/or sensory neurones is of concern and largely unknown. Moderate titers of IgM (natural or vaccine induced) against GD2 have not been associated with toxicity, but administration of high doses of one (but not other) IgG mAbs against GD2 have been associated with peripheral neuropathy in melanoma patients (Cheung *et al.*, 1987; Saleh *et al.*, 1992). Similarly, high but not lower doses of anti Le^Y mAb BR96 conjugated to doxorubicin resulted in vomiting and hematemesis in many patients (Giantonio *et al.*, 1996). BR55, a second mAb against Le^Y studied by the same investigators, resulted in no such toxicity. With regard to vaccines, ongoing trials with vaccines against GD2, Fucosyl GM1 and Le^Y have addressed these questions more directly. Moderate titers of IgM and IgG antibodies have been induced with no evidence of autoimmunity (Dickler *et al.*, 1999; Sabbatini *et al.*, 1999).

The relatively short half-lives of administered mAbs may also make treatments against several of the differentiation antigens on leukemias and lymphomas more practical with mAbs than vaccines. Intermittent treatment [with mAbs] against differentiation antigens such as CD20 on B cells has proven highly effective (Kwak and Grossbard, 1995) in a setting where long-term antibodies that might be induced by treatment with a vaccine against CD20 would prove toxic. Anti-idiotype vaccines against the unique lymphoma cell antibody, which is different for each B-cell lymphoma patient, is an approach to overcoming this handicap.

An entirely new approach to detecting antibody-defined tumor antigens was reported by Sahin *et al.* (1995); this is based on the use of autologous patients' sera to screen expression cDNA libraries from human tumors. Such an approach (SEREX) allowed the discovery of a large number of antigens, some of which were already known also to elicit a T-cell response (e.g. MAGE-1). These studies confirmed that human neoplasms can induce multiple, specific immune responses in the autologous host and indicate, at least for the cancer/testis antigen NY-ESO-1, that the antibody response may correlate with the evolution of antigen-positive tumors (Jäger *et al.*, 1999).

THE BASIS FOR ANTIBODY-MEDIATED THERAPY OF CANCER

Antibodies are the primary mechanism for eliminating infectious pathogens from the bloodstream. The effect of all commonly used vaccines against infectious agents is thought to be primarily a consequence of antibody induction. Antibodies are also ideally suited for elimination of circulating tumor cells and micrometastases (see Table 4.4). The importance of antibodies in mediating protection from tumor recurrence is well documented in experimental animals (reviewed in Livingston, 1998). Experiments involving the administration of mAb 3F8 against GD2 or induction of anti-GD2 antibodies by vaccination are two examples. Administration of 3F8 prior to intravenous tumor challenge or as late as 4 days after tumor challenge results in complete protection of a majority of mice (Zhang *et al.*, 1998b). Comparable protection was induced by immunization with a GD2 conjugate vaccine. This timing may be comparable to antibody induction, or administration, in patients in the adjuvant setting after surgical resection of the primary or lymph node metastases in cancers such as melanoma or colon cancer and after response to chemotherapy in cancers such as small cell lung cancer (SCLC) and breast cancer. In both cases the targets may be circulating tumor cells and micrometastases. Administration of 3F8 seven or more days after tumor challenge had little impact on tumor progression.

There is also evidence in cancer patients that natural or passively administered antibodies in the adjuvant setting are associated with a more favorable prognosis (Table 4.4).

1. Natural antibodies (antibodies present in patient sera prior to vaccination) have been correlated with an improved prognosis. This is true for patients with paraneoplastic syndromes where high titers of antibodies against onconeural antigens expressed on particular cells in the nervous system and certain types of tumors have been associated both with debilitating autoimmune neurologic disorders and with delayed tumor progression and prolonged survival. Also, patients with AJCC Stage III melanoma and natural antibodies against GM2 ganglioside treated at two different medical centers have had an 80–100% five-year survival compared to the expected 40% rate (Jones *et al.*, 1981; Livingston *et al.*, 1989, 1994).
2. Tumor vaccine induced antibodies in the adjuvant setting against GM2 and several other melanoma antigens at four different medical centers, and against sialyl Tn antigen in adenocarcinoma patients, have correlated with a prolonged disease-free interval and survival (reviewed in Livingston, 1995).
3. Patients with Dukes C colon cancer treated with mAb 17-1A in the only randomized mAb trial in the adjuvant setting had a significantly prolonged disease-free and overall survival compared to controls (Riethmuller *et al.*, 1994).

Hence, in the adjuvant setting, passively administered and vaccine-induced antibodies have been shown to correlate with improved disease-free and overall survival in mouse and

TABLE 4.4
The basis for administration of mAbs, or cancer vaccines that induce antibodies, in the adjuvant setting

Animal models:	Antibodies eliminate micrometastasis
Natural antibodies:	Correlated with improved prognosis • GM2 Abs in melanoma patients • Paraneoplastic syndrome due to natural antibodies
Tumor-vaccine-induced Abs correlate with prolonged survival in patients with melanoma and adenocarcinomas	
17-1a mAb administration in Dukes C colon carcinoma increased overall survival	

man. Since the great majority of cancer patients are initially rendered free of detectable disease by surgery and/or chemotherapy after initial diagnosis, administration of mAbs or vaccines inducing antibodies may have broad applicability. There are advantages to each approach. Titers of anti-cancer antibodies are generally higher after administration of mAbs, and mAbs can be generated against virtually any antigen. On the other hand, human anti-mouse and anti-idiotype antibodies may limit the usefulness of continued administration of mAbs, and maintenance of antibody titers with vaccines is more practical and less expensive than with mAbs.

CONSTRUCTION OF CANCER VACCINES THAT AUGMENT THE ANTIBODY RESPONSE

VACCINES AGAINST GANGLIOSIDES

A variety of approaches for augmenting the antibody response against gangliosides and related antigens have been compared in the mouse and in melanoma patients. These approaches range from the use of vaccines containing irradiated cultured tumor cells to vaccines containing purified or synthetic antigens. Initially mixture of gangliosides with BCG was found to be optimal. While this approach was not able to induce antibodies against the major melanoma ganglioside, GD3, it was more successful against the two more minor melanoma gangliosides, GM2 and GD2. Antibodies against GD2 were induced in 25% of patients and against GM2 in 85% of vaccinated patients, and the presence of GM2 antibodies correlated significantly with an improved disease free and overall survival. Consequently, we conducted a randomized trial comparing vaccination with BCG versus BCG with GM2 adherent to the BCG surface (GM2/BCG) in the adjuvant setting in 122 patients with AJCC stage III melanoma (patients who are free of detectable melanoma after surgical dissection of lymph node metastases). The results after a 4-year follow-up demonstrated improved disease-free survival for patients receiving the GM2/BCG vaccine compared to those receiving BCG (48% versus 30%), but this result did not achieve statistical significance (Livingston *et al.*, 1994).

Subsequently, covalent attachment of gangliosides, other carbohydrate antigens and mucins to the immunogenic carrier protein KLH and use of the potent immunological adjuvant QS-21 were identified as a superior approach to vaccine construction in experimental animals. The rational for this approach is reviewed in the second paragraph of this chapter and in Table 4.5. Based on this background, GM2-KLH plus QS-21 (termed GMK) was tested in patients. It induced 8 times higher titers of IgM antibody which lasted twice as long compared to the GM2/BCG vaccine and for the first time GMK induced consistent IgG antibodies as well (Helling *et al.*, 1995). Antibodies were induced in >95% of patients vaccinated with GMK instead of 85% as seen with the GM2/BCG vaccine.

Consequently, a randomized multicenter Phase III trial comparing GMK to high dose interferon alpha was conducted by Progenics Pharmaceuticals Inc. (Tarrytown, NY) in the intergroup setting with ECOG, SWOG, NCCTG, CALGB, MD Anderson Cancer Center and Memorial Sloan-Kettering Cancer Center (MSKCC) in Stage III and high risk Stage II melanoma patients. Previous trials comparing high dose interferon alpha to no treatment,

TABLE 4.5
Conjugate vaccine components and probable role in antibody induction against cancer antigens

Antigen	*Carrier (KLH)*	*Adjuvant (QS-21)*
1) Antigen configuration must mimic expression on tumor cell. Site of conjugation and tertiary structure are key.	1) Carrier immunogenicity results in cytokine release. Foreign, highly immunogenic carrier molecule is key, especially for overcoming tolerance.	The mechanism of action for most adjuvants is largely unknown but is assumed to include: • Activation of APCs
2) High antigen/carrier ratio is required, suggesting high density of single antigen per carrier molecule.	2) Sequence of cytokine release may be important so an immunogenic carrier is better than a cytokine, cytokine mixture or cytokine inducer	• B cell activation • T cell activation • Depot effect

and GM2/BCG to BCG, resulted in comparable benefit for interferon and GM2/BCG, but the timing of the benefits was quite different. The beneficial effect of interferon was during the initial 6 months while the effect of GM2/BCG was not clearly evident until after two years. An early look in the Phase III trial after eighteen months median follow-up has demonstrated a significantly prolonged disease free survival for the patients receiving interferon, and the trial has been stopped, though follow-up continues. If the late benefit of GMK is not seen with further follow-up, a possible explanation is low or heterogeneous expression of GM2 in many melanomas. The solution might be a polyvalent vaccine.

VACCINES AGAINST OTHER ANTIGENS AND POLYVALENT VACCINES

The KLH conjugate plus QS21 vaccine approach has also been applied to other antigens. Antibody induction against Fucosyl GM1, GD2 and sTn in essentially all vaccinated patients and against Globo H and GD3 in over 50% of patients has been observed. In each case the antibody response with these -KLH plus QS21 conjugate vaccines has been significantly higher than with the use of BCG, other carriers or other adjuvants. Immune sera reacted with tumor cells expressing these antigens by flow cytometry, and antibodies against the gangliosides and Globo H have effectively induced complement-mediated lysis. The IgG subclasses in all trials have been restricted to IgG1 and IgG3, the two subclasses known to mediate complement lysis and ADCC. Trials with MUC1, MUC2, KSA, Le^Y, Tn, TF and polysialic acid conjugate vaccines are ongoing.

A randomized adjuvant multicenter trial with a vaccine against sTn has also recently been initiated. The vaccine contains sTn disaccharide (also referred to as TAG-72) covalently linked to KLH and mixed with immunological adjuvant Detox, and is prepared by Biomira Inc. (Edmonton, Alberta). Biomira is conducting the trial in patients with high-risk breast cancer at multiple centers in Canada, the USA and Europe. This trial is based on the high-titer antibodies induced by this vaccine in this patient population, the correlation between expression of sTn on tumors and a more aggressive phenotype and the correlation between antibody induction against sTn and longer disease-free and overall survival (MacLean *et al.*, 1996).

Heterogeneity of antigen expression in different cancers of the same type, as well as different cells of the same cancer, and heterogeneity of immune response in different patients make it likely that maximal benefit may not result from immunization against a single antigen. Consequently, immunization with polyvalent vaccines containing several of the antigens shown in Table 4.3 is the goal. The use of tumor cells, tumor cells genetically transduced to produce cytokines and adhesion factors, or tumor cell extracts is one approach to this end. However, these approaches, while having the potential for inducing T-cell responses against protein antigens and antibodies against other yet to be identified antigens, are not nearly as effective at inducing antibodies against known antigens as the conjugate vaccine described above. Other approaches to vaccine construction such as expression of antigen in viral or bacterial vectors, DNA vaccines or the use of heat shock protein vaccines each have unique advantages but are designed primarily to induce T-cell immune responses. The use of purified or synthetic antigens in conjugate vaccines with a potent immunological adjuvant is the optimal approach for antibody induction. This is especially true with tumor antigens, since most tumor antigens are autoantigens or slightly modified autoantigens and antibody induction involves overcoming some level of tolerance.

PREPARATION OF MONOCLONAL ANTIBODIES THAT RECOGNIZE CANCER

In the antibody heavy and light chain variable regions (Fv) there are three hypervariable regions called complementarity-determining regions (CDR1, CDR2 and CDR3) within four regions of more limited variation (Clark *et al.*, 1995). The CDR regions are principally responsible for contact with the antigen (see Figure 4.1). In mAbs as opposed to immune sera, every antibody molecule contains the same variable region and CDRs. mAbs are generally of murine or human origin (originating from murine or human B cells), or chimerized (or humanized) to contain the murine variable region (or CDRs) and the remainder of the antibody of human origin (see Figure 4.3). In the past, immune B cells from immunized mice were fused to a mouse myeloma cell line as originally described by Kohler and Milstein using Sendai virus (Kohler and Milstein, 1976) or more recently polyethylene glycol. This approach to cell fusion is far more successful in murine than human systems. However, the use of murine mAbs in the clinic is generally restricted to a 2–3-week period before human anti-mouse antibodies (HAMA) are produced, which effectively inactivate the murine mAb. Consequently, a variety of approaches have been used to prepare antibodies which are less immunogenic.

Human mAbs can be derived from human B-lymphocytes which have been transformed by viruses such as the Epstein-Barr Virus, but these transformed cells are generally not stable for long-term production of high levels of antibody. Murine antibodies can be humanized using recombinant DNA technology. One advantage of this approach is that the human constant region utilized can be selected based on the properties desired. IgG1 and IgG3 antibodies have the advantage of activating human complement and mediating opsonization and ADCC, but these reactions are likely to be undesirable if the antibody is to be used for imaging or targeting cytotoxic agents, in which case IgG2 or IgG4 may be preferable. Other approaches to improved imaging include the use of Fab', $F(ab')_2$, single chain antibodies or single chain fv (scfv) in which the heavy and light chain variable

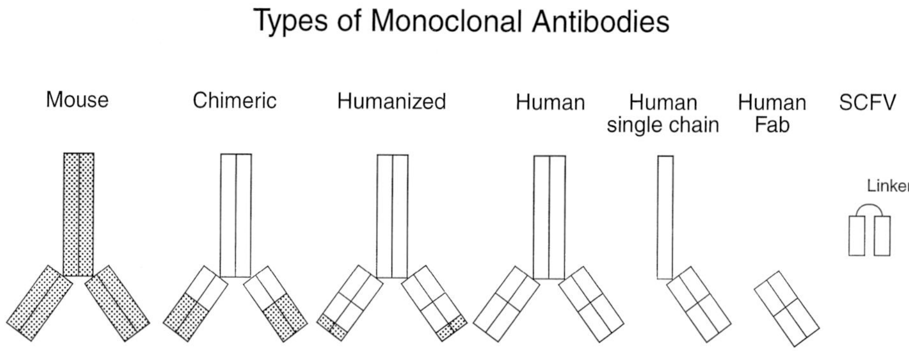

Figure 4.3 Monoclonal antibody preparations used in clinical trials. Inked-in portions of antibodies are of murine origin.

regions are connected with a linker in a single small chain (see Figure 4.3). These smaller molecules are more rapidly cleared and have better penetration of tumor tissue, though binding avidity and stability are decreased (Scheinberg and Chapman, 1995; Schlom, 1995). Overall, these smaller molecules have not yet lived up to their promise.

Recombinant DNA technology can be used to genetically engineer almost any antibody and to produce it to high levels (Clark *et al.*, 1995). This approach can also be used to prepare fully humanized chimeric antibodies with only the CDR regions of murine origin. Widely used methods for preparing high affinity recombinant antibody genes now involve the use of combinatorial and phage display libraries. In the Kohler and Milstein technology (Kohler and Milstein, 1976) once the immortalized hybridoma cells are established, culture supernatants from each well are assayed for the presence of the desired antibody reactivity and the resulting cultures are then grown, cloned and recloned based on production of the antibody of interest. The same procedure needs to be adopted for the production of antibody fragments in bacteria. This can be performed by lysing the genetically engineered bacteria and detecting antigen-specific Fab fragments by immunoassay. Phage display libraries are an alternative approach to this end. The Fab or Fv fragments can be expressed as fusion proteins with a bacteriophage coat protein such that each phage carries surface Fv fragments and internally, the cloned DNA for that fragment. These can then be affinity purified. Affinity maturation can be mimicked by using phage display libraries in which the heavy and light chains are allowed to randomly re-assort and further by artificially mutating the CDR sequences with random oligonucleotide primers. It is even possible to completely eliminate the Kohler-Milstein fusion technology (which initially was needed to expedite the derivation of high affinity antibodies) by extensive application of these approaches, resulting in high affinity human mAbs. All of these approaches are currently being used for the production of genes for high affinity mAbs. Once the desired recombinant antibody genes have been prepared, they are generally placed into myeloma, B cell or CHO cultured lines because immunoglobulins must be processed and glycosylated appropriately and the appropriate disulfide bonds formed.

mAbs have a variety of uses ranging from research reagents to diagnostics, imaging and therapy. The many clinical trials with mAbs used as imaging or therapeutic agents have been reviewed (Scheinberg and Chapman, 1995; Schlom, 1995). Several of these mAbs

TABLE 4.6
FDA approved mAbs for imaging or therapy

mAbs (label)	*Company*	*Class*	*Antigen*	*Indications*
Imaging				
CEA scan (Tc-99m)	Immunomedics	Murine Fab′	CEA	Colon cancer
Oncoscint (in-111)	Cytogen	Murine IgG_1	sTn	Colon and ovarian cancer
Prostascint (in-111)	Cytogen	Murine IgG_1	PSMA	Prostate cancer
Verluma (Tc-99m)	NeoRx	Murine Fab′	KSA	Small cell lung cancer
Therapy				
Herceptin	Genentech	Humanized IgG	$HER2/_{neu}$	$HER2^+$ breast cancers
Rituxan	IDEC/Genentech	Chimerized IgG	CD20	B cell lymphoma
Panarex (approved in Europe only)	Centocor	Murine IgG_{2a}	KSA	Colon cancer (adjuvant treatment)

have recently been approved by the Food and Drug Administration (FDA) for clinical use and are becoming increasingly common components of the oncologist's armamentarium (see Table 4.6).

THERAPY WITH MONOCLONAL ANTIBODIES

A variety of clinical trials with mAbs have been conducted in patients with advanced solid tumors. The target antigens have included CEA, KSA, HER2/neu, TAG-72, Le^y, Le^x, Globo H, GD2, GD3 and ferritin (reviewed in Scheinberg and Chapman, 1995; Schlom, 1995; Jurcic *et al.*, 1998). Only occasional evidence of anti-tumor efficacy was seen in most cases. The exceptions are the following:

1. Herceptin, a mAb against HER2neu, inhibits epidermal growth factor binding by cell surface receptors and so mediates an antitumor effect at least partially through a non-immunological pathway. Herceptin has resulted in clinical responses in patients with HER2/neu positive cancers and has been especially effective in combination with Taxol or other systemic chemotherapy (Mendelsohn and Baselga, 1995; Pegram *et al.*, 1998).
2. While anti-GD2 mAb 3F8 has resulted in occasional clinical responses in patients with melanoma, clinical responses in patients with neuroblastoma have been more frequent. Radiolabeled and unlabeled 3F8 are part of the current combination treatment regimen involving high-dose chemotherapy in patients with poor-prognosis progressive neuroblastoma. An increase in the long-term response rate from 15% to 49% has been associated with the addition of 3F8 (Cheung *et al.*, 1998).
3. ^{135}I-radiolabeled immune serum against ferritin has resulted in shrinkage of tumors in 29 of 43 patients with a hepatocellular carcinoma (Tang *et al.*, 1993).
4. There has been only one published randomized trial involving mAbs in the adjuvant setting, the use of mAb 17-1a against the panepithelial antigen KSA in patients with resected Dukes C colon cancer. After a median follow-up of 7 years (Riethmuller

et al., 1998), treatment with 17-1a reduced the overall death rate by 30% and so has been approved for use for this purpose in Europe. Confirmatory trials are ongoing in the USA. It is important to note that treatment with 17-1a, like the other antibodies mentioned above, resulted in only occasional responses when used in the advanced disease setting.

The use of mAbs for the treatment of patients with advanced lymphomas and leukemias has been more successful than was the case with advanced solid tumors. mAbs against B-cell antigens have been especially effective. CD-20 is a B-cell differentiation antigen. The CD-20 mAb Rituxan and several ^{135}I-labeled CD-20 mAbs, including Lym-1 and OKB-7, have each resulted in evidence of therapeutic effect in over 50% of treated patients (Kwak and Grossbard, 1995; Schlom, 1995; Jurcic *et al.*, 1998). Rituxan is now FDA approved in the USA for treatment of patients with B-cell lymphoma. This is a mouse/human chimeric antibody which binds complement and induces ADCC and which was shown, as a single agent, to be safe and to have a significant clinical activity in patients with bulky relapsed or refractory low-grade follicular B-cell lymphomas (Davis *et al.*, 1999). This antibody also increases the clinical response when given in combination with CHOP in patients with B-cell lymphoma (Czuczman *et al.*, 1999). CD33 is a differentiation antigen of the myelocytic lineage. Treatment of minimal disease acute promyelocytic leukemia (APL) patients with regimens containing humanized M195 mAb against CD33 has resulted in more complete elimination of APL cells, documented by RT-PCR assays for the t(15;17) marker (Jurcic *et al.*, 1998). A multicenter phase II/III trial of HuM195 in patients with acute myelocytic leukemia in first remission has recently been initiated.

mAbs have also been used for therapy coupled to chemotherapeutic agents, radioactive isotopes, toxins or cytokines. Several limitations to antibody therapy have been identified. Antibody penetration into large tumor metastasis is generally limited and so smaller versions of antibodies have been used such as Fab or single chain antibodies or scfv chains in an attempt to overcome this limitation. mAbs may be inhibited by circulating soluble antigen or the development of antibodies against the mAbs, especially if the mAb is of murine origin or carries foreign components such as drugs or toxins. A variety of approaches have been pursued to overcome the limitation imposed by the anti-mouse immunoglobulin response (see Table 4.6). Of the three mAbs approved for therapy, one is murine, the second is chimerized and the third is humanized. Radiolabeled humanized and murine CD-20 mAbs are likely to be the next mAbs approved for therapy.

DIAGNOSTIC APPLICATIONS OF MONOCLONAL ANTIBODIES

Most tumor antigens are expressed on subpopulations of normal cells as well. Nevertheless, antibodies against these antigens can be useful for tumor diagnosis by identifying increased quantities of antigen or antigen at abnormal locations. Antibodies may be used for imaging *in vivo* or for immunodiagnosis *in vitro*.

A variety of radiolabeled antibodies against tumor antigens have been used for imaging tumors but these have seldom proved more sensitive than computerized tomography (CT) or nuclear magnetic resonance imaging (reviewed in Scheinberg and Chapman, 1995;

Schlom, 1995; Jurcic *et al.*, 1998). Furthermore, imaging with radiolabeled antibodies is cumbersome because antibodies need to be freshly labeled for each patient. Nevertheless, four murine antibodies or Fab fragments labeled with Indium 111 or technetium 99m have been approved for human use (see Table 4.6). The most widely used have been antibodies against TAG-72.3 (sTn antigen), including phase III multi-center trials demonstrating that Oncoscint could increase detection of colorectal cancer lesions to 88% from 49% for CT alone in TAG-72 positive tumors. In occult ovarian cancer, metastases undetectable by CT were identified in 27% of cases. Higher affinity mAbs against TAG-72 such as CC-49 are currently being studied. Newer approaches to the use of radiolabeled mAbs include the use of smaller, more rapidly cleared recombinant immunoglobulin molecules and the use of a hand-held probe at definitive surgery one or two weeks after administration of radiolabeled mAbs. This approach with radiolabeled CC-49 has recently shown that surgical management was altered in over 40% of cases. The implications of this in terms of disease-free and overall survival remains to be determined.

Pathologists now commonly use antibodies for identifying the cell of origin of undifferentiated tumors and for detection of micrometastasis in the bone marrow and lymphoid organs. Immunohistology plays a critical role in the identification of micrometastasis after sentinel lymph node biopsies in patients with breast cancer and melanoma, though the clinical consequences of micrometastasis in bone marrow or lymph nodes is unclear. Also widely used are immunoassays that determine the presence and extent of tumor antigens in the serum as a surrogate marker of tumor burden. These include carcinoembryonic antigen (CEA), alpha fetal protein (AFP), prostate-specific antigen (PSA), CA125, CA15-3 and TAG-72. The use of mAbs for prognostication is also assuming greater importance. Identification of HER2/neu and TAG-72 on tumor cells is correlated with a more ominous prognosis. The use of mAbs for typing hematopoietic tumors has become routine and is the basis for both prognostic and therapeutic decisions.

CONCLUSION

Antibodies are increasingly important components of the oncologist's diagnostic and therapeutic armamentarium. mAbs are already widely used for immunodiagnosis. Antibodies, actively induced by vaccines or mAbs passively administered, against cell surface antigens are able to eliminate early cancer metastases in experimental animals. Their presence in cancer patients in the adjuvant setting correlates with an improved prognosis. Several mAbs have been approved for clinical use. Drawing on evidence concerning the role of antibodies in protection against infectious diseases, the presumed role of antibodies in immunotherapy of cancer is induction of complement activation, Fc-mediated opsonification and antibody-dependent cell-mediated cytotoxicity against circulating tumor cells and micrometastases. If antibodies of sufficient titer can be induced or administered, and maintained, against cell surface tumor antigens to eliminate tumor cells from the blood and lymphatic system, and to eradicate micrometastases, this would dramatically change our approach to treating the cancer patient. With repeated showers of metastases no longer possible, aggressive local therapies of established cancers, including surgery, radiation therapy, chemotherapy and intralesional treatments, might result in long-term control of even metastatic cancers. Several clinical trials designed to test this hypothesis are in progress.

REFERENCES

Capurro, M., Bover, L., Portela, P., Livingston, P.O., and Mordoh, J. (1998) FC-2.15, a monoclonal antibody active against human breast cancer specifically recognizes Lewis X hapten. *Cancer Immunol. Immunother.*, **45**, 334–339.

Cheung, N.-K.V., Lazarus, H., Miraldi, F.D., Abramowsky, C.R., Kallie, S., Saarinen, U.M., Spitzer, T., Strandjord, S.E., Cocci, P.F., and Berger, N.A. (1987) Ganglioside GD2 specific monoclonal antibody 3F8: a phase I study in patients with neuroblastoma and malignant melanoma. *J. Clin. Oncol.*, **5**, 1430–1440.

Cheung, N.-K.V., Kushner, B.H., Cheung, I.Y., Kramer, K., Canete, A., Gerald, W., Bonilla, M., Finn, R., Yeh, S.J., and Larsen, S.M. (1998) Anti-GD2 antibody treatment of minimal residual stage IV neuroblastoma diagnosed at more than 1 year of age. *J. Clin. Oncol.*, **16**, 3053–3060.

Clark, M. (1995) General introduction. Monoclonal antibodies. In J.R. Birch, and E.S. Lennox, (eds.), *Princ. Appl.*, **1**, 1–43.

Czuczman, M.S., Grillo-Lopez, A.J., White, C.A., Saleh, M., Gordon, L., Lo Buglio, A.F., Jonas, C., Klippenstein, D., Dallaire, B., and Varus, C. (1999) Treatment of patients with low-grade B-cell lymphoma with the combination of chimeric anti-CD20 monoclonal antibody and CHOP chemotherapy. *J. Clin. Oncol.*, **17**, 268–276.

Davis, T.A., White, C.A., Grillo-Lopez, A.J., Velasquez, W.S., Link, B., Maloney, D.G., Dillman, R.O., Williams, M.E., Mohrbacher, A., Weaver, R., Dawden, S., and Levy, R. (1999) Single-agent monoclonal antibody efficacy in bulky non-Hodgkin's lymphoma: results of a phase II trial or Rituximab. *J. Clin. Oncol.*, **17**, 1851–1857.

Dickler, M.N., Ragupathi, G., Liu, N.X., Musselli, C., Martino, D.J., Miller, V.A., Kris M.G., Brezicka, F.T., Livingston, P.O. and Grant, S.C. (1999) Immunogeneticity of the fucosyl-GM1-keyhole limpet hemocyanin (KLH) conjugate vaccine in patients with small cell lung cancer. *Cancer Research* **5**: 2773–2779.

Fearon, D.T., Kelsoe, G., Kinef, J.P., MacLennan, I., Parham, P., and Rajewsky, K. (1997) The humoral immune response. In *Immunobiology the Immune system in Health and Disease (3rd edn)*. Janeway, Travers, **8**, 1–54.

Giantonio, B.J., Gilewski, T., Bookman, M.A., Norton, L., Kilpatrick, D., Dougan, M.A., Sliehenmyer, W.J., Onetto, N.M., and Canetta, R.M. (1996) A phase I study of weekly BR96-doxorubicin in patients with advanced carcinoma expressing the Lewis (Le^y) antigen. *Proc. Am. Soc. Clin. Oncol.*, **15**, 53.

Hamilton, W.B., Helling, F., Lloyd, K.O., and Livingston, P.O. (1993) Ganglioside expression on human malignant melanoma assessed by quantitative immune thin layer chromatography. *Int. J. Cancer*, **53**, 566–573.

Helling, F., Zhang, A., Shang, A., Adluri, S., Calves, M., Koganty, R., Longenecker, B.M., Oettgen, H.F., and Livingston, P.O. (1995) GM2-KLH conjugate vaccine: increased immunogenicity in melanoma patients after administration with immunological adjuvant QS-21. *Cancer Res.*, **55**, 2783–2788.

Jäger, E., Stockert, E., Zidianakis, Z., Chen, Y.-T., Karbach, J., Jäger, D., Araud, M., Ritter, G., Old, L.J., and Knuth, A. (1999) Humoral immune responses of cancer patients against ''cancer/testis'' antigen NY-ESO-1: correlation with clinical events. *Int. J. Cancer*, **84**, 506–510.

Jones, P.C., Sze, L.L., Liu, P.Y., Morton, D.L., and Irie, R.F. (1981) Prolonged survival for melanoma patients with elevated IgM antibody to oncofetal antigen. *J. Natl. Cancer Inst. USA*, **66**, 249–254.

Jurcic, J.C., Scheinberg, D.A., and Houghton, A.N. (1998) Monoclonal antibody therapy of cancer. *Cancer Chemother. Biol.*, **17**, 195–216.

Kohler, G., and Milstein, C. (1976) Derivation of specific antibody-producing tissue culture and tumour cell lines by cell fusion. *Eur. J. Immunol.*, **6**, 511–519.

Kwak, L.W., and Grossbard, M.L. (1995) Clinical applications of monoclonal antibodies in cancer. In V.T. DeVita Jr., S. Hellan, and S.A. Rosenberg, (eds.), *Biologic Therapy of Cancer (2nd edn)*, J.B. Lippincott Company, New York, pp. 553–565.

Livingston, P.O., Ritter, G., Srivastava, P., Padavan, M., Calves, M.J. Oettgen, H.F., and Old, L.J. (1989) Characterization of IgG and IgM antibodies induced in melanoma patients by immunization with purified GM2 gangliosic. *Cancer Res.*, **49**, 7045–7050.

Livingston, P.O., Wong, G.Y.C., Adluri, S., Tao, Y., Padavan, M., Parente, R., Hanlon, C.M.J., Helling, F., Ritter, G., Oettgen, H.F., and Old, L.J. (1994) Improved survival in AJCC stage III melanoma patients with GM2 antibodies: A randomized trial of adjuvant vaccination with GM2 ganglioside. *J. Clin. Oncol.*, **12**, 1036–1044.

Livingston, P.O. (1995) Immunization with synthetic or highly purified tumor antigens. In V.T. DeVita Jr., S. Hellan, and S.A. Rosenberg, (eds.), *Biologic Therapy of Cancer (2nd edn)*, J.B. Lippincott Company, New York, pp. 680–690.

Livingston, P.O. (1998) The case for melanoma vaccines that induce antibodies. In J.M.. Kirkwood, (ed.), *Molecular Diagnosis. Prevention and Treatment of Melanoma*, Marcel Dekker Inc., pp. 139–157.

MacLean, G.D., Reddish, M.A., Koganty, R.R., and Longenecker, B.M. (1996) Antibodies against mucin-associated sialyl-Tn epitopes correlate with survival of metastatic adenocarcinoma patients undergoing active specific immunotherapy with synthetic STn vaccine. *J. Immunother Emph. Tumor Immunol.*, **19**, 59–68.

Mendelsohn, J., and Baselga, J. (1995) Antibodies to growth factors and receptors. In V.T. DeVita Jr., S. Hellan, and S.A. Rosenberg, (eds.), *Biologic Therapy of Cancer (2nd edn)*, J.B. Lippincott Company, New York, pp. 607–623.

Merritt, W.D., Taylor, B.J., Der-Minassian, V., and Reaman, G.H. (1996) Coexpression of GD_3 ganglioside with CD45RO in resting and activated human T lymphocytes. *Cell. Immunol.*, **173**, 131–148.

Pegram, M.D., Lipton A., Hayes, F., Weber, B.L., Baselga, J.M., Tripathy D., Baly D., Baughman, S.A., Twaddell, T., Glaspy, J.A., and Slamon, D.J. (1998) Phase II study of receptor-enhanced chemosensitivity using recombinant humanized anti-p$185^{HER2/neu}$ monoclonal antibody plus cisplatin in patients with HER2/*neu*-overexpressing metastatic breast cancer refractory to chemotherapy treatment. *J. Clin. Oncol.*, **16**, 2659–2671.

Riethmuller, G., Holz, E., Schlimok, G., Schmiegel, W., Raab, R., Hoffken, K., Gruber, R,, Funke, I., Pichlmaier, H., Hirche, H., Buggisch, P., Witte, J., and Pichlmayr, R. (1998) Monoclonal antibody therapy for resected Dukes' C colorectal cancer: seven-year outcome of a multicenter randomized trial. *J. Clin. Oncol.*, **16**, 1788–1794.

Sabbatini, P., Kudryashov, V., Danishefsky, S., Livingston, P.O., Ragupathi, G., Bornmann, W., Spassova, M., Spriggs, D., Aghajanian, C., Soignent, S., Peyton, M., O'Flaherty, C., Curtin, J. and Lloyd, K.O. (2000) Immunization of ovarian cancer patients with a synthetic Lewis Y – protein conjugate vaccine: clinical and serological results. *Int. J. Can* **87**: 79–85.

Sahin, U., Tureci, O., Schmitt, H., Cochlovius, B., Johannes, T., Schmits, R., Stenner, F., Luo, G., Schobert, I., Pfreundschuh, M. (1995) Human neoplasms elicit multiple specific immune responses in the autologous host. *Proc Natl Acad Sci USA*, **92**, 11810–11813.

Saleh, M.N., Khazaeli, M.B., Wheeler, R.H., Dropcho, E., Liu, T., Urist, M., Miller, D.M., Lawson, S., Dixon, P., Russell, C.H., and LoBuglio, A.F. (1992) Phase I trial of the murine monoclonal anti-GD2 antibody 14G9a in metastatic melanoma. *Cancer Res.*, **52**, 4342.

Scheinberg, D.A., and Chapman, P.B. (1995) Therapeutic applications of monoclonal antibodies for human disease. In J.R. Birch, and E.S. Lennox (eds.) *Monoclonal Antibodies. Principles and Applications*, **2**, 45–105.

Schlom, J. (1995) Monoclonal antibodies in cancer therapy. In V.T. DeVita Jr., S. Hellan, and S.A. Rosenberg, (eds.), *Biologic Therapy of Cancer (2nd edn)*, J.B. Lippincott Company, New York, pp. 507–521.

Tang, Z.-H., Liu, K.-D., Fan, Z., *et al.* (1993) A decade's studies on the immunotargeting therapy of hepatocellular carcinoma. *Antibody Immunoconj. Radiopharm.*, **6**, 155–165.

Zhang, S., Cordon-Cardo, C., Zhang, H.S., Reuter, V.E., Adluri, S., Hamilton, W.B., Lloyd, K.W., and Livingston, P.O. (1997a) Selection of carbohydrate tumor antigens as targets for immune attack using immunohistochemistry. I. Focus on Gangliosides. *Int. J. Cancer*, **73**, 42–49.

Zhang, S., Zhang, H.S., Cordon-Cardo, C., Reuter, V.E., Singhal, A.K., Lloyd, K.O., and Livingston, P.O. (1997b) Selection of tumor antigens as targets for immune attack using immunohistochemistry. II. Blood group-related antigens. *Int. J. Cancer*, **73**, 50–56.

Zhang, S., Zhang, H.S., Cordon-Cardo, C., Ragupathi, G., and Livingston, P.O. (1998a) Selection of tumor antigens as targets for immune attack using immunohistochemistry: protein antigens. *Clin. Cancer Res.*, **4**, 2669–2676.

Zhang, H., Zhang, S., Cheung, N.-K., Ragupathi, G., and Livingston, P.O. (1998b) Antibodies can eradicate cancer micrometastases. *Cancer Res.*, **58**, 2844–2849.

5 Immunotherapy of Cancer

Peter Hersey and Francesco M. Marincola

ABBREVIATIONS

APC	Antigen-presenting cell
BCG	Bacillus Calmette-Guérin
CT	Cancer-testis
CTL	Cytotoxic T lymphocytes
DC	Dendritic cells
FNA	Fine needle aspiration
GM-CSF	Granulocyte-macrophage colony-stimulating-factor
IFN-α, -β, -γ	Interferon-alpha, -beta, -gamma
IL-. . .	Interleukin-2, -4, -5, -6, -10, -12
LAK	Lymphokine activated killer
MAA	Melanoma associated antigens
PBL	Peripheral blood lymphocytes
PBMC	Peripheral blood mononuclear cells
PCR	Polymerase chain reaction
rIL-	recombinant interleukin-
TC	T cytotoxic
TCR	T cell receptor
TH	T helper
TIL	Tumor-infiltrating lymphocytes
TNF	Tumor necrosis factor

Cancer Vaccines

1. **In cancer, the aim of immunization is to eradicate the disease, rather than to prevent it as is the case with other vaccines.**
2. **Cancer vaccines are used to induce effector mechanisms against cancer cells and to maintain them for periods of time sufficient to fight the tumor e.g. 6 months or longer.**
3. **Establishment of memory is critical so that reappearance of the cancer will be met with a rapid expansion of the chosen effector mechanisms.**
4. **Clinical, histopathological and laboratory evidence supports the theory that tumor regression is mediated by immune responses. This provides a basis for the development of a therapeutic approach against cancer.**
5. **A major advancement in the field of tumor immunology will be the identification of those patients who are likely to respond to this form of therapy.**

INTRODUCTION

Treatment of cancer by immunization with vaccines dates from the beginning of the twentieth century at a time when immunologists were making huge gains in the control of infections, such as tetanus and diphtheria, by immunization with bacterial products. The vaccines employed were autologous or allogeneic tumor cells or extracts and as early as 1914 physicians were suggesting that the success of this approach was related to a small tumor burden and an increase in leukocyte counts in the patients (Vaughan, 1914). By 1929, however, Woglom (1929) was writing that resistance was "not connected with any neoplastic qualities of the graft" and that "while a selective cytolysin for the malignant cell may some day be found, the chances of its discovery are remote."

Since this period there have been a number of advances, not least being the advances made in conduction of clinical trials. The idea that cancers were foreign tissue has been replaced by knowledge that most cancer antigens are also expressed in normal tissue, albeit at different levels or at different developmental stages. It is also clear that exposure to antigen may not lead to an immune response but inactivate or tolerize lymphocytes. If an immune response does occur it may take several forms, such as antibody production or induction of cytotoxic T cells. The type of antigen, its physical form and route of presentation appear critical in determining the type of response. This information about immunoregulatory mechanisms is gradually being incorporated into design of new cancer vaccines. These new developments, together with evidence of clinical responses in some patients treated with cancer vaccines, is encouraging enough to suggest that Woglom was too pessimistic and that cancer vaccines may be a valuable additional modality against cancer. An overview of important events in development of cancer vaccines is given in Table 5.1.

The following sections describe some of the basic considerations involved in design and use of cancer vaccines. Where possible, past or present clinical studies are described to illustrate the principles involved.

TABLE 5.1
Highlights in the evolution of cancer vaccine therapy

1895–1929	Immunization with autologous and allogeneic cancer cells or extracts. Passive transfer of antisera.
1960–1970s	Autologous tumors or extracts as vaccines. Non-specific immunotherapy with bacterial products – BCG and *C. Parvum* (Hersey and Balch, 1984).
1970s	Helper effects by T cells (Mitchison, 1970).
1976	Discovery of MHC restriction of T cell responses (Doherty *et al.*, 1976).
1986	T cells recognize peptides from within the cell in association with MHC antigens (Townsend *et al.*, 1986).
1986	Different subsets of helper T cells direct antibody or cell mediated responses (Mosmann and colleagues).
1980's–Present	Specific cancer vaccines back in vogue.
1989–Present	Randomized trials with first generation vaccines (Hersey *et al.*, 1996; Wallack *et al.*, 1998).
1991	Description of the first human tumor antigen recognized by CTL (MAGE-1) (by Boon and colleagues).
1995–Present	Phase I studies with second generation vaccines.

SOME GENERAL PRINCIPLES

Differences in Therapeutic versus Preventive Vaccines

Immunization of patients with cancer differs from immunization against most infectious disease in several respects. Firstly, immunization against infectious organisms is mostly used to prevent the disease whereas in cancer the aim is to eradicate existing disease and not to prevent it, i.e. the vaccines are intended to be therapeutic not preventive. In certain infections, such as malaria and leprosy, vaccines may also be used with therapeutic intent (Ponnighaus *et al.*, 1992; Nosten *et al.*, 1996).

Secondly, vaccines used for prevention are designed principally to establish memory in the immune system so that subsequent exposure to the infection will lead to rapid expansion of effector mechanisms such as cytotoxic T cells, macrophages and antibodies against the organisms. In patients with cancer the vaccine is used to induce effector mechanisms against cancer cells and to maintain them for periods of time sufficient to eradicate the tumor, e.g. for periods of 6 months or more. When cancer vaccines are used in an adjuvant setting (i.e. treatment of patients after surgical removal of all clinically evident disease) the aim is similar but the vaccinations are carried out over a more protracted period such as 1–3 years. Establishment of memory is also critical in cancer patients so that reappearance of the cancer will be met with a rapid expansion of effector mechanisms. These considerations have resulted in protocol designs that include repeated immunization in the first 6 months and less frequent injections in the remainder of year 1 and 2. There is, however, no agreement as to the optimal frequency or for how long the vaccines should be administered (Hersey, 1997) (Table 5.2; see also Table 5.6).

TABLE 5.2
General principles in use of cancer vaccines

- Differences in therapeutic vs. preventative vaccines
- Reduce tumor bulk and immunize away from site of tumor.
- Reset the immune response to cell mediated pathways.
- Select antigens with high expression and with high frequency of precursor T cells.
- Provide helper components in the vaccine.
- Use adjuvants that increase numbers of APC and processing by APC.

Reduce Tumor Bulk and Immunize away from the Tumor

It is now clear that tumors evade or inhibit immune responses against them by a number of different mechanisms, as shown in Table 5.3. Some of the factors involved are reviewed elsewhere (Hersey, 1998) and include IL-10, TGF-β_2, hydrogen peroxide and FasL (see also Chapter 6 of this book).

Specific inhibitors of some of these factors may be determined over the next few years but until more is known about the inhibiting factors, it appears appropriate to reduce the negative effects of tumors on immune responses by surgical removal of as much tumor as possible and immunization at sites removed from negative effects of the tumor.

Switching Immune Responses from TH2 to TH1 and Cell Mediated Responses

It has been known for some time that certain antigens produce predominantly cell mediated responses or antibody responses (Parish, 1972; Parish, 1996). This phenomenon was poorly understood until the description by Mossman of T helper subsets which made different combinations of cytokines that mediated help (Mosmann and Sad, 1996). So-called TH1 subsets made IL-2 and IFN-γ, which amplified macrophage and CTL responses, and TH2 subsets made IL-4, IL-5 and IL-10. IL-4 and IL-5 played a key role in antibody production. Since then it has become evident that CD8 T cells also exist as T cell subsets (TC_1 and TC_2) (Seder and Le Gros, 1995) which have cytotoxic or immunoregulatory effects on macrophages and surrounding CD8 and CD4 T cells. Rejection of tumor cells is dependent on cell mediated responses and in view of this, procedures which induce TH_1 TC_1 responses form a key part of new vaccine strategies.

TABLE 5.3
Mechanisms involved in inhibition of immune responses to tumors

Mechanism	*Factors involved*
Inhibition of antigen presentation	VEGF, IL-10
Inhibition of cytokine production	IL-10, TGF-β, α-MSH
Tolerance/anergy of T-cells	H_2O_2, TGF-β, Muc-1, α-MSH
Shift of TH_1 TC_1 to TH_2 TC_2	IL-10, TGF-β, ?FasL
Inhibition of migration of leukocytes from blood vessels	PGE_2, tumor matrix, P16E
Tumor-mediated destruction of T-cells	FasL, Muc-1
Resistance of tumor cells to killing	IL-10, immunoselection of HLA and antigen loss variants

For references see Hersey (1998).

Prolonged exposure to antigen or other factors from tumors is believed to result in switch of immune responses to the TH_2 pathway, resulting in antibody production rather than cell mediated responses (Guilloux *et al.*, 1994). Attempts to switch the response back to cell mediated responses include use of the cytokine IL-12 as TH_1 but not TH_2 cells express receptors for IL-12 (Rogge *et al.*, 1997). In past studies low dose cyclophosphamide has been used to remove conditioned (?suppressor T cells, ?TH_2) T cells and B cells (Berd and Mastrangelo, 1988). Evidence for the effectiveness of these approaches is not yet available.

Select Antigens Expressed at High Density on Tumor Cells Which Have High Numbers of Precursor T Cells Against Them

The immune system has the capacity to reject large numbers of tumor cells provided there is a high frequency of T cells against the antigen on the tumor cells. An example of this is shown by Figures 5.1(a) and (b), which are chest X-rays of a renal transplant patient who received by accident a donor kidney containing melanoma cells (Elder *et al.*, 1997). Figure 5.1(b) illustrates clearing of the metastases six weeks after cessation of immunosuppression. In this case the remission was most probably on the basis of recognition of alloantigens on the donor melanoma cells against which a high frequency of pre-existing precursor T cells are known to be present.

Another example of rapid generation of high numbers of specific T cells is that reported to occur after infection with EBV where up to 50% of CD8 T cells were specific for the virus (McMichael and O'Callaghan, 1998). Presumably, the infection of large numbers of B cells acts to produce large numbers of APC and thereby with EBV, generation of large numbers of CD8 T cells against the virus. Clearly one of the aims in the use of cancer vaccines is to achieve similarly high numbers of reactive CTL against the cancer. Available information indicates precursor frequencies against some cancer antigens (e.g. MAGE) are low (Chaux *et al.*, 1998), though recent studies with HLA-2/Melan-A/MART-1 tetramers suggest a relatively high frequency of anti-Melan-A/MART-1 memory CTL in metastatic melanoma patients (Romero *et al.*, 1998; Anichini *et al.*, 1999).

The antigen density on tumor cells is also critical for mediating rejection. In the case of one of the MAGE-3A2 peptides, CTL were generated against it but antigen expression on several melanoma cells was too low to induce killing (Valmori *et al.*, 1997). Similarly, induction of IL-2 production from T cells was shown to be dependent on the level of antigen expression (Labarriere *et al.*, 1997).

"Helper" Molecules are Needed to Generate Optimal Immune Responses

The design of cancer vaccines has to a large extent changed in parallel with advances in understanding of immune responses. In the 1960s and 70s the concept of T and B cells was introduced (Raff, 1973). It was then shown that T cells consisted of CD4 "helper" and CD8 cytotoxic T cells (CTL). CD4 T cells provided "help" to B cells, macrophage responses, cytotoxic and $CD8^+$ T cells. These discoveries led to the development of vaccines which incorporated components to stimulate T helper cell responses. These included viruses such as vaccinia (Hersey *et al.*, 1987), and Newcastle disease virus (Cassel and Murray, 1992). Other helper strategies included use of chemical haptens such as dinitrochlorobenzene (Berd *et al.*,

(a)

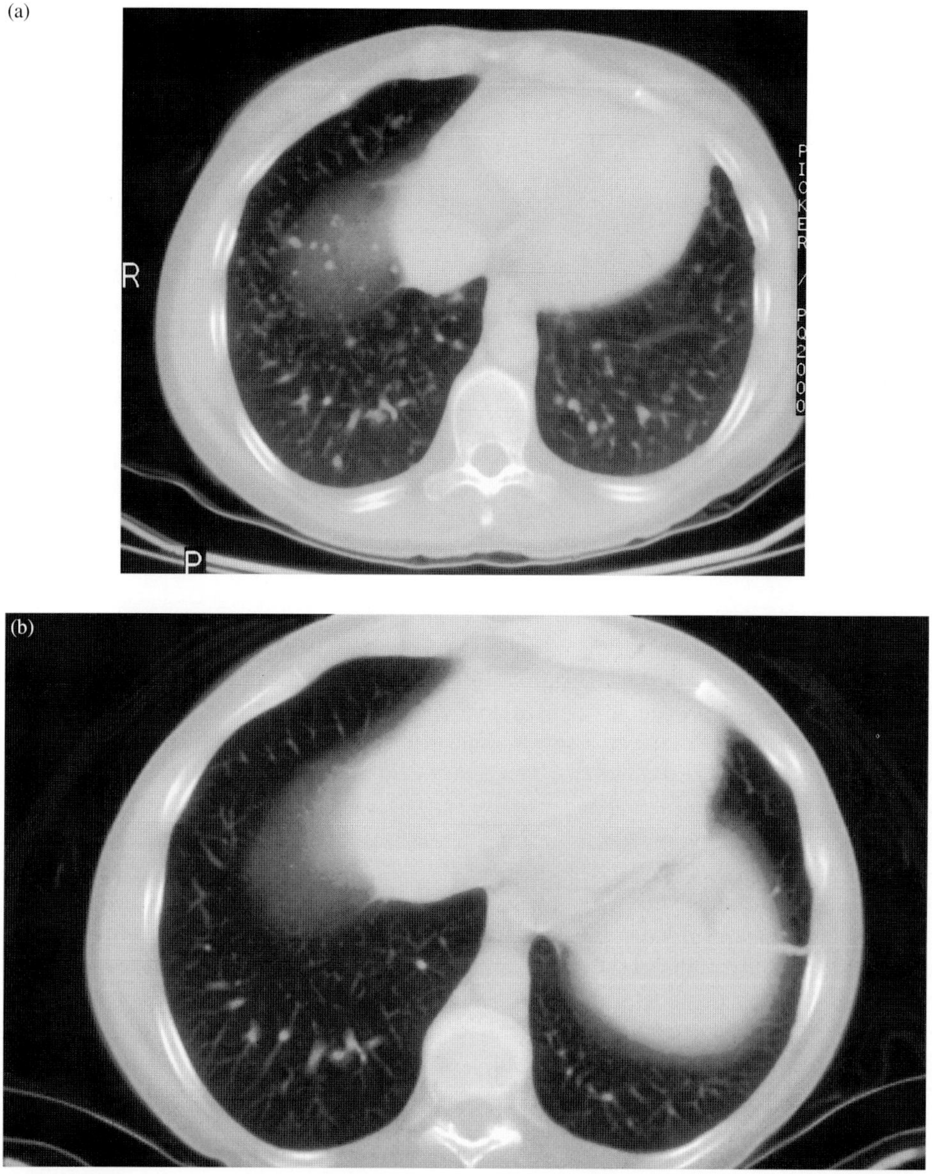

Figure 5.1 Regression of multiple lung metastases from a melanoma transplanted with the donor kidney after cessation of immunosuppression. (**a**) CAT scan of the chest of a 21-year-old woman showing multiple metastases from melanoma transplanted with the donor kidney. (**b**) CT of chest of the same patient 6 weeks after cessation of immunosuppression. The donor graft expressed A29 and B45 that was not shared by the recipient.

1991) and foreign proteins such as keyhole limpet hemocyanin (KLH) (Livingston, 1995), tetanus toxoid (Vitiello *et al.*, 1995; Livingston *et al.*, 1997) and purified protein derivative (PPD) of BCG. Vaccines including helper components remain under evaluation but helper components may differ in their ability to induce cell mediated responses to tumors. Viruses usually induce strong cell mediated responses but heterologous proteins such as tetanus toxoid may induce help for antibody rather than cell mediated responses.

Certain proteins, such as tetanus toxoid, contain epitopes which bind to practically all DR class II antigens and are referred to as universal helper epitopes (O'Sullivan *et al.*, 1991). The PADRE peptide is another example (Alexander *et al.*, 1994). They can be synthesized to contain class I restricted epitopes and so provide ''help'' at the site of interaction with CD8 T cells. There is also interest in using modified class II invariant chain peptides to provide help to CD8 T cells (Sinigaglia and Hammer, 1995). Helper components in vaccines should also (when possible) be present in the tumor so that the helper response can be restimulated on reappearance of the tumor. Unless the helper component is expressed by the tumor there will be no recall and the tumor may escape detection (Ossendorp *et al.*, 1998). Several $CD4^+$ Th cell epitopes have been recently reported to be expressed in melanomas and other human tumors, though none of them has been tested yet in vaccination protocols (see Chapter 1).

The most recent ideas concerning activation of CTL by helper cells is shown in Figure 5.2. This model suggests that CD40 Ligand on activated helper T cells activates dendritic or other APC and this enables the APC to activate CTL (further details in Chapter 2).

Selecting the Right Adjuvants

Vaccines are frequently given with an adjuvant to boost the strength of the response. They may do this by acting as a depot for release of antigen or by attraction of APC to the site. A detailed discussion of adjuvants is beyond the scope of this chapter but those commonly used with cancer vaccines are listed in Table 5.4. QS21 was reported to be very effective in inducing IgG antibody to the ganglioside GM2 (Helling *et al.*, 1995) and may have T cell stimulatory properties (Rhodes, 1996). BCG has been used as an adjuvant in several studies of Morton *et al.* (1992) and Detox as an adjuvant to a melanoma vaccine prepared from an ultrasonicate of three melanoma cell lines (Mitchell *et al.*, 1990). It has cell walls from a mycobacterium and monophosphoryl lipid A from Salmonella, which may activate macrophages. Montanide ISA720 is a water in oil adjuvant containing a metabolizable oil, which was shown to be effective in induction of T cell responses to cytomegalovirus (CMV) peptides in murine models and to proteins from malaria in human studies (Scalzo *et al.*, 1995; Lawrence *et al.*, 1997). The water in oil composition was found to be important in induction of CTL. Incomplete Freund's (IFA) is composed of mineral oil and Arlacel A (emulsifier) and pristine oil. Although widely used for induction of immune responses to peptides (Salgaller *et al.*, 1996), it induces granuloma formation and skin reactions at the site of injections. MFS9 is an oil in water biodegradable adjuvant which has been used as an adjuvant to increase immune responses to peptides (O'Hagan *et al.*, 1997). GM-CSF is used to increase the number of APCs at the injection site and was found by Knuth *et al.* to increase responses to melanoma peptides (Jäger *et al.*, 1996b).

TUMOR ANTIGENS RECOGNIZED BY THE IMMUNE SYSTEM OF HUMANS

Antigens Recognized by T Cells

Our understanding of antigens recognized by T cells developed firstly from the observation by Doherty *et al.* (1976) that recognition of viral antigens required the target cells to

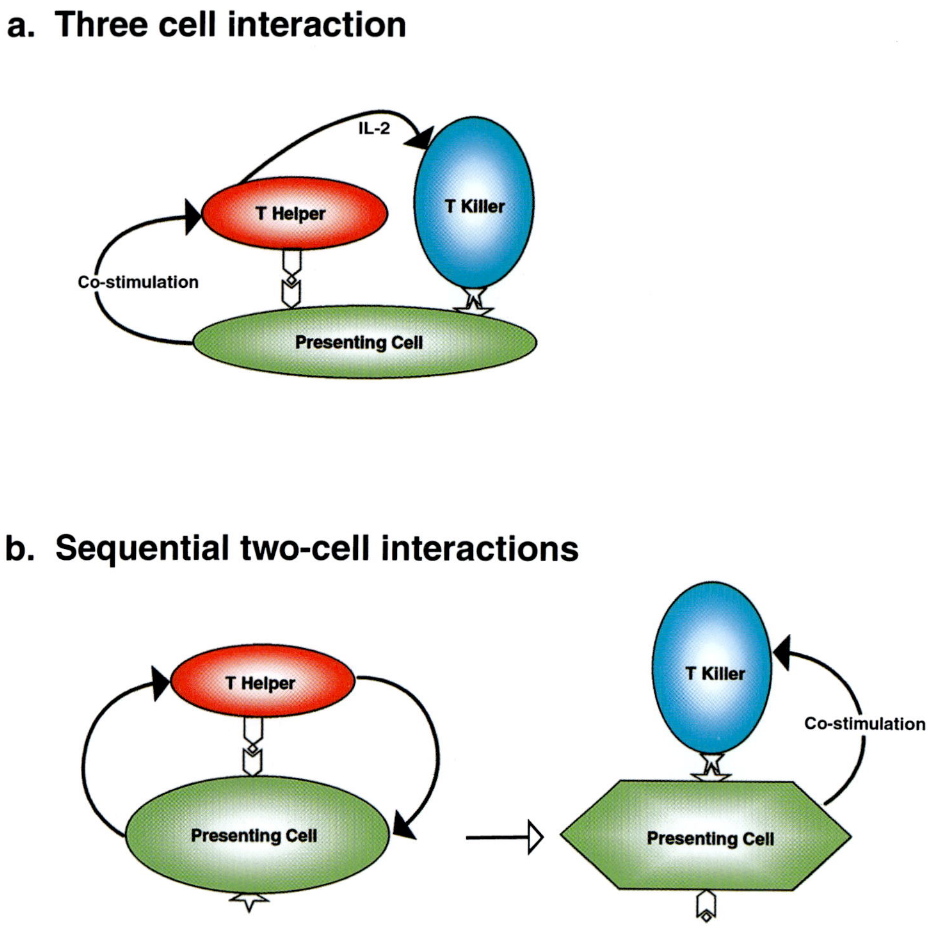

Figure 5.2 Two models of the delivery of help to $CD8^+$ killers. (**a**) The ''passive'' model in which the dendritic (presenting) cell presents antigen to both the T helper and the killer but delivers co-stimulatory signals only to the helper, which is thereby stimulated to produce IL-2 for use by the nearby killer. (**b**) The ''dynamic'' model in which the dendritic cell offers co-stimulatory signals to both cells. It initially stimulates the T helper (left), which, in turn, stimulates and ''conditions'' the dendritic cell to differentiate to a state (right) where it can now directly co-stimulate the killer. Reprinted with permission from Ridge *et al.* (1998).

express the same MHC antigens as the effector T cells. This puzzling finding was made clear when Alain Townsend reported that T cells recognized proteins that were processed within the cell and exported to the cell surface as peptides of 9–10 amino acids bound to class I MHC antigens (Townsend *et al.*, 1986). Subsequent studies showed that antigens external to the cell were processed within lysosomes within the cell and exported as peptides of 10–14 amino acids in association with MHC class II antigens. Helper T cells appeared to recognize antigens associated with MHC class II antigens and cytotoxic T cells recognized antigens associated with MHC class I antigens.

TABLE 5.4
Adjuvants for cancer vaccines

Compound	*Available from*
Incomplete Freund's (IFA)	Seppic
DeTox	Ribi
QS21	Cambridge Biotech
Montanide ISA 720	Seppic
MF59	Chiron Corporation
BCG	Different companies
GM-CSF	Different companies

Until the early 1990s information about human tumor antigens was largely confined to antigens recognized by antibodies such as those described against the gangliosides GM2, GD2 and acetylated GD3. The nature of antigens recognized by T cells remained elusive until Thierry Boon in Brussels introduced gene transfection and limiting dilution techniques to analyze the specificity of clones of T cells isolated from a patient with melanoma. Subsequent studies by this group and others using peptide elution techniques (Castelli *et al.*, 1995) have led to the discovery of a number of antigens, some of which are listed in Table 5.5 (see also Chapter 1 for more details).

In addition to the gene transfection approach, antisera from patients have been used to screen cDNA libraries from tumor cells. This approach, referred to as the SEREX approach (serological screening of expression libraries), depends on the molecule expressing determinants recognized by antibodies and helper T cells. This is usually the case but the molecule may not necessarily have determinants recognized by CTL. A large number of antigens have been detected using this approach (Old and Chen, 1998) and those referred to as cancer-testes (CT) antigens appear particularly attractive as candidates for cancer vaccines (see also Chapter 4).

TABLE 5.5
Human cancer antigens

		Antigen category		
Tumor-specific (cancer testis) antigens	*Differentiation antigens*	*Mutation of normal genes or alteration in splicing*	*Overexpressed genes*	*Viral antigens*
– MAGE 1–4	– Tyrosinase	– K ras (12, 13 or 61)	– P53	– HPV16, E6 and E7 oncoproteins
– MAGE C1	– MART-1	– p53	– Her-2/neu	
– BAGE	– gp100	– CDK4	– CEA	
– GAGE	– gp75 (TRP-1)	– Caspase 8	– Carbamic anhydrase	
– DAM	– TRP-2	– HLA-A2	– Galactin 9	
– NY-ESO-1	– Mucin 1	– β-Catenin	– Aldolase	
– SSX2		– N acetylglucosaminyl transferase	– elf-4y	
– SCP1				
– CT7		– TRP-2/INT2		

Additional references to the above antigens are given in Hersey (1997) and Old and Chen (1998). See also Chapter 2 of this book.

Another approach to identify tumor antigens has been to examine known oncogene protein products for epitopes recognized by T cells. Vaccines against Ras with mutations at position 12 or 61 were reported to be effective against murine tumors (Fenton *et al.*, 1995; Gjertsen and Gaudernack, 1998) and vaccines against peptides from (overexpressed) HER-2/neu were protective against tumors in rats (Disis *et al.*, 1996). One of the HER-2/neu peptides (p369–377) was found to be immunogenic *in vitro* but CTLs raised against the peptide did not kill carcinoma cells (Zaks and Rosenberg, 1998). The tumor suppressor protein p53 is also frequently overexpressed and mutated in cancers. CTL produced against wild type p53 were shown to be effective against murine cancers but not against normal tissues (Vierboom *et al.*, 1997).

Selection of Antigens for Cancer Vaccines

Several criteria are used in selection of antigens for cancer vaccines. Firstly, antigens that are recognized by $CD4^+$ helper T cells and $CD8^+$ CTL need to be included in the vaccine (Ossendorp *et al.*, 1998). Helper T cell antigens are needed which will recall an effector response against recurrent tumor whereas antigens recognized by CTL are needed for destruction of the tumor. In some instances CD4 T cells may also mediate destruction of tumor cells by non-secretory pathways mediated by ligands of the tumor necrosis family, such as FasL or TRAIL (tumor necrosis related apoptosis inducing ligand). Our recent studies suggest the latter is particularly important against melanoma (Thomas and Hersey, 1998).

Secondly, the antigens need to be expressed widely on tumor cells and in sufficient concentration to be recognized by T cells, i.e. expression needs to be at high enough levels to trigger cytotoxic T cell responses (Valmori *et al.*, 1997). Thirdly, the antigens need to be recognized by a high proportion of patients. This may require that the antigens have binding motifs for MHC antigens that are commonly expressed in human subjects such as HLA-A2, A3, A24, B7, B8, B12, DR3 and DR4. This increases the proportion of patients who can be treated with the antigen. Fourthly, the host T cells should not be tolerant of the antigens. Many of the tumor antigens described so far are found in varying degrees in normal cells (see also Chapter 1 of this book). It is therefore possible that prior exposure of the immune system to the antigens may have deleted high affinity T cells and left low affinity cells that have low capacity to kill the tumor cells (Toes *et al.*, 1996). In view of this it may be preferable to utilize antigens that have had low exposure to the immune system (i.e. cryptic antigens). The MAGE-antigens and other CT antigens are examples of such antigens in that the genes are methylated and not expressed in normal tissues except the testes. In melanoma and a variety of other cancers the genes are demethylated and expressed to varying degrees. Some of the other tissue-specific antigens may fulfil these criteria in that they are expressed at very low levels in normal tissue but become expressed at high levels in tumor tissue (e.g. gp 100, Her-2/neu). In the case of peptide vaccines, it may be possible to recruit high affinity T cells by modifying the MHC peptide binding sites to produce peptides with high affinity to the MHC antigens. There are now many examples of melanoma peptides that have been modified to increase their affinity and immunogenicity (Parkhurst *et al.*, 1996; Romero *et al.*, 1997); Rivoltini *et al.*, 1999).

An antigen which possesses most of the above requirements for making it an excellent immunogen in vaccination is the Ig idiotype expressed by B cell lymphomas. In fact, the idiotype determinant is clonally expressed by the large majority of tumor cells, it is hardly selected against during natural tumor growth and can be recognized both by the T and B cell components of the immune system (Kwak *et al.*, 1992). The only major drawback of this antigen is its uniqueness, since the idiotype sequence may be different for each lymphoma patient.

VACCINE DELIVERY SYSTEMS FOR GENERATION OF IMMUNE RESPONSES AGAINST TUMORS

The different vaccine approaches to treat cancer are shown in Figure 5.3. The following are short descriptions of these approaches.

Whole Cells and Cell Fragments

Most of the whole cell or particulate vaccines have been given subcutaneously with or without adjuvants such as BCG or Detox. Viral lysates have been given either subcutaneously or intradermally and have not been given with adjuvants. There has been some controversy as to whether whole cancer cells are recognized directly by T cells. This led to suggestions that the tumor cells in the vaccine should share HLA antigens with those of the patient. Experimental evidence suggests, however, that immune responses to whole cells, as for cell fragments, depends on uptake of the injected material by host APC and presentation to T cells of the recipient (Huang *et al.*, 1994). This process, referred to as

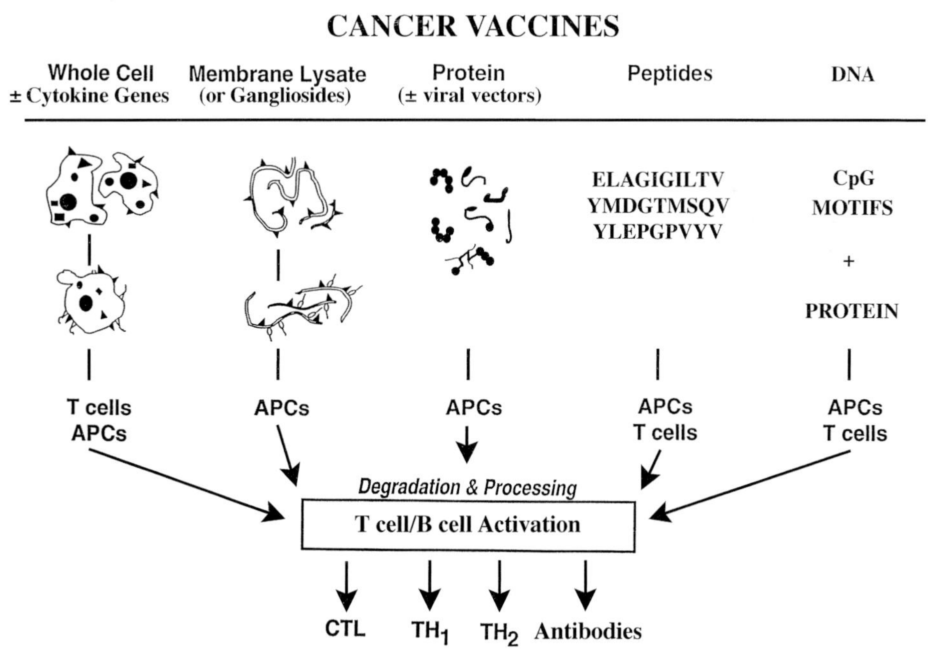

Figure 5.3 Diagrammatic representation of different vaccine approaches used in treatment of cancer. The APCs referred to in the diagram may be those naturally occurring in the patient or dendritic cells generated *ex vivo* and primed with the antigen preparations shown in the figure.

"cross presentation", appears to apply not only to generation of MHC class II helper responses by CD4 T cells, but also to MHC class I restricted responses by CD8 T cells (Carbone *et al.*, 1998).

Whole cell or cell fragment vaccines have the potential to express a wide range of antigens to the immune system and limit the opportunity for escape due to generation of antigen loss variants. The disadvantage of this approach is that the tumor antigens represent a small fraction of the protein from the cell and APC may be saturated by irrelevant peptides. In the eventuality that the vaccine is shown to have therapeutic effects, it is also difficult to evaluate which components of the vaccine were responsible. It is therefore not easy to build more effective vaccines by this approach. These considerations have led many investigators to use subunit vaccines. It can be expected that these may not be as effective as the crude vaccines in initial studies but correlation of immune responses with clinical outcomes should be possible and allow stepwise development of more effective vaccines.

A summary of current trials with these "first generation" vaccines is shown in Table 5.6.

Cytokine Gene Transfected Cancer Cells

Studies in a number of animal models suggested that immunization with cancer cells containing genes for cytokines led to protection against transplanted cancers and in some models rejection of established tumors (reviewed elsewhere (Tepper and Mulé, 1994). Tumor cells transfected with genes for GM-CSF appeared particularly effective (Dranoff *et al.*, 1993). These studies led to a number of trials in patients with cancer, as reviewed elsewhere (Parmiani *et al.*, 1997). Autologous melanoma transfected with genes for GM-CSF induced dense infiltrates with T cells and mixed tumor responses in some patients (Soiffer *et al.*, 1998). However, the technical difficulty involved in producing autologous vaccines has so far limited this approach. Clinical trials based on immunization with IL-2 or IL-4 genes have induced limited responses (Belli *et al.*, 1997; Arienti *et al.*, 1999) and there is a general impression that delivery of cytokines to the local site of vaccination by other means may be as effective as transfection of genes into tumors (Pardoll, 1998).

Proteins and Peptides as Vaccines

Information about binding epitopes within proteins has made it possible to produce relatively short peptides of 9–10 amino acids that are recognized by CTL. One question is whether immunization with peptides is preferable to using the whole protein. Immunization with recombinant whole proteins has the potential to include epitopes for both helper T cells and CTL. This appears to be the case for tyrosinase, MAGE-3 and NY-ESO-1 (Stockert *et al.*, 1998) for which HLA-class II epitopes have been defined (see Chapter 1). Whole proteins may also express binding sites for a larger range of MHC antigens than exist with purified peptides. This is shown from studies on tyrosinase, gp100 and MAGE-3 (reviewed in Hersey, 1997). In studies against some viral antigens, however, peptides have proven more effective than whole protein (Disis *et al.*, 1996). This may be because the peptides may occupy more MHC antigens on APC and hence be more effective in triggering T cell responses. Whether this will apply against tumor cells which have a wider array of tumor/MHC antigen complexes is not known. Peptides are easier to

TABLE 5.6
Randomized trials with melanoma vaccines

*Investigator/ Clinical stage of trial**	*Melanoma vaccine*	*Trial design*	*Protocol*	*Number of patients/status*
Hersey *et al.* (21, 22) IIB and III	Vaccinia lysates of one allogeneic melanoma cell	Control untreated	i.d. q2w × 4, then q3w × 6, then q4w × 18	700 (closed 2/98) In progress
Wallack *et al.* (17) III	Vaccinia lysates of three allogeneic melanoma cells	Control vaccinia alone	i.d. q1w × 13, then q2w × 40	250 Non-significant trend
Livingston *et al.* (18) III	GM2 + Cyclo and BCG vaccine	Control BCG/ Cyclo	4–5 × over 6 months	122 Non-significant trend
ECOG-1694 (20) Schering/Bristol Myers IIB and III	GM2-KLH/QS21	Control HDI	sc. qlw × 4, then each 12 weeks for 2 yrs	851 (closed 11/99) Significant difference in favor of HDI p. 009 for survival, p. 0015 for DFS
EORTC 18961 (28) Bristol Myers IIA, IIB	GM2-KLH/QS21	Control untreated	sc. qlw × 4, then each 12 weeks for 2 yrs 6 monthly Year 3	1300–1500 (projected)
NCI/Morton *et al.* (23) IIB and III	Three allogeneic melanoma cells + BCG vaccine	Control HDI or BCG alone	i.d. q2w × 3, then monthly × 12, then 3 monthly × 4, then 6 monthly × 6	825 (projected) In progress
NCI/Morton *et al.* (23) IV	Three allogeneic melanoma cells + BCG vaccine	Control HDI or BCG alone	id. q2w × 3, then monthly × 12, then 3 monthly × 4, then 6 monthly × 6	420 projected In progress
Corixa/Schering (24) Mitchell *et al.* IIB and III	Two allogeneic melanoma cells + 'Detox' + IFN 5×10^6	Control HDI	sc. qlw × 4, then q2w × 1, then monthly with repeat courses 6 mthly	315/400 accrued as of 2/2000 In progress
SWOG 9035/Ribi/ Corixa IIA (19)	Two allogeneic melanoma cells + 'Detox'	Control untreated	sc. qlw × 4, then q4w × 1, then q8w × 5, then 6 monthly to 2 yrs	689 (closed 11/96) n.s. overall but in subset <3 mm significant prolongation of DFS (p. 04)
Avax/Berd *et al.* (26) (26) III	Cyclo Autol Mel/DNP/ BCG	Control HDI	sc. qlw × 6 booster at 6 months	400 (25 sites) Projected
Bystryn (46) III	Shed antigens from 4 melanoma + alum.	Placebo (Alb) + Alum.	id. q3w × 4 then monthly × 3, then to 5 yrs	36 Sig. DFS Non-sig. Survival

* American Joint Committee on Cancer (AJCC) stages III and IV refer to patients with lymph node metastases and disseminated metastases, respectively. Stage IIA, IIB refers to localised melanoma >1.5 and >4.00 mm thick respectively.

BCG: Bacillus Calmette-Guerin; Cyclo: Cyclophosphamide; i.d.: intradermal; IFN: Inteferon: HDI: high dose IFN-α2b; KLH: Keyhole limpet haemocyanin; qxw: every × weeks; s.c.: subcutaneous; DNP: Dinitrophenyl; DFS: Disease free survival.

produce than recombinant proteins, which require production in fermentation vessels and purification from bacterial products.

Both proteins and peptides have the advantage of being safe, relatively cheap to produce and sterilize. They suffer, however, from being poorly immunogenic. For this reason it is necessary to use adjuvants to enhance their immunogenicity. Adjuvants have a number of roles in enhancing immune responses to these products, such as attraction of APC to the site of vaccination, facilitation of uptake into APC and in some instances, modulation of responses by causing local release of cytokines that stimulate TH_1 TC_1 responses.

Some of the clinical trials in progress using melanoma peptides or proteins are summarized in Table 5.7. The studies by Boon and colleagues (Marchand *et al.*, 1999)

TABLE 5.7
Current melanoma peptide trials

Investigator or reference	*Peptide*	*Adjuvant**	*Number of patients*	*Clinical response*
Marchand *et al.*, 1999	MAGE-3A.1	Nothing	25	3 CR, 4 PR
Marchand, Van Baren, Boon	MAGE-3A.1	MPL & QS21	7	1 PR
(Ludwig Institute, Brussels)	MAGE-3A.2	Nothing	17	1 CR, 1 PR, 2 SD
	MAGE-3 protein	MPL & QS21	Ongoing	–
	MAGE-1.A1	Nothing	Ongoing	–
	MAGE-1.A1 + MAGE-3A.1	Nothing	Ongoing	–
Cormier *et al.*, 1997b	MART-1	IFA	18	None
Rosenberg *et al.*, 1998b	gp100 154, 209, 280	IFA	28	None
Rosenberg *et al.*, 1998a	gp100 209 2M	IFA	11	3 mixed
		IF + IL-2	31	1 CR, 12 PR
Jäger *et al.*, 1996b	MART-1, gp100, tyrosinase 1, 368	GM-CSF (3 pts)	10	1 CR, 2 PR
Weber *et al.*, 1999	MAGE-3.A1 and PADRE†	IFA	18	Not available
Wang *et al.*, 1999	MART-1	IFA	25	Not available
Cebon *et al.*, 1999	MART-1	IL-12	20	1 CR, 1 PR
Schmittel *et al.*, 1999	Tyrosinase 234, 368, 206, 192	GM-CSF	18	1 MR, 2SD
Hersey (University of	MART-1, 26 2L	–	16	2 SD
Newcastle, Australia)	Tyrosinase, MAGE-3A.2	Montanide ISA720	Ongoing	
	gp100 209, 2M; 280, 9V	PPD ± GM-CSF	Ongoing	

* GM-CSF, granulocyte-macrophage colony-stimulating-factor; IFA, incomplete Freund's adjuvant; MPL, monophosphoryl lipid A (modified LPS); QS21, carbohydrate extract of Quillaja Saponaria; Montanide ISA720, water in (metabolisable) oil emulsion.

† PADRE (Pan DR Epitope) is a 13-mer peptide which can stimulate class II-restricted Th cells.

continue to puzzle many clinicians in that impressive results (7 responses, most durable, in 25 patients) have been achieved by injection of MAGE-3A1 peptides alone without adjuvants, albeit over long periods. However, no clear evidence of clinical response in 18 high-risk melanoma patients was observed when MAGE-3.A1 peptide was given in incomplete Freund's adjuvant (IFA), though 5 of 14 patients showed a specific CTL response to MAGE-3 targets (Weber *et al.*, 1999). The studies of Rosenberg and colleagues with the modified gp100 209 2M peptide are also impressive, with 13 responses in 31 patients (42%) (Rosenberg *et al.*, 1998a). The latter trial is, however, difficult to evaluate because of the concomitant use of high dose IL-2.

In one trial, patients were immunized intradermally with the MART-1 peptide as well as the 2 HLA-A2 binding tyrosinase peptides in a soluble form (Jäger *et al.*, 1996a). Although tumor regression was not observed in this trial, delayed type hypersensitivity responses directed against the tyrosinase signal peptide were observed in some patients. In addition, immunization appeared to enhance the responses generated to the MART-1 and tyrosinase signal peptides following a single *in vitro* stimulation with peptide pulsed cells. Immunization of HLA-A2 patients with the MART-1 and gp100:209–217 peptides in IFA appeared to result in modest enhancement in the ability to induce tumor reactive T cells in bulk cultures following *in vitro* stimulation with peptides (Salgaller *et al.*, 1996; Cormier *et al.*, 1997b). Significant clinical responses, however, have only been seen in small numbers of patients in these trials.

An unresolved issue remains the relationship between *in vitro* immune response to the vaccine and the clinical response. In fact, one should mention that the *ex vivo* CTL response of these patients failed to match their clinical response. In fact, none of the clinically responding patients in the MAGE study showed a detectable, anti-MAGE-3.A1 CTL in the blood and a similar finding was reported for most of the clinically responding patients in the gp100 2092M trial of Rosenberg's group. However, gp100 2092M or Melan-A/MART1$_{27-36}$ peptides were able to generate detectable CTL responses in melanoma patients who failed to respond clinically (Rosenberg *et al.*, 1999a). This discrepancy has not been clearly explained but it could be due to accumulation of antigen-specific CTL at tumor site (see also the subchapter on ''Adoptive Immunotherapy'').

A remarkable success is that reported by vaccinating follicular (B-cell) lymphoma patients, made apparently tumor-free by chemotherapy, with their own idiotype protein bound to KLH and given with GM-CSF (Bendandi *et al.*, 1999). In fact, this vaccine resulted in molecular complete and durable response in $\frac{8}{11}$ (recent update 14 out of 14) patients, such responses being associated with a strong T cell specific activity (Bendandi *et al.*, 1999).

Viral Vectors

Over the past few years a number of alternative ways of immunizing with purified antigens have become available. Viral vectors, such as adenovirus, avipox virus and vaccinia, are some of those in use. Viral vectors have the advantage of introducing the antigens into both the MHC class I and class II pathways so that T cells with both helper and CTL activity may be induced. Most viruses are immunogenic and the cytokines released may favor induction of TH_1 TC_1 pathways. However, their immunogenicity reduces their infectivity and hence their effectiveness with repeated immunization (Hodge *et al.*, 1997). This is of little concern in immunization against infective organisms where only 2 or 3 immunizations are needed but may become a problem in cancer patients where frequent immunization over long periods may be needed. There are also ethical concerns about use of viruses because of the risk of generation of pathogenic mutants and insertional mutation of normal genes in the host resulting from insertion of viral genes into the host genome. Viral vectors can be engineered to express cytokines and thereby modulate responses towards TH_1 TC_1 pathways. IL-12 is favored for this purpose. Immune responses against the virus, however, may limit their production of cytokines. Table 5.8 summarizes some of the clinical trials with viral vectors.

TABLE 5.8
Immunotherapy with viral vectors: human studies

Tumor	*Antigen*	*Vector*	*References*
Colon carcinoma	CEA	rVV-CEA	Cole *et al.*, 1996
Colon carcinoma	Col7-1A/GA733	rAd-GA733	Li *et al.*, 1997
Melanoma	p97	rVV-p97	Estin *et al.*, 1988
Carcinoma cervix	HPV16/18,E6/E7	rVV-E6/7	Borysiewicz *et al.*, 1996
Melanoma	MART-1 ± IL-2 ± IL-12	rAd-V2CMV	Rosenberg *et al.*, 1998b
Melanoma	gp100 ± IL-2 ± IL-12	rAd-V2CMV Avipox	Rosenberg *et al.*, 1998b

"Naked" DNA Vaccines

More recent studies have shown that plasmids engineered to contain genes for antigens behind strong promoters can result in the production of proteins when injected directly into skin or muscle. This means that it may not be necessary to utilize viral vectors for entry into cells and so avoid many of the concerns expressed about safety of viral vectors. An unexpected benefit from use of DNA vaccines was the discovery that the plasmids induced strong TH_1 TC_1 responses. This was found to be due to immunostimulatory (CpG) motifs consisting of cytosine flanked on the 5′ end by two purines and the 3′ end by two pyrimidine bases (Chu *et al.*, 1997). These short DNA sequences stimulate IL-6, IL-12 and IFN-γ production from lymphoid cells and result in the skewing of immune responses to the TH_1 TC_1 pathway (Klinman *et al.*, 1997). Subsequent studies have shown that similar effects could be obtained by injection of the immunostimulatory sequences with protein antigens (Chu *et al.*, 1997). There is as yet no published experience with this approach in cancer patients but immunization with DNA for gp100 was found to be effective in animals (Schreurs *et al.*, 1998).

Dendritic Cells

Studies over the past decade have shown that it is possible to produce large numbers of DCs from blood lymphocytes by culture in cytokines such as GM-CSF, IL-4 and TNF-α (Tjandrawan *et al.*, 1998). A large variety of different protocols have been used to generate DCs *in vitro*. The starting population may be either $CD34^+$ cells from blood or bone marrow or adherent cells (monocytes) from blood. Requirements for the *in vitro* generation of DCs include cytokines that induce proliferation of DCs like GM-CSF and Flt-3 ligand (McBride, 1997) and agents which induce differentiation of DCs such as TNF-α and CD40L (Morse *et al.*, 1998). The latter appears to be a key molecule in induction of functional ability to stimulate CTL activity (Bennett *et al.*, 1998).

It is beyond the scope of this chapter to discuss the different type of DCs that are produced *in vitro* (Banchereau and Steinman, 1998) (see also Chapter 2 of this book). The availability of DCs, however, provides the opportunity of using them to immunize against tumor antigens. This may be by addition of peptides or protein antigens directly to DCs (Tjandrawan *et al.*, 1998) or by transfection of the DCs with genes for the tumor antigens (Tuting *et al.*, 1998). Other approaches have been to incubate the DCs with extracts of the tumor or RNA from the tumors (Ashley *et al.*, 1997; Celluzzi and Falo, 1998). Table 5.9 summarizes some of the clinical studies in progress but this is not a comprehensive list of the many trials in progress or about to be initiated. The two most relevant studies, at the moment, are those carried out by Nestle *et al.* (1998) and Thurner *et al.* (1999). In the first one, metastatic melanoma patients were vaccinated with autologous DC pulsed with either HLA-A2 binding peptides (tyrosinase, gp100, Melan-A/MART-1) or HLA-A1 binding peptides MAGE-1 or -3. Some patients also received DC pulsed with proteic tumor lysate. Responses were found in 5 out of 16 patients which were accompanied by DTH responses to the given peptide (Table 5.9). The second study also used DC pulsed with the MAGE-3.A1 peptide that were shown to expand specific CTL in 8 out of 11 patients while inducing regression of individual metastases in 6 patients (minor or mixed responses).

Advantages of DC-based vaccines are the known ability of DCs to prime and initiate immune responses to tumors and the ability to provide these in sufficient numbers to create a

TABLE 5.9
Dendritic cells in immunotherapy of cancer patients

Investigator or reference	*Source of antigen*	*Route*	*No. of patients*	*Clinical response*
Mukherji *et al.*, 1995	MAGE-3.A1	s.c.	3	0
Nestle *et al.*, 1998	Melanoma tumor lysates or peptides + KLH helper protein	Lymph nodes	16	2 CR 3 PR
Hu *et al.*, 1996	MAGE-1	i.d. & i.v.	3	0
Chakraborty *et al.*, 1998	Melanoma lysates	i.d.	15	1 PR
Ranieri *et al.*, 2000	gp100, MART-1, tyrosinase	i.v.	N. A.	N. A.
Murphy *et al.*, 1998	Prostate PSMA peptides P1 or P2	i.v. × 6	33	2 CR, 6 PR
Thurner *et al.*, 1999	MAGE-3.A1	i.d. & i.v.	11	0
Gajewski T. (University of Chicago)	MAGE-3.A2, MART-1 + IL-2	s.c.	8	2 PR

s.c. = subcute; i.d. = intradermal; i.v. = intravenous.

wave of T cell responses to the tumor. The need for *in vitro* cultures to produce DC is currently a limitation to this approach but there is some hope that the use of cytokines such as Flt-3 ligand (Lynch *et al.*, 1997; McBride, 1997; Esche *et al.*, 1998) may enable production of large numbers of DCs *in vivo* and hence avoid the need for production *in vitro*.

CONCLUSIONS

The history of immunotherapy is characterized by waves of enthusiasm and pessimism. Clinical, histopathological and laboratory evidence for tumor regression mediated by immune responses provides a sound basis for attempting to develop this therapeutic approach against cancer. The potential limitations of this approach are, however, many and enthusiasm needs to be tempered with a long-term view of its development. A major advance will be identification of patients who are likely to respond to this form of therapy. At present selection of patients is largely on the basis of clinical stage of the disease and tumor burden. Apoptosis research may provide another measure of likely response in that our recent studies have shown that responses of melanoma to killing by CD4 T cells can be correlated to their susceptibility to apoptosis induced by TRAIL. Other measures of responsiveness may include MHC antigen expression on the tumor cells. Loss of MHC antigens may, however, not be as serious as thought, as the immune system appears to employ multiple mechanisms against cancers and can still destroy MHC loss variants. There is also considerable research to be carried out in the use of chemotherapeutic agents as an adjunct to immune therapy. This may be to modulate immune responses or to ''condition'' the tumor. An example of the latter may be to reduce the levels of inhibitors of apoptosis such as FLIP. The decade ahead promises to be most challenging.

CYTOKINE THERAPY

FRANCESCO M. MARINCOLA

Cytokine Therapy of Cancer

1. ***Cytokines already assessed for the systemic treatment of patients with metastatic cancer.***
   - IFN (interferons): IFN-α, IFN-β, IFN-γ.
   - IL-2 (interleukin-2).
   - CSF (colony stimulating factors): granulocyte-CSF, platelet-CSF, macrophage-CSF.
   - IL-4 (interleukin-4).
   - IL-6 (interleukin-6).
   - IL-12 (interleukin-12).
   - TNF (tumor necrosis factor): TNF-α.
   - Combination therapy with multiple cytokines, with other biologic agents or in association with chemotherapy.
2. ***Mechanisms of action.* Although tumor regressions have been noted after systemic administration of cytokines the mechanisms mediating them have not been identified. At least three mechanisms can be postulated:**
   - Direct effect of tumor cell growth (e.g. IFN, IL-10, TNF).
   - Direct effects of various immune cells such as T cells or antigen presenting cells (e.g. IL-2, IL-12, GM-CSF, IL-4, TNF, etc.).
   - Direct effect of the tumor blood vessels (e.g. TNF).
3. ***Future questions.***
   - Why are a few tumor types (melanoma, renal cell cancer) more sensitive to cytokine therapy?
   - Can cytokine therapy effectively enhance TAA (tumor associated antigen)-mediated CTL responses observed in patients with metastatic cancer?
   - Could effectiveness of cytokine therapy be enhanced without enhancing its toxicity?

About 15 years have passed since the first administration, with therapeutic intent, of the T cell growth factor IL-2 to cancer patients. Since then, IL-2 and other cytokines with pure immune modulatory and no direct antitumor effects have been used for the treatment of patients with cancer. As a consequence, a large number of clinical studies involving the administration of these cytokines alone or in combination with other agents have been reported. In 1992 IL-2 received approval from the U.S. Food and Drug Administration (FDA) for the treatment of patients with renal cancer and in 1998 for the treatment of patients with metastatic melanoma. Improved understanding of the immune biology of cancer that was concurrently achieved during the last decade has provided better characterization of the mechanisms leading to tumor rejection in response to immunologic manipulation. As the sophistication of the understanding of the mechanisms leading to immune-mediated rejection of cancer has improved, more complex and specific forms of treatments were added. Yet, as we will see, none of them seem to achieve effectiveness unless it is associated with the systemic administration of IL-2. Similarly to IL-2, several immune reagents have shown effectiveness and have been (IFN-α) or are being (antibodies) approved for the treatment of cancer with adjuvant or therapeutic purposes. Furthermore, cytokine therapy has been associated with multiple other forms of biological therapy (anti-angiogenesis therapy, gene therapy, etc.) whose complicated scientific rationale is often confusing for the general practitioner and the general oncologist. As the field of cancer immunotherapy is experiencing an exponential growth, treating cancer with biologic agents is therefore becoming a discipline in itself, deserving special training for its rationale and safe administration. In this section we will review some of the basic principles of cytokine administration with particular attention to safety guidelines for its administration and treatment efficacy evaluation.

In reality exploitation of the immune system to eliminate neoplastic growth was suggested a long time ago (Burnet, 1970). However, it was only after the identification and use of cytokines such as Interferons and Interleukins that reproducible responses against selected cancers could be observed with a high enough frequency to warrant clinical use and increasing research efforts. A large proportion of interest in tumor immunobiology is focused on the understanding of T cell mediated recognition of cancer. This bias is derived from pre-clinical studies suggesting that tumor-bearing animals can reject syngeneic tumors through cellular rather than antibody-mediated mechanisms (Restifo and Wunderlich, 1996). During the past decade the field of tumor immunotherapy has evolved rapidly, particularly in the context of metastatic melanoma, due to the identification of tumor antigens recognized by TIL or other tumor-reactive T cells (Boon *et al.*, 1997; Rosenberg, 1997a). Therefore the theoretical basis for the relevance of immune stimulatory cytokines (in particular IL-2) in cancer treatment was strengthened. Furthermore, the identification of T cell epitopes responsible for recognition of MAA led to the development of vaccination protocols based on the administration of short peptides representing such epitopes to patients with metastatic melanomas in combination with various cytokines. As a consequence the combination of antigen-specific vaccination with the supporting administration of molecules with general immune stimulatory effects is providing a new exciting tool for the study of immunologic principles beyond the direct scope of cancer treatment. Recent work at the Surgery Branch of the National Cancer Institute (NCI, Bethesda, MD) has revealed that peptide-based immunization when given in association with high-dose IL-2 may lead to clinical responses in a limited but significant number of patients. It is not clear, however, why clinical responses to vaccination occur in some but not in the majority of patients. More importantly it is not known why cytokine therapy remains a general requirement for clinical responses in spite of the demonstration of a strong effect of the immunization on T cell induction *in vivo* (Salgaller *et al.*, 1996; Cormier *et al.*, 1997b; Rosenberg *et al.*, 1998a). Future work should focus on this question if further improvement in vaccination strategy is to be achieved.

INTERFERONS

Interferons represented the first biologic molecules to be introduced in the clinic to treat cancer patients. IFN-α was originally described as a factor that could mediate the ability of a virus to interfere with the replication of another virus (Isaacs and Lindenman, 1957). This factor was subsequently recognized to include a family of polypeptides with broad biological properties, including several immunological effects or direct effects on cellular proliferation. For this reason IFNs have been studied extensively for the treatment of patients with proliferative diseases and have demonstrated significant effectiveness for some of them, including hairy cell leukemia, chronic myelogenous leukemia and other myeloproliferative disorders (Foon *et al.*, 1986; Talpaz *et al.*, 1986). The anti-neoplastic activity of IFN-α for the treatment of these diseases appeared to be, at least in part, directly related to its anti-proliferative effects. Because of the usefulness of this agent for the treatment of these hematologic disorders, attempts were made to use IFN-α for the prevention or treatment of advanced solid cancers. Some randomized trials have been published in the past few years addressing the effectiveness of IFN-α as adjuvant for the prevention of metastatic recurrences from loco-regional melanoma (Cascinelli, 1995; Creagan *et al.*, 1995; Kirkwood *et al.*, 1996; Rusciani *et al.*, 1997; Pehamberger *et al.*, 1998). These studies suggest a survival benefit with IFN-α either in patients with loco-regional node involvement or in patients without nodal involvement but at high risk of recurrence because of the stage of their primary tumor. IFN-α and IFN-β have also been used for the treatment of metastatic melanoma and renal cell cancer and their therapeutic effectiveness has been extensively discussed for metastatic melanoma (see Kirkwood, 1995) and for renal cell cancer (Savary, 1995). In either disease clinical responses were noted when these cytokines were used systemically. A compilation of a total of 1608 patients treated with various dosage schedules of single agent IFN suggested a 15% response rate, 36 complete and 199 partial responses (Savary, 1995).

Interferons have been used in combination with other biologic substances or chemotherapeutic agents for the treatment of renal cancer; however, results have not appeared to be better than the results obtainable with either agent alone with the possible exception of IL-2 (see ''Combination treatments with IL-2'' section). Similar results were collected for metastatic melanoma (Kirkwood, 1995). A very interesting analysis was recently published by Gleave and co-workers which compared in a randomized trial the efficacy of IFN-γ with a placebo for the treatment of metastatic renal cell carcinoma (Gleave *et al.*, 1998). One hundred and eighty-one patients were randomized to receive either IFN-γ1b 60 $\mu g/m^2$ subcutaneously once a week or placebo. Response rates were similar with 4.4% responses in the treatment group and 6.6% responses in the placebo group. Interestingly, complete remissions could be observed in the placebo group, emphasizing the necessity of conclusively evaluating the efficacy of immune modulators only with randomized studies. This type of study also emphasizes the difficulty in evaluating objectively the efficacy of immune modulators over a background of spontaneously regressing tumor deposits. Although spontaneous regression is not frequently observed in patients not undergoing cancer treatment, most of these patients are not followed as aggressively as patients undergoing experimental protocols. Therefore, the rate of spontaneous regression in the untreated population might be higher than predicted by retrospective analyses. This consideration should be kept in mind while reading the rest of this chapter. **To our knowledge, no controlled studies have been performed comparing other cytokines with placebo and, as a consequence, judgment about treatment efficacy should take into account a non well characterized, yet significant, number of spontaneous regressions**. Unfortunately the study by Gleave *et al.*, analyzed IFN-γ (as shown by the low response rates observed in the treatment group), which may have lower response rates than other cytokines. A similarly interesting study could be considered to compare the administration of IL-2 or IFN-α to placebo. However, the ethical consideration of offering placebo to patients with an expected three-month median survival has generally limited the enthusiasm for such studies, even if the patient is given the option to receive treatment after assessment of the placebo.

INTERLEUKIN-2

A growth factor able to maintain and expand T cells *in vitro*, named IL-2, was purified from normal lymphocytes and given to two patients with melanoma in 1983 (Bindon *et al.*, 1983). The principle of using IL-2 for the treatment of cancer patients was quite different from the rationale for the use of IFN. While the anti-tumor effect of IFN could partly be attributed to a direct anti-proliferative activity (Kirkwood, 1995), IL-2 did not have any direct effect on cancer cells and its antitumor activity was mediated by stimulation of various components of the immune system (Lotze, 1991). Therefore, it was hoped that IL-2 could enhance naturally occurring immune defenses against cancer. In 1984, after the identification of the DNA sequence coding for the expression of IL-2 and the application of recombinant technology for large-scale production of cytokines in *Escherichia coli*, sufficient amounts of IL-2 became available for clinical studies (Lotze *et al.*, 1985). On May 5, 1992, almost 10 years after the first *in vivo* administration of IL-2, the U.S. Food and Drug Administration (FDA) licensed IL-2 for the treatment of patients with metastatic renal cell cancer. In 1998 the FDA licensed IL-2 also for the treatment of metastatic melanoma. The approval of IL-2 corresponded to the first recognition of the effectiveness of a biologic agent acting against cancer purely by enhancing the host immune resistance. Therefore it was a milestone in the recognition of a fourth modality for the treatment of cancer patients after surgery, radiation therapy, and chemotherapy (Marincola, 1994).

Administration of high-dose rIL-2 resulted in durable complete responses in patients with metastatic renal cell cancer and metastatic melanoma. Treatment of 283 consecutive patients in the Surgery Branch, NCI between September 1985 and December 1992 with high-dose bolus rIL-2 (720,000 IU/kg every 8 hours) resulted in complete responses in 7% of patients with metastatic melanoma and 9% of patients with renal cell cancer. An additional 10% and 11% of patients, respectively, achieved a partial response. Complete responses were most often durable with several patients remaining disease-free more than five years from their initial treatment (Rosenberg, 1997b). Many other clinical trials have been reported with the administration of high-dose bolus IL-2 for the treatment of metastatic melanoma (Table 5.10) or metastatic renal cell cancer (Table 5.11). Although treatment of other solid tumors has been reported with similar regimens, results have not been comparable to those obtained in the case of these tumors and will not be reviewed here.

TABLE 5.10
Administration of IL-2 as an intravenous bolus for the treatment of patients with metastatic melanoma

Investigator	*Year*	*Dose regimen per cycle*	*No. patients*	*Responses*		
				Complete (CR)	*Partial (PR)*	*% CR + PR*
Parkinson *et al.*	1990	600,000/kg tid* × 5 days	46	2	8	22
Demchak *et al.*	1991b	600,000/kg tid × 5 days	27	0	4	26
Rosenberg *et al.*	1994a	720,000/kg tid × 5 days	134	9	14	17
Hersh *et al.*	1989	0.001–14 MU/m^2 daily dose	26	0	3	12
Budd *et al.*	1990	0.1–22 MIU/m^2 daily dose	23	0	5	22
Whitehead *et al.*	1991	36–60 MIU/m^2 daily dose	42	0	4	10
Sparano *et al.*	1993	6 MU/m^2 tid × 5 days	44	0	2	5
Total responses			**342**	**11**	**40**	**15**

*tid = three injections/day.
N.B. For more information about the exact schedule of administration of cytokine source we refer the reader to the reference cited.

TABLE 5.11
Administration of IL-2 as an intravenous bolus for the treatment of patients with metastatic renal cell cancer

Investigator	*Year*	*Dose regimen per cycle (tid* × 5 days)*	*No. patients*	*Responses*		
				Complete (CR)	*Partial (PR)*	*% CR + PR*
Rosenberg *et al.*	1994a	720,000/kg	134	9	14	17
Atkins *et al.*	1993	600,000/kg	71	4	8	17
McCabe *et al.*	1991	600,000/kg	37	1	2	8
Abrams *et al.*	1990	600,000/kg	16	0	0	0
Poo *et al.*	1991	600,000/kg	15	0	4	27
Fyfe *et al.*	1995	6–700,000/kg	255	12	24	14
Total responses			528	26	52	15

*tid = three injections/day.
N.B. For more information about the exact schedule of administration of cytokine source we refer the reader to the reference cited.

Administration of IL-2 was associated with high systemic toxicity (capillary leak syndrome) in the first 155 patients treated with high bolus rIL-2. Major toxicity and death were usually due to cardiac or septic complication. However, in the next 310 patients treatment-related mortality dropped to 1.5%. White and collaborators analyzed cardiopulmonary toxicity in 199 patients receiving 310 courses of high-dose IL-2 (White *et al.*, 1994). Although no deaths occurred in this cohort of patients, multiple types of cardiopulmonary toxicity were observed, including respiratory failure, cardiac arrhythmia, creatinine phospho-kinase elevation and most frequently hypotension. Interestingly, response to treatment was associated with the development of hypotension requiring vasopressor treatment (23% vs. 6.5% response, P_2 = 0.037). After cardiac screening of patients and aggressive use of prophylactic antibiotics were instituted, no treatment-related mortality occurred in the next 775 consecutive patients who received high-dose bolus rIL-2 (Marincola, 1994; Rosenberg, 1997b). Indeed, safety of high-dose IL-2 bolus administration has improved over the past decade as recently reported by Kammula *et al.*, (1998). Progressive reduction in morbidity and mortality was found over the 12-year period studied. The improvement in safety most likely reflected the development of strategies to screen eligible patients, optimize therapeutic conditions and determine limiting toxicity. Despite these changes in treatment strategy leading to reduced toxicity, no changes were noted in overall response rates. These trends suggested that high-dose rIL-2 can be considered extremely safe when appropriate management skills and patient-selection are applied. An interesting characteristic of IL-2 treatment is the decreased tolerance of patients to this cytokine with progressive cycles of therapy. Marroquin and co-workers analyzed patient tolerance to IL-2 over multiple courses of therapy and the factors that affected the number of doses delivered (Marroquin *et al.*, 2000). In this study the median number of doses tolerated during the first course of therapy was significantly higher than the doses tolerated during the subsequent second course of therapy (15 vs. 12 doses, P_2 = 0.0001). Earlier creatinine elevation was found to be the most common reason for reduced tolerance to IL-2 with subsequent cycles. Other variables associated with reduced tolerance included being male (P_2 = 0.006), older age (P_2 = 0.0055) and having received prior nephrectomy (P_2 = 0.001). Low (renal) dose intra-venous dopamine has been used to enhance kidney perfusion and avoid the acute renal failure associated with IL-2 therapy. A recently reported prospective randomized evaluation of the benefit of prophylactic use of low-dose dopamine during IL-2 therapy failed, however, to demonstrate a beneficial effect of this drug to prevent renal toxicity (Cormier *et al.*, 1997a). Patients were randomized either to receive dopamine before starting high-dose IL-2 therapy or to receive dopamine during therapy upon marked reduction of renal output. The study was performed with the secondary purpose of evaluating whether reduced renal toxicity could lead to administration of more doses of IL-2 and consequently to enhance response rates. Although differences were noted in urine flow and weight gain, no significant differences were observed in creatinine elevation and most importantly in the number of doses received. Similarly, no differences in response rate were noted between the two cohorts.

Because of the severe toxicity associated with the administration of IL-2 and the consequent intensive and costly monitoring, alternate routes of administration have been explored. Although animal models suggested a direct relationship between tumor regression and dose of IL-2 systemically administered (Rosenberg *et al.*, 1985) **no clinical study has been able to conclusively show a higher efficacy of high (and toxic) dose intravenous of IL-2 over less intensive dosage schedules**. Original treatments of patients with cancer with IL-2 used the rapid infusion of boluses of IL-2. These were characterized by particularly high toxicity and therefore alternative routes were explored. Another commonly used schedule of administration has been the continuous intravenous

TABLE 5.12
Administration of IL-2 as a continuous intravenous infusion for the treatment of patients with metastatic melanoma

Investigator	*Year*	*Dose regimen per cycle*	*No. patients*	*Responses*		
				Complete (CR)	*Partial (PR)*	*% CR + PR*
Thompson *et al.*	1988	0.3–3 MU/m^2 daily	15	0	0	0
Creekmore *et al.*	1989	0.001–30 MU/m^2	12	0	2	17
Richards *et al.*	1990	3 MU/m^2 daily × 5 days	33	0	3	9
Perez *et al.*	1991	17–72 MIU/m^2 daily	17	0	1	7
Dorval *et al.*	1992	16–24 MIU/m^2 daily × 3–5 days	37	0	8	22
Vlasveld *et al.*	1992	0.2–9 MIU/m^2 daily	13	0	1	8
Legha *et al.*	1996 a	12 MIU/m^2 daily	31	1	6	22
Total responses			158	1	21	16

N.B. For more information about the exact schedule of administration of cytokine source we refer the reader to the reference cited.

TABLE 5.13
Administration of IL-2 as a continuous intravenous infusion for the treatment of patients with metastatic renal cell cancer

Investigator	*Year*	*Dose regimen per cycle (daily)*	*No. patients*	*Responses*		
				Complete (CR)	*Partial (PR)*	*% CR + PR*
Negrier *et al.*	1989	18 MIU/m^2	32	2	4	19
Bajorin *et al.*	1990	9 MIU/m^2	24	1	2	13
Geertsen *et al.*	1992	18 MIU/m^2	30	1	4	20
Sorio *et al.*	1992	18 MIU/m^2	30	5	3	27
Escudier *et al.*	1992	24 MIU/m^2	88	0	16	18
Negrier *et al.*	1998	18 MIU/m^2	138	2	7	6.5
Gold *et al.**	1997	18–88 MIU/m^2	173	9	17	19
Whitehead *et al.*†	1995	4.5–6 MU/m^2	45	0	6	13
Total responses			560	20	59	14

* In this study 76 patients received also LAK cells.
† This treatment was followed by outpatient therapy with lower doses of IL-2.
N.B. For more information about the exact schedule of administration of cytokine source we refer the reader to the reference cited.

infusion of IL-2, which appeared to result in reduced acute toxicity compared to the bolus administration. Results are summarized in Tables 5.12 and 5.13 for melanoma and renal cell cancer respectively with overall similar results. IL-2 was also administered in lower doses with the intent of decreasing systemic toxicity and the hope of achieving similar response rates. Several groups suggested that tumor reductions can be observed with the administration of low-dose IL-2, particularly in the context of renal cell carcinoma, and recommend route and dosages of administration compatible with out patient treatment (Angevin *et al.*, 1995; Guida *et al.*, 1996; Tourani *et al.*, 1996). To address these issues Yang *et al.* (1995) published interim results of a randomized, triple-arm trial in which IL-2 was given either as high-(720,000 IU/kg tid) or low-(72,000 IU/kg tid) dose intravenous bolus or intermediate-dose via subcutaneous route. Intravenous administration consisted of standard dose intravenous injections every 8 hours for a maximum of 15 doses or earlier in case of limiting toxicity. Subcutaneous administration consisted of a first week in which IL-2 was administered at the dose of 250,000 IU/kg/day for 5 of 7 days followed by 5 weeks in which IL-2 was given at the dose of 125,000 IU/Kg/day for 5 of 7 days (Yang and Rosenberg, 1997). In the two-arm comparison of high-dose versus low-dose intravenous IL-2 it was noted (at 52 months follow-up) a significantly decreased toxicity in the low doses cohort (less hypotension, thrombocytopenia, malaise, pulmonary toxicity and neurotoxicity). The overall response rate (partial plus complete responses) was 19% with high dose and 10% with low dose, and responses with the high-dose dose regimen were more durable and, with higher frequency, complete. Response rates with subcutaneous administration were intermediate between the high and low dose while toxicity was minimal. This study is still ongoing and although suggestive of a better anti-cancer effect of high-dose IL-2, the number is not high enough to reach significance. Similar conclusions were reached by a recent report by the Cytokine Working Group experience (Dutcher *et al.*, 1997). Review of the experience of several clinical trials conducted by this group suggested that high-dose IL-2 induces a higher frequency of complete responses and that these responses are more sustained. Other approaches aimed at reduction of IL-2 toxicity by decreasing the dosage of administration or altering the route or schedule have been suggested. Yang's group used polyethylene glycol-modified IL-2 (PEG-IL-2) for the treatment of patients with metastatic melanoma or renal carcinoma (Yang *et al.*, 1995). PEG-IL-2 is a compound with similar *in vivo* and *in vitro* effects of IL-2 but exhibits longer circulating half-life. In mice, one dose of PEG-IL-2 resulted in tumor regression comparable to those obtained by multiple bolus doses of IL-2. Based on these pre-clinical studies a phase-I study was conducted in which the antitumor effects and toxicity of PEG-IL-2 were tested. Although overall this treatment was well tolerated, no significantly improved antitumor activity was noted compared with high-dose IL-2 alone. Furthermore, because of the delayed type of toxicity caused by the longer circulating half-life of PEG-IL-2, patient management was not simplified but was found to be rather more complex and unpredictable as several types of toxicity manifested after patient discharge from the hospital several days following the discontinuation of treatment.

Royal analyzed correlates of response to IL-2 therapy in a series of 509 consecutive patients with metastatic renal cancer or melanoma (Royal *et al.*, 1996). Patients with renal cancer responded more frequently if they had not previously failed other immunotherapy. Response also correlated with thrombocytopenia during the first cycle of therapy. In patients with melanoma, response was found to correlate with disease in the subcutaneous tissues. Furthermore, clinical responses were more frequently observed in patients who could receive more doses of IL-2 in their first course of therapy and exhibited a more profound lymphocytosis following treatment. Although several correlates of response could be identified by this analysis there was much variability and a reliable predictive model of response to therapy could not be formulated. More importantly, the significance of these correlates was difficult to assess as to possible cause–effect relationship.

In summary, IL-2 has been shown by different groups to have reproducible antitumor effect against metastatic melanoma and renal cell carcinoma (Marincola, 1994). At present, IL-2 should be considered a significant component of a multi-modality approach for the treatment of these two cancers for which no recognized standard treatment is available.

ADOPTIVE THERAPY AND INTERLEUKIN-2

The identification of tumor reactive lymphocytes responsible for partial or complete responses in patients treated with IL-2 involved the growth in rIL-2 of lymphocytes that were infiltrating into tumor deposits (Itoh *et al.*, 1986; Rosenberg *et al.*, 1986). TIL from approximately half the individuals with melanoma exhibited specific *in vitro* reactivity against the autologous melanoma as well as against allogeneic melanoma cell lines expressing appropriate HLA-class I molecules (Rosenberg, 1997b). Adoptive transfer of LAK therapy in combination with systemic IL-2 administration has also been extensively analyzed. Studies in which the administration of IL-2 alone or in combination with LAK cell was directly compared failed to demonstrate any benefit of the combined approach over IL-2 alone and demonstrated increased toxicity (Rosenberg *et al.*, 1993b; Law *et al.*, 1995). Adoptive therapy of cancer is discussed more extensively in the next section of this chapter.

TUMOR ANTIGENS AND INTERLEUKIN-2

Several tumor-associated antigens have been identified with a high predominance of MAA (Rosenberg, 1997a; Boon *et al.*, 1997). Since most tumor antigens have been identified in the context of melanoma, treatment of patients with this disease with antigen-specific therapy has taken the lead over other tumor histologies. Thus melanoma has become a model for the immunotherapy of cancer and principles can be learned from the experience gained that can be applied more broadly in the context of other tumors. Among the MAA, MART-1 and gp100 are widely expressed in melanoma lesions and are predominantly recognized by CTL in the context of HLA-A*0201, which is present in about half of the melanoma population (Marincola *et al.*, 1995a; Player *et al.*, 1996). In addition, MART-1 and gp100 are recognized by the majority of HLA-A*0201-restricted melanoma-specific CTL generated from TIL. *In vitro* studies led to the identification of T-cell epitopes for both of these MAA, which in turn led to active specific immunotherapy of melanoma patients using MART-1_{27-35}, peptide as a vaccine against melanoma. Cormier *et al.* (1997b) compared CTL reactivity *in vitro* from PBMC pools obtained before and after vaccination with MART-1_{27-35} administered to HLA-A*0201 melanoma patients subcutaneously (4 times at 3-week intervals) in an emulsification with incomplete Freund's adjuvant. This analysis demonstrated that peptides alone can generate strong CTL responses *in vivo*. These results were subsequently confirmed in the context of a phase I active immunization protocol in which the ability of the MAA gp 100 in eliciting cellular immune responses *in vivo* was analyzed (Salgaller *et al.*, 1996). Several clinical trials involving the vaccinations of melanoma patients with peptides derived from MAA were conducted to ascertain the effectiveness of vaccination with the MAA gp100 and its derivative peptides (Rosenberg *et al.*, 1998a). Nine HLA-A*0201+ patients with metastatic melanoma were treated with the native g209–217 nine amino acid peptide and then 11 patients were treated with its synthetic variant, g209-2M. The 209-2M peptide, a single residue variant of gp100 209-217, was identified as one of the immunodominant HLA-A*0201 restricted CTL epitopes of gp100 (Kawakami *et al.*, 1995). G209-2M is characterized by a higher affinity for the HLA-A*0201 allele than the naturally occurring gp209 and by a higher efficiency of CTL induction *in vitro* (Parkhurst *et al.*, 1996) and *in vivo* (Salgaller *et al.*, 1996). Thirty-one additional patients were treated with the g209-2M peptide plus adjuvant IL-2. In each trial immunologic responses were evaluated as originally described by Cormier *et al.* (1997b) and lymphocytes were collected from patients before and after immunization for immunologic testing of reactivity against peptide and tumor (Rosenberg *et al.*, 1998a). Using an immunologic assay based on the ability of peptides to elicit specific cytokine release from circulating lymphocytes, 2 of 8 (25%) patients that received the native g209–217 peptide exhibited successful immunization compared to 10 of 11 (91%) patients successfully immunized with the modified g209-2M peptide ($p = 0.006$). Recognition of peptide *in vitro* correlated with recognition of tumor cells *in vitro* and was far greater in patients receiving the modified peptide. Interestingly, only one of the 20 patients immunized with peptide alone (g209) achieved objective tumor regression. However, 13 of 31 patients (42%) receiving the synthetic g209-2M peptide plus IL-2 had objective cancer responses and four additional patients had mixed responses (Rosenberg *et al.*, 1998a). The high response rate (42%) noted in patients who received the combination of vaccine and IL-2 was higher than the 17% response rate previously seen in 134 consecutive patients treated at the Surgery Branch (NCI) with the same dose of IL-2 alone (Rosenberg *et al.*, 1994a). This suggested that the enhancement of CTL reactivity *in vivo* might not be sufficient to induce clinical effects and the additional proliferative effects of IL-2 may be required. This could explain why the combination of the two treatments may increase response rates compared with IL-2 alone. However, the absence of randomization in this phase I study could not prove this point. To conclusively analyze whether the addition of peptide vaccination to high-dose IL-2 bolus treatment of patients with metastatic melanoma can result in increased clinical response rates a multi-institutional randomized study of immunization with gp209-2M followed by high-dose IL-2 vs. high dose IL-2 alone is planned (for more information contact Dr. Douglas Schwartzentruber, at djs@pop.nci.nih.gov). Other cytokines have been used at the NCI in association with epitope-specific vaccination. IL-12 and GM-CSF were used for patients with metastatic melanoma, which received the same treatment schema of patients subsequently treated with IL-2. In contrast to the high response rates observed with IL-2, no responses were noted in the cohort of patients treated with the other two cytokines (Rosenberg *et al.*, 1999a).

CHEMOTHERAPY AND INTERLEUKIN-2

IL-2 has also been used in combination with other cytokines or with chemotherapy. Although some studies have reported additional advantage of combination therapy, overall the results do not support this conclusion (Marincola, 1994). In particular, several studies reported a high response rate when IL-2 administration is combined with chemotherapy. However, the results have been compared to historical controls. Few randomized studies in which the administration of chemotherapy alone was compared to the administration of IL-2 plus chemotherapy have been performed. In a recently completed study at the Surgery Branch (NCI) **no significant differences in response rates or survival were noted between the chemotherapy alone or the chemotherapy plus immunotherapy cohorts** (Rosenberg *et al.*, 1999b). In this study patients were randomized to receive chemotherapy with cis-platinum, dacarbazine and tamoxifen or the same chemotherapy regimen followed after a one-day interval by the standard NCI high-dose IL-2 regimen plus IFN-α. It is possible that the concomitant administration of chemotherapy (which has an immuno-suppressive effect) inhibited the immunostimulatory effect of IL-2. Furthermore, it was noted that IL-2 enhanced the frequency of allergic reactions toward the chemotherapeutic agents used (in particular dacabazine). Anaphylactic reactions were noted in some patients and rashes in others, which resulted in a lower amount of chemotherapy received by the combination therapy patients. Similarly Johnston *et al.* (1998) compared in a randomized study the treatment of patients with metastatic melanoma with chemotherapy (carmustine, cisplatin, dacarbazine and tamoxifen) vs. treatment with the same chemotherapy regimen in combination with IL-2 and IFN-α. This study also failed to demonstrate a response rate or survival advantage of the combination therapy and rather demonstrated increased toxicity compared to chemotherapy alone. At present no studies are under way comparing the efficacy of IL-2 alone with the efficacy of IL-2 administered in combination with chemotherapy.

The lack of better results with combination chemo-immune therapy is difficult to explain. It is possible that the combined administration has more deleterious than positive effects and an alternative strategy could be the distanced administration of either therapy to allow recovery of the patient from either therapy toxic effects. Legha (Legha *et al.*, 1996b) noted that the sequential administration of chemotherapy followed by biotherapy resulted in higher response rates (69%) than the combined administration (50%) and significantly prolonged survival. Atzpodien *et al.* (1995a) and Guida *et al.* (1996) reported similar results.

OTHER CYTOKINES

Human GM-CSF was utilized in a clinical phase I trial of continuous intravenous infusion (50, 100, 150 μg/kg over 24 hours for seven days). This study demonstrated minimal toxicity of GM-CSF at the maximum tolerated dose of 100 μg/kg (Cole *et al.*, 1998). However, no objective responses were observed. IL-6 was tested by various groups for treatment of patients with advanced renal cancer (Weiss *et al.*, 1995; Schuler *et al.*, 1998). IL-12 has been used for the treatment of melanoma (no clinical responses in 10 patients treated) (Bajetta *et al.*, 1998) and renal cancer (1 response among 51 patients treated)

(Motzer *et al.*, 1998). The maximum tolerated dose corresponded to 1.0 mg/kg and dose limiting toxicity included increase in transaminase concentration in serum, pulmonary toxicity and leukopenia. IL-4 has also been used for the treatment of metastatic renal cancer (1 response out of 18 evaluable patients) (Stadler *et al.*, 1995) and of other solid tumors such as lung cancer (1 response out of 55 patients treated) (Vokes *et al.*, 1998). Janik *et al.* (1996) reported the use of IL-1 in combination with indomethacin for the treatment of metastatic melanoma with 11% response rate among patients without visceral metastases. Overall the use of cytokines other than IL-2 did not yield response rates comparable to the administration of IL-2.

COMBINATION TREATMENTS WITH INTERLEUKIN-2

The most commonly used cytokine combination is IL-2 and IFN-α (Tables 5.14 and 5.15) because of the synergistic effect believed to occur between the two agents and the demonstrated effectiveness as single agents. However, **there is no consistent evidence that the combination of the two cytokines improves results obtainable with either agent alone**. Jayson and co-workers (1998) reported the result of a randomized trial in which treatment with IL-2 alone (18 MU subcutaneous injection, Monday through Friday for three weeks) was compared with the combination of IL-2 and IFN-α (9 MU IFNα-2b). With a total accrual of 60 patients, no significant difference in survival or response rates

TABLE 5.14
Administration of IL-2 in combination with IFN-α for the treatment of patients with metastatic melanoma

Investigator	*Year*	*Dose regimen IL − 2 per cycle*	*Dose regimen IFN − α per cycle*	*No. Patients*	*Responses*		
					Complete (CR)	*Partial (PR)*	*% CR + PR*
Kruit *et al.*	1991	4.5 MU/m^2 ivb* tid × 5	3 MU/sq	9	1	4	56
Budd *et al.*	1992	4–26 MU/m^2 ivb daily	10 MU/im	17	2	3	29
Sparano *et al.*	1993	4.5 MU/m^2 ivb tid × 5	3 MU/iv	41	0	4	10
Marincola *et al.*	1995b	3–16 MU/m^2 ivb tid × 5	3–6 MU/iv tid × 5†	82	6	14	24
Karp *et al.*	1998	60,000 IU/kg ivb tid × 5	10 MU/sq	38	1	5	16
Lee *et al.*	1989	3–16 MU/m^2 ci^c	6 MU/sq	15	1	2	20
Kruit *et al.*	1991	3 MU/m^2 ci × 4	6 MU/sq	54	1	10	20
Mittelman *et al.*	1990	0.5–7 MU/m^2 ci × 4	6–12 MU/im	14	0	0	0
Budd *et al.*	1990	3–4.5 MU/m^2 ci	0.1–10 MU/im	13	0	2	15
Bergmann *et al.*	1990	18 MIU/m^2 ci × 6	10 MU/sq	11	0	3	27
Keilholz *et al.*	1993	1–4 mg/m^2 ci × 5	10 MU/sq	54	4	12	30
Whitehead *et al.*	1993	2 MU/m^2 ci	6 MU/im or sq	14	0	0	0
Kruit *et al.*	1996	7.8 MU/m^2 ci × 4	6 MIU/m^2 sq	51	1	7	16
Eton *et al.*	1996	9 MIU/m^2 ci	5 MU/m^2 im	23	0	2	8
Total responses				422	17	68	20

*tid = thrice injections daily; ivb = intravenous bolus; iv = intravenous; ci = continuous infusion; im = intra-muscle.
† At the highest doses IFN-α was given once a day.
N.B. For more information about the exact schedule of administration of cytokine source we refer the reader to the reference cited.

TABLE 5.15
Administration of IL-2 in combination with IFN-α for the treatment of patients with metastatic renal cell cancer

Investigator	*Year*	*Dose regimen IL − 2 per cycle*	*Dose regimen IFN − α per cycle*	*No. Patients*	*Responses*		
					Complete (CR)	*Partial (PR)*	*% CR + PR*
Atkins *et al.*	1993	600,000 IU/kg ivb* tid	3 MU/iv tid	28	0	3	11
Sznol *et al.*	1990	7–22 MIU/m^2 ivb tid	10 MU/im tid	14	1	2	21
Marincola *et al.*	1995b	3–16 MU/m^2 ivb tid × 5	3–6 MU/iv tid × 5†	75	12	9	28
Karp *et al.*	1998	60,000 IU/kg ivb tid × 5	10 MU/sc	14	0	1	1
West *et al.*	1990	18 MU/m^2 ci × 5	3 MU/sc qod	41	0	5	12
Ilson *et al.*	1991	3 MU/m^2 ci	5 MU/iv	32	0	3	9
Mittelman *et al.*	1990	0.5–7 MU/m^2 ci × 4	6–12 MU/im	18	0	4	22
Bartsch *et al.*	1990	18 MIU/m^2 ci	10 MU/sc	19	0	3	16
Demchak *et al.*	1991a	5 MIU/m^2 ci × 5	9 MU/sc	29	0	5	17
Bergmann *et al.*	1993	18 MIU/m^2 ci × 6	10 MU/sc	30	2	7	30
Besana *et al.*	1993	18 MIU/m^2 ci	9 MU/sc	14	1	4	36
Lipton *et al.*	1993	1–4 MU/m^2 ci	3–12 MU/im	31	6	7	42
Jayson *et al.*	1998	18 MU sc × 5 days/w	9 MU sc × 3 days/w	29	0	0	0
Negrier *et al.*	1998	18 MIU/m^2 daily	18 MIU/m^2 daily	140	1	25	19
Bukowski *et al.*	1997	9 MIU/m^2 ci × 5	10 MU/m^2 tiw	36	3	3	17
Atzpodien *et al.*	1995b	5–20 MIU/m^2 sq tiw	2.6 MU/m^2 sq tiw	152	9	29	25
Total responses				702	35	110	21

*tid = three injections/day; ivb = intravenous bolus; iv = intravenous; ci = continuous infusion; im = intra muscle; qod = quadruple on day; sc = subcutaneous; tiw = three injections/week.
† At the highest doses IFN-α was given once a day.
N.B. For more information about the exact schedule of administration of cytokine source we refer the reader to the reference cited.

was noted. Furthermore, the toxicity observed with the combination therapy was severe when high doses of both agents were used (Marincola *et al.*, 1995b; Jayson *et al.*, 1998) limiting the usefulness of this approach. Other two randomized trial in which the combination of IL-2 plus IFN-α was compared with IL-2 alone were discontinued after the first interim analysis since IFN-α failed to show any benefit when added to IL-2 therapy alone (Atkins *et al.*, 1993; Sparano *et al.*, 1993). Others have noted a benefit of the combination therapy over either agent alone. For instance Negrier and collaborators (1998) recently reported the results of a large study in which patients were randomized to receive either IL-2 or IFN-α alone or the combination of both. In this study a significant increase in response rate and in disease survival was noted in the combination group compared with either treatment alone. However, overall survival was not improved in the combination arm. It is difficult to judge the overall effectiveness of this combination therapy. On one hand the largest randomized study published (Negrier *et al.*, 1998) suggests a benefit over the administration of either cytokine alone. On the other hand, other randomized (Atkins *et al.*, 1993; Sparano *et al.*, 1993; Jayson *et al.*, 1998) Jayson *et al.*, 1998) and non-randomized studies (Oldham *et al.*, 1992; Marincola *et al.*, 1995b) (Oldham *et al.*, 1992; Marincola *et al.*, 1995b) did not show a clear benefit that could justify the increased toxicity. Compilation of available reports (Tables 5.14 and 5.15) suggests a slightly higher response rate in melanoma (20%) and renal cancer (21%) with the combination treatment compared with the approximately 15% response rates observed with IL-2 alone whether administered as intravenous bolus or continuous infusion (see previous tables). It is possible that some studies did not have sufficient power to exclude a minor but significant synergistic effect of the two cytokines and this possibility should not be totally discounted. Ravaud *et al.* (1998) have reported the results of a multicentric phase II clinical trial in which administration of IFN-α and IL-2 was combined with the continuous infusion of fluorouracil for the treatment of metastatic renal cancer. Their conclusion was that this treatment was ineffective (1.8% response rate). Similar conclusions were reached by others for this (Ellerhorst *et al.*, 1997; Tourani *et al.*, 1998) and other cancers (Goey *et al.*, 1996). IL-2 and IFN-α administration has also been evaluated in combination with Tumor Necrosis Factor-α (Eskander *et al.*, 1997), retinoic acid (17% response rate) (Stadler *et al.*, 1998), tamoxifen (Henriksson *et al.*, 1998), and vinblastine (38.7% response rate) (Pectasides *et al.*, 1998). With few exceptions, however, these trials failed to suggest additional therapeutic benefits. The combination of IL-2 and IFN-α has also been used for cancers other than renal and melanoma. Chang *et al.* (1995) reported a 14% response rate in patients with metastatic colorectal carcinoma. This experience may be of particular interest because neither IL-2 nor IFN-α has known significant antitumor activity in the context of colorectal cancer. However, a similar study performed by another group failed to demonstrate clinical responses in the context of the same disease (Hjelm *et al.*, 1995).

Other combination treatments with IL-2 and other cytokines have been reported. Witte *et al.* (1995) suggested efficacy of the combination treatment with IL-2 and IFN-β for the treatment of renal cell carcinoma. We have analyzed the usage of high-dose IL-2 bolus in combination with IFN-γ (Kim *et al.*, 1996). This cytokine has several immunologic effects, which could be considered complementary to the effects of IL-2. In particular, IFN-γ induces the expression of HLA class I and class II molecules in cancer cells *in vitro* (Marincola *et al.*, 1994). Most tumors express little amount of HLA class I (in particular HLA-B and -C alleles) and HLA class II and the reduced expression of HLA is correlated with decreased recognition of target cells by MAA-specific CTL (Rivoltini *et al.*, 1995a). Thus, it was hypothesized that the systemic administration of IFN-γ before the systemic administration of IL-2 could have a beneficial effect by enhancing the sensitivity of tumor cells to the lytic activity of T cells expanded and activated by IL-2 at the tumor site. Escalating doses of IFN-γ (0.1, 0.2, 0.3 and 0.5 mg/m^2 once a day for seven consecutive days) were administered to patients with metastatic melanoma followed by IL-2 (720,000 IU/kg) intravenously (Kim *et al.*, 1996). The maximal tolerated dose was 0.3 mg/m^2. The dose limiting toxicity was hepatotoxicity. **Immunohistochemistry failed to demonstrate enhancement of HLA class I expression in the majority of samples analyzed** (HLA up-regulation was noted only in one of 12 patients tested). The lack of effect of IFN-γ in inducing expression of HLA class I and II antigens was attributed to the low concentration of IFN-γ achieved *in vivo* compared with the concentration needed to achieve HLA up-regulation *in vitro* (Marincola *et al.*, 1994). Although IFN-γ was well tolerated, no clinical responses were noted with this combination treatment. From those findings we concluded that further studies looking at this combination treatment were not warranted. Similar results were reported by Reddy *et al.* (1997) in a cohort of patients with metastatic cancers of different histology.

Other combination treatments have been reported. Curti *et al.* (1998) have recently reported the results of a phase I trial of anti-CD3-stimulated CD4+ T cells, IL-2 and cyclophosphamide for the treatment of patients with advanced cancer. This treatment resulted in objective clinical responses. TNF-α was administered in sequence with IL-2 for the treatment of patients with advanced cancer and 2 out of 14 patients (both with metastatic melanoma) responded to this treatment (Krigel *et al.*, 1995). The number of combinations and treatments attempted is enormous and beyond the scope of this chapter. In general, however, these therapies, although often based on a sound biological rationale derived from pre-clinical experimentation, tend to address the problem of cancer immune biology in an equivalent and non-specific way. In particular, these studies do not consider that an antitumor specific immune response generated in animal models by administration of cytokines is often obtained with immunogenic tumors transplanted into healthy individuals, whereas these crucial factors are not evaluated in clinical trials. Therefore, it is unlikely that new frontiers will be opened by these approaches. New strategies encompassing agents with broader biologic activity, such as anti-angiogenesis factors, may have a new impact on the treatment of advanced cancer or may enhance the effect of the presently used biological agents.

CONCLUSIONS

Over the years, the availability of IL-2 has played a major role in helping clinicians and scientists understand and observe the fascinating phenomenon of tumor–host interactions. IL-2 has allowed *in vitro* expansion of immunological reagents with direct anti-cancer properties and at the same time has demonstrated indirect anti-tumor effectiveness when systemically administered to patients with metastatic cancer. Although the overall clinical benefit is still limited, for poorly understood reasons, the immunological basis for tumor rejection has been strongly supported by these experiences. The recent identification of tumor antigens recognized by autologous T cells has further strengthened the support for a T-cell mediated rejection of tumors. Future studies should be devoted to the development of strategies to broaden the effectiveness of these treatments to more patients with the same histology and to more cancers of different histology. This result is likely to be achieved by increasing the understanding of the basic immunologic principles governing T-cell mediated recognition of tumors and conversely tolerance mechanisms.

ADOPTIVE IMMUNOTHERAPY

FRANCESCO M. MARINCOLA

Evolution of Adoptive Cellular Immunotherapy

1. ***T cell infusions*. Small numbers of lymphocytes could be expanded *in vitro* and given *in vivo* in humans.**
2. ***PAK* (phytohemagglutinin-activated killer) cells. Large numbers of PAK cells could be expanded that could be administered safely to patients.**
3. ***LAK* (lymphokine activated killer) cells. LAK could be expanded with IL-2 (interleukin-2) and given to patients with metastatic cancer in combination with the systemic administration of IL-2. Total regression of disease was occasionally noted that could be attributed to the LAK cells or the IL-2 or their combined effects. Toxicity was significant.**
4. ***TIL* (tumor-infiltrating lymphocytes). TIL are expanded *in vitro* with cytokines such as IL-2 and noted to recognize specifically TAA (tumor associated antigens), which were shared among tumors and were expressed on the cell surface in associated with HLA (human leukocyte antigen) molecules. TIL were given to patients with metastatic melanoma and other cancers in combination with IL-2 and appeared to increase response rates compared with IL-2 alone.**
5. ***Gene modified TIL*. TIL engineered to express cytokines such as TNF-α were given to patients in an attempt to enhance their effectiveness at tumor site. No additional benefits over TIL were noted by introducing these genes, however, the feasibility of genetic therapy was established.**
6. ***TAA epitope-specific CTL*. After the identification of TAA and their T cell epitope it was possible to expand in large numbers CTL specific for such antigens to enrich the population of adoptively transferred T cells. Transfer of epitope-specific CTL, however, did not prove to enhance response rates over TIL plus IL-2 therapy.**
7. ***TAA epitope-specific CTL clones*. Improvement in T cell culture technology allowed the large-scale expansion of CTL clones that could be selected for their TAA specificity and their effectiveness in recognizing and killing tumor cells. Trials are ongoing evaluating the efficacy of these CTL populations selected according to their ability to kill tumor cells.**

INTRODUCTION

Adoptive immunotherapy is defined as the passive transfer in the tumor-bearing host of immune cells activated *ex vivo* and characterized by antitumor activity in *in vitro* assays. The principle behind this treatment strategy rests on the assumption that immune competent cells can be more efficiently produced *ex vivo* than in the organism from which they were derived. Due to the availability of the T cell growth factor IL-2 (Knuth *et al.*, 1984) T-lymphocytes are more readily grown *in vitro* than B-lymphocytes. Thus, adoptive therapy has been limited to the transfer of T-lymphocytes which can be considered the counterpart to the infusion of immune sera for the passive enhancement of humoral immune responses.

Individuals become immune resistant to external pathogens by developing humoral (B cell) as well as cellular (T cell) responses. The level of immune competence of an organism against a particular pathogen will, therefore, depend upon the efficiency of the combined humoral and cellular responses and the behavior of the pathogen in the extra and intra-cellular domains respectively (Zinkernagel, 1996).

Tumor antigens consist almost exclusively of intra-cellular proteins and, therefore, it is in general assumed that cellular immune responses are the prevalent immunological defense of the organism against tumors (Yewdell and Bennink, 1990). Although serological analysis of recombinant cDNA expression libraries has shown that the host can promote humoral responses against cancer-specific proteins, the antitumor role of these antibodies recognizing intra-cellular proteins remains unclear (Old and Chen, 1998). Indeed most experimental models support a predominant role of the cellular rather than the humoral arm of the immune response in cancer: the adoptive transfer of T lymphocytes from immune animals can induce resistance to tumor in the recipient animal (Restifo and Wunderlich, 1996). Furthermore, an extensive analysis of primary melanoma lesions suggested a strong correlation between brisk infiltration of T cells and long-term survival (Clemente *et al.*, 1996). For this reason, tumor immunology is focused largely on the enhancement of cellular responses and as a consequence adoptive transfer of immune cells plays a prominent role in cancer.

Contrary to the passive infusion of antibody-containing sera, whose kinetics of tissue distribution and function are well understood, the transfer of immune T cells leaves several questions open. It is yet not clear whether the function of the transfused cells is maintained once introduced in the host. It is possible for T cells to become inactivated in the host circulation. Furthermore, localization studies with ^{111}Indium labeled T cells have shown that most infused T cells are trapped in lungs, liver, spleen and other organs with an abundant Reticular Endothelial System (Pockaj *et al.*, 1994). Trapping could prevent the localization of effector cells at tumor site where their action is supposed to occur. Furthermore, the long-term fate of the infused lymphocytes and their proliferative potential *in vivo* when exposed to the target antigen are largely unknown. For these reasons, adoptive therapy with cancer-specific T cells may yield important information about target/T cell interactions *in vivo* besides providing possible therapeutic benefits.

LAK AND TILS AS EFFECTORS OF ADOPTIVE IMMUNOTHERAPY

With the identification of IL-2 as a human T cell growth factor (Morgan *et al.*, 1976), stable T cell lines could be expanded that could recognize autologous tumor cells (Knuth *et al.*, 1984). Two categories of tumor-reactive T cells were identified: LAK cells and tumor specific CTL. LAK cells were generated by culturing PBMC in IL-2 (6,000 IU/ml)

(Grimm *et al.*, 1983). Tumor-specific CTL were obtained from TIL expanded in IL-2 from single cell suspensions of tumors (Rosenberg *et al.*, 1986). LAK cells are not tumor-antigen specific and killing of ''abnormal'' cells is not MHC-restricted. Although able to kill tumor targets *in vitro*, LAK cells did not prove useful for the treatment of patients with metastatic melanoma and renal cancer. A randomized trial, in which IL-2 was administered alone or with LAK cells (Rosenberg *et al.*, 1993b), failed to show significant differences in response rates or survival.

Pre-clinical models and *in vitro* experiments with human T cells suggest that TIL recognize tumor targets 100 fold more efficiently than LAK cells (Rosenberg *et al.*, 1986; Spiess *et al.*, 1987). Administration of TIL in combination with high-dose intravenous IL-2 (720,000 IU/kg every 8 hours) is associated with regression of metastatic lesions in patients with melanoma (Rosenberg *et al.*, 1988). From 1987 through 1992, 86 consecutive patients with metastatic melanoma (145 treatment courses) were treated at the Surgery Branch, NCI with autologous TIL plus high-dose, bolus intravenous IL-2 (Rosenberg *et al.*, 1994b). One course of treatment with TIL plus IL-2 consisted of two cycles separated by an approximately 2-week interval. Patients received IL-2 at 8-hour intervals until dose limiting toxicity or a maximum of 15 doses was reached. Fifty-seven of the 86 patients also received 25 mg/kg cyclophosphamide before the first infusion of TIL plus IL-2. The response rates were 34% and not significantly different in patients who had received or not received cyclophosphamide (31 vs. 35%). Previous failure to response to IL-2 alone did not affect response rates (32% vs. 34). The frequency of response to treatment was greater in patients treated with TIL that grew more briskly in culture ($P = 0.0001$). A strong predictor of response was also the ability of TIL to lyse autologous tumor ($P = 0.0008$) and the origin of TIL from subcutaneous rather than lymph nodal metastases ($P = 0.006$). There were no treatment-related deaths although the toxicities noted were significant and required continuing monitoring of the patients in Intensive Care Unit settings. A similar study, carried out in a smaller number of melanoma patients and using a lower dose of IL-2 both to select TILs *in vitro* and to treat patients, yielded a response rate of 33% in 12 evaluable patients (Arienti *et al.*, 1993). Overall, the results suggested a potential value of immune lymphocytes for the treatment of patients with melanoma.

In the majority of cases, therapeutic administration of TIL consisted of $CD8^+$ CTL, which could readily kill HLA-matched tumor cells in *in vitro* assays. Although occasionally TIL cultures with predominantly T-helper-cell phenotype ($CD4^+$) were observed, administration of pure $CD4^+$ cultures failed in all instances to produce clinical responses. Furthermore, the ability of $CD8^+$ TIL to recognize and kill autologous or HLA-matched tumor targets *in vitro* was found to be predictive of clinical response (Rosenberg *et al.*, 1994b). These observations suggested that tumor regression is a direct consequence of CTL/tumor interaction. The empirical observation, on the other hand, that the combined administration of TIL and IL-2 only modestly enhances the frequency of tumor regression over the administration of IL-2 alone has cast doubt on the relevance of specific CTL/tumor interactions *in vivo* over the broader immunologic effects of IL-2. A definitive demonstration of the additional benefit of TIL administration over IL-2 alone for the treatment of patients with melanoma is lacking. The cost of large-scale TIL expansion *ex vivo* for clinical use and the relatively low percentage of successful TIL cultures (40–50% of attempts) has made it impractical to perform a definitive clinical study randomizing patients to receive IL-2 alone or in combination with TIL. Infusion of TIL for the treatment of patients with metastatic melanoma has been the most extensively studied form of adoptive therapy during the past decade. Although efforts to treat patients with melanoma using TIL are languishing due to the high cost, high toxicity and relatively minor therapeutic advantage over IL-2 alone, significant information was gathered by these trials which strongly influences present approaches for the biologic therapy of cancer.

TIL have also been expanded in the context of cancers different from melanoma and several clinical studies of infusion of TIL in patients with cancers other than melanoma have been reported (Belldegrun *et al.*, 1996; Freedman and Platsoucas, 1996; Melioli *et al.*, 1996; Ratto *et al.*, 1996; Figlin *et al.*, 1997). The immunologic characteristics of these effectors, however, have been more elusive since TIL include mixed populations of $CD4^+$ and $CD8^+$ cells and often it is difficult to identify the cancer-related epitope responsible for their presence in tumors. Furthermore, clinical trials did not yield results comparable to those obtained in the melanoma settings. For this reason this chapter will discuss TIL (and more broadly CTL) responses in the context of melanoma as a model that could help establish immunological principles perhaps useful in the context of other cancers.

Adoptive Immunotherapy with TIL in Melanoma Patients

Because of their high effectiveness in pre-clinical models and the ease with which tumor-specific TIL could be expanded from patients with metastatic melanoma, this particular cancer has served as the prototype model for human tumor immunology, in particular for adoptive transfer studies. The observation in animal models (Spiess *et al.*, 1987) and perhaps in humans (Rosenberg *et al.*, 1994b) that treatment with TIL plus IL-2 is of additional benefit over the administration of IL-2 alone raises the possibility that T cells are less easy to activate *in vivo* than *in vitro*. IL-2 might expand and activate T cells *in vivo* less efficiently than *in vitro*. For instance, concentrations of IL-2 necessary for the expansion of T cells might be unachievable *in vivo* without excessive toxicity but can easily be maintained in culture. Therefore efforts have continued to improve methods for expansion of large numbers of tumor-specific T cells *ex vivo* where the immune stimulatory conditions can be more easily controlled than *in vivo*. The *ex vivo* expansion of immune cells has the additional advantage of allowing targeted modifications of T cells by the addition (or removal) of beneficial characteristics. *Ex vivo* genetic manipulation of TIL resulted in one of the first examples of genetic therapy in humans (Rosenberg *et al.*, 1990; Culver *et al.*, 1991; Rosenberg *et al.*, 1993a) by the addition of a marker gene into TIL. This study was aimed at the evaluation of long-term localization and survival of adoptively transferred TIL. Localization studies using ^{111}Indium-labeled TIL had previously shown that the majority of TIL are trapped in the lung, liver and spleen of the recipient. However, in a smaller proportion of cases TIL could localize at tumor site and this localization was necessary to mediate tumor regression. None of the patients whose ^{111}Indium-labeled TIL failed to localize at tumor site responded to TIL infusion (Pockaj *et al.*, 1994). Localization, however, was not absolutely predictive of response and several cases were noted in which TIL could be demonstrated to home at tumor site yet no clinical response was observed. The limited half-life of ^{111}Indium (2.8 days) and the spontaneous release by TIL had, however, precluded long-term studies on survival and distribution of adoptively transferred T cells in humans. A breakthrough that circumvented this problem was the development of strategies, that allow stable expression of marker genes using retro-viral vectors (Aebersold *et al.*, 1990; Culver *et al.*, 1991).

TIL were modified by the introduction of a gene coding for neomycin phosphotransferase, an enzyme that induces resistance to neomycin *in vitro* allowing selection of TIL which had successfully integrated the transduced gene. When the gene-modified TIL were administered to patients their trafficking and survival *in vivo* could be monitored by PCR as the neomycin resistance gene is not part of the human genome. The infusion of the gene-modified TIL was well tolerated without any toxicity related to the gene transfer. In each of the five patients infused it was possible to demonstrate that the gene had been integrated into the TIL and was expressed. The gene-modified TIL could be recovered from PBMC of patients up to 200 days after transfer and in tumor deposits up to two months after transfer (Aebersold *et al.*, 1990). Others reported similar studies in the context of other cancers and other routes of TIL administration (Freedman *et al.*, 1996). These experiments were important because they suggested that immune cells could be expanded and genetically manipulated ex vivo before being returned into the host.

Around the same time it was noted that the effectiveness of adoptively transferred TIL correlated with the capacity of these cells to secrete tumor necrosis factor-α (TNF-α) and other cytokines in response to autologous tumor challenge (Schwartzentruber *et al.*, 1991). Pre-clinical models suggesting that cytokine release by T cells was a better correlate of response than cytotoxic activity (Asher *et al.*, 1989) also supported this clinical correlation. Although it is presently believed that these associations simply reflected a higher avidity of these CTL for their epitope (Gervois *et al.*, 1996), it was then concluded that TNF-α represented an important mediator of tumor regression. Thus the possibility of introducing functional (rather than marker) genes into TIL to enhance their antitumor activity was entertained. A small series of patients was treated with TIL genetically modified to secrete TNF-α. However, the efficiency of transduction of TIL was low and the clinical effectiveness of this technologically challenging strategy did not bear the results hoped (Rosenberg *et al.*, 1990). Nevertheless, these first attempts at the adoptive transfer of T cells modified to express functionally relevant genes solidified the concept that *ex vivo* manipulation of TIL was possible and potentially useful if the appropriate genetic strategy could be identified. Similar approaches have since been followed for the treatment of diseases other than cancer. An example is the *ex vivo* expansion of epitope-specific CTL for the treatment of opportunistic infections in immune suppressed hosts such as patients with HIV (Riddel and Greenberg, 1994). Furthermore, $CD4^+$ T cells could be made resistant to viral infection through the retro-viral transduction of anti-sense vectors directed to the HIV-1 *tat* gene. In pre-clinical models, adoptive transfer of these T cells enhanced the host resistance to HIV load (Manca *et al.*, 1997). These approaches are presently under investigation for safety and feasibility in humans (Walker, 1996).

Overall, adoptive transfer of bulk TIL populations provides minor therapeutic (if any) advantage over the administration of IL-2 alone. The discrepancy between the strong antitumor activity demonstrated by TIL *in vitro* and their limited effectiveness *in vivo* has fostered a large number of studies aimed at the understanding of the immunobiology of the TIL phenomenon. Bulk TIL cultures often consist of heterogeneous populations of which only a minority of cells recognize tumor. TIL often preferentially recognize one over another MAA in the context of a particular HLA. The preferential expansion of epitope-specific TIL is taken by some as *pro forma* evidence of immunodominance of one MAA over another. For instance, TIL derived from metastases of melanoma patients with the HLA-A*0201 phenotype recognize MART-1 in the vast majority of cases (Kawakami *et al.*, 1994). As a consequence MART-1 seems to play an immunodominant role in the context of HLA-A*0201. The same TIL cultures, however, can recognize alternative MAA on several occasions and the clinical relevance of one versus another TIL specificity is not yet clear. Kawakami *et al.* (1994) noted that while MART-1 is the most commonly recognized MAA in the context of HLA-A*0201, gp100 is the most commonly recognized MAA among TIL that, when adoptively transferred, are associated with clinical response. This observation suggests that one MAA may function as a better immunologic target for adoptive transfer efforts although, at present, the biologic reasons for such an event are obscure.

TILs Specificity and the Antigenic Heterogeneity of Target Cells

The basis for the heterogeneous specificity of TIL is not clear. It may reflect the heterogeneity of the tumor microenvironment from which TIL are generated or subtle variability of the stimulatory conditions to which TIL cultures are subjected *in vitro*. Heterogeneity of tumor microenvironment could in turn be related to variability of expression of HLA (Ferrone and Marincola, 1995; Garrido *et al.*, 1997) or MAA (Chen *et al.*, 1995; Jäger *et al.*, 1996; Cormier *et al.*, 1998; Cormier *et al.*, 1999) or other mechanisms leading to tumor tolerance *in vivo* (Marincola, 1997). Synchronous metastases are comprised of cell populations with often dramatically different patterns of expression of MAA. Furthermore, intra-lesional heterogeneity is commonly observed whereby only a portion of cancer cells express detectable levels of MAA (Cormier *et al.*, 1998). Presently it is not known what consequence tumor heterogeneity may have on the natural history of melanoma or to influence response to immunologic therapy. However, it is logical to expect that tumor heterogeneity may modulate the tumor microenvironment to a point where TIL with different specificity might be noted in different metastatic deposits or in heterogeneous areas within the same metastasis.

Molecular analysis of TCR utilization suggests an oligoclonal repertoire of TIL. TIL from different lesions from the same patient are often similar, suggesting a common systemic origin with a relative enrichment at tumor site related to the presence of an appropriate antigenic stimulus (Puisieux *et al.*, 1996; Hishii *et al.*, 1997; Clemente *et al.*, 1998). Similar conclusions can be drawn by the analysis of TCR usage in TIL after epitope-specific vaccination (Cole *et al.*, 1997; Sensi *et al.*, 1998). Furthermore, oligoclonality of TIL is supported by the observation that TIL from different metastases recognize the same epitope (Yannelli *et al.*, 1995). A predominantly monomorphic response of TIL in a particular patient suggests that adoptive transfer is likely to be broadly effective. However, these studies did not address the heterogeneity of tumor cells in synchronous metastases and variation of tumor characteristics with time. The interactive nature of tumor/T cell interactions, however, need to be taken into account in the context of tumor characterization. For example, clonal T cell responses in TIL from regressive and progressive regions of primary human melanoma demonstrate significant differences in TCR utilization (tor Straten *et al.*, 1996). Given that TIL specificity may reflect the immunogenic potential of the tumor from which they originated, lack of effectiveness of TIL could be partly related to the variability of target metastases. Synchronous metastases differing in MAA or HLA expression may demonstrate various levels of sensitivity to TIL originated from a previously removed lesion (Cormier *et al.*, 1998). Furthermore, tumors may vary with time. Excisional biopsy of tumors and subsequent expansion of TIL/tumor pairs has been used for the analysis of tumor–host interaction (Pandolfi *et al.*, 1991). However, these studies assume homogeneity among tumors in order to take the excised lesion as representative of other metastases left *in vivo*, whereas synchronous metastases are often heterogeneous in expression of MAA and HLA (Cormier *et al.*, 1998). Furthermore, the removal of the tumor excludes comparative studies of the same lesion at different points in time in relation to the natural progression of the disease or in response to immune pressure. To overcome the limitations posed by excisional biopsy, we have been following metastases by serial FNA biopsies. With this technique it is possible to evaluate tumors at various time-points for the expression of MAA, HLA and other markers with accuracy comparable to frozen section material (Marincola *et al.*, 1996). By following the same lesion serially, heterogeneity among tumors can be avoided as a confounding factor. The ability to expand TIL and autologous tumor from the FNA permits the analysis of CTL localization and function at tumor site. This strategy was tested on a melanoma patient with a metastasis of particular interest: the mass had shrunk after vaccination with a gp100 epitope (see later), suggesting effectiveness of treatment (Lee *et al.*, 1998). gp100-reactive CTL were identified in post-but not pre-vaccination PBL. Limiting dilution analysis identified one predominant CTL clone recognizing gp100 expressing targets in association with HLA-A*0201. Additionally, two autologous melanoma lines (F001TU-3 and -4) and 20 separate TIL cultures were generated from a fine needle aspirate of the metastasis at the time of progression after initial response. Both F001TU did not express gp100 and were not recognized by C1-35. Loss of gp100 by F001TU correlated with a marked reduction of gp100 expression in the same metastatic lesion compared to pre-vaccination. Thus, ineffectiveness of C1-35 and tumor progression could be best explained by loss of target antigen expression. Interestingly, 12 of 20 TIL cultures recognized F001TU but none demonstrated g209/g209-2M reactivity, suggesting a functional dissociation between systemic and local antitumor response. This example underscored the variability of the tumor microenvironment with time and its potent effects on the local immune response. Subsequent studies done in a large cohort of patients are presently ongoing and are demonstrating a strong variability in the immune response of patients related to tumor heterogeneity (Panelli *et al.*, 2000).

Identification of Relevant Epitopes Recognized by TIL

The tumor microenvironment can powerfully modulate CTL responses as elegantly demonstrated by DeBruyne *et al.* (1996). Metastatic melanoma nodules were directly injected with a vector encoding for the allogeneic HLA class I molecule HLA-B7 in the context of a vaccination protocol. The authors noted that the direct transfer of foreign MHC into human melanoma altered TCR usage in TIL (DeBruyne *et al.*, 1996). Thus TIL can be considered as the mirror image of the immunogenic potential of a tumor. Therefore, identification of the MAA recognized by TIL might yield the critical information about relevant *in vivo* epitopes. Indeed the identification of human tumor regression antigens was a direct consequence of the availability of TIL, which had been associated with antitumor responses. Kawakami and collaborators had convincingly shown that the majority of TIL recognize ''shared'' antigens in an HLA class I restricted fashion (Kawakami *et al.*, 1992). Most frequently TIL could recognize and kill not only the autologous melanoma but also most other melanoma cells originated from other patients as long as appropriately HLA matched. Furthermore, TIL could also recognize normal melanocytes (Anichini *et al.*, 1993). This observation suggested that MAA include not mutated, lineage-specific normal molecules expressed in the large majority of melanomas and therefore their identification could potentially lead to a broad application of anti-melanoma immunization strategies.

TIL lines were used to clone the genes that encoded the MAA that they recognized. cDNA libraries were developed from autologous and allogeneic HLA-matched tissue culture lines of melanoma, and these cDNA libraries were screened for recognition by TIL after transfection of cDNA into target cells expressing the appropriate MHC class I allele (Rosenberg, 1997a). Several MAA have been identified to date by this approach. While most MAA recognized by TIL are melanosomal protein remainders of the melanocytic origin of melanoma cells, some TIL recognize proteins related to the neoplastic process or mutated proteins overexpressed by cancer cells. Other TIL recognize proteins expressed differentially by cancer cells or protein products of an alternative open reading frame transcript of a non-mutated gene (see also Chapter 1).

The identification of MAA recognized by CTL and their respective epitopes led to the development of anti-melanoma vaccines, which sensitize T cells *in vivo* against specific MAA (Boon *et al.*, 1997; Rosenberg, 1997a). Among ten HLA-A2-restricted melanoma-specific TIL lines examined at the Surgery Branch of NCI, nine reacted with MART-1 and all these anti-MART-1 TIL lines recognized the same peptide, MART-1_{27-35} (AAGIGILTV). The immunodominance of MART-1_{27-35} appears to be restricted to the HLA-A*0201 phenotype as no recognition of the MAA in association with HLA alleles other than HLA-A*0201 has been described either naturally in TIL or in experimental models (Bettinotti *et al.*, 1998). A panel of ten MART-1-derived 9-mer peptides containing the HLA-A*0201 binding was screened for their ability to induce *in vitro* specific CTL with antitumor reactivity by repeated *in vitro* stimulation of PBMC. Among the ten peptides tested, MART-1_{27-35} was the only one that could induce CTL reactivity against melanoma cells, yielding more evidence for the immunodominance of this epitope in the context of HLA-A*0201. These observations suggested that MART-1_{27-35} was an ideal candidate for MAA-specific immunotherapy of melanoma patients (Rivoltini *et al.*, 1995b).

$MART\text{-}1_{27-35}$, was therefore the first peptide used for the active immunization of patients with metastatic melanoma.

In vitro Selection and Expansion of Antigen-specific TIL

The inability of *in vivo* sensitization trials to produce dramatic enhancement of clinical outcomes over IL-2 (see also the previous section "Cancer Vaccines") has re-proposed the usefulness of an *ex vivo* strategy for expansion and activation of tumor-reactive CTL. As Rivoltini and co-workers had previously shown, repeated *in vitro* stimulation of PBMC with $MART\text{-}1_{27-35}$ could generate powerful CTL capable of recognizing tumors with an efficiency 100 fold higher than TIL (Rivoltini *et al.*, 1995b). This observation provided a proof of principle that CTL reactivity against MAA could be elicited by the simple use of HLA class I restricted epitopes and suggested the utilization of this method for *ex vivo* expansion of tumor-reactive cells for adoptive transfer. Preliminary attempts to expand epitope-specific CTL *ex vivo* were, however, frustrated by limitations in achieving the number of cells believed to be necessary for adoptive transfer. It became subsequently clear that the expansion of epitope-specific CTL was more effective if T cells were elicited from PBMC obtained after successful vaccination with the same epitope. Therefore, CTL were expanded from patients that had shown powerful sensitization to gp100-209-2M (the prevalently used epitope at the Surgery Branch, NCI). Patients received leukapheresis and the whole PBMC were stimulated *in vitro* with gp100-209-2M. After 10–12 days of culture in IL-2 (300 IU/ml) CTL were tested for tumor recognition and then transfused into the patients. Using this procedure it was possible to expand epitope-specific CTL that could recognize autologous tumors in numbers comparable to those used for the administration of TIL ($1\text{–}10 \times 10^{11}$). The availability of such CTL allowed subsequent administration for therapeutic purposes. Only a few patients have been treated so far with such a protocol, due to the complexity of obtaining the CTL. Among the patients treated, one experienced a dramatic response that included the disappearance of a large number of cutaneous tumor deposits. The other patients treated with this protocol were, however, refractory to response. This method for the *ex vivo* expansion of CTL was limited by the short-term ability to expand reactive T cells. The large number of CTL obtained could be sustained only because of the large number of PBMC used to start the cultures ($2\text{–}4 \times 10^9$). Furthermore, most CTL populations used for adoptive transfer were noted to be quite heterogeneous in MAA specificity.

Recently a new technique for CTL expansion was described by Riddell and co-workers, which allows for large-scale expansion of CTL (Riddell and Greenberg, 1994; Yee *et al.*, 1996). Cultures are plated in the presence of OKT3 (anti-TCR monoclonal antibody), irradiated allogeneic PBMC and irradiated EBV-B cells in the presence of IL-2. Preliminary attempts at expansion of epitope-specific CTL bulk cultures suggested, however, that OKT-3 driven expansion, while representing a powerful stimulus, also has the potential disadvantage of stimulating a broad T cell population irrelevant to the target epitope. This strategy could be best suited for the expansion of clonal populations with antigen specificity relevant to the therapeutic aims. Based on the principle that a given MAA is recognized by a limited array of T cell clones demonstrating often preferential

TCR β-chain utilization, Maccalli *et al.* (1997) have suggested TCR β-chain driven expansion of antitumor T cells. Monoclonal antibodies recognizing predominant beta-chain expressed in 4-week mixed lymphocyte – tumor cultures were utilized to drive expansion of highly reactive CTL that could recognize autologous tumor. This approach may allow for the rapid expansion of clinically relevant T cells that could be utilized for the adoptive treatment of patients with cancer.

The use of MHC/peptide tetramers now allows a better approach to the selection and expansion of antigen (epitope)-specific T cells. In fact, either CTL clones were obtained by this technology from peripheral blood and TIL which could be characterized in a relatively short time (< 6 weeks) or sub-populations of high avidity anti-melanoma antigens (MART-1, gp100) could be isolated that lend themselves, once expanded to 10^{11-12}, as therapeutic effectors in adoptive therapy of metastatic melanoma patients (Dunbar *et al.*, 1999; Yee *et al.*, 1999).

In the NCI experience it was noted that in a significant proportion of cases CTL generated by epitope sensitization *in vitro*, although able to recognize the target cells pulsed with the relevant epitope, often could not recognize autologous (when available) or HLA matched tumors. In a significant proportion of cases the *in vivo* immunization followed by the *in vitro* sensitization of CTL with peptide had stimulated CTL with a broad TCR repertoire often characterized by low avidity for the HLA–peptide complex. Limiting dilution cloning of these CTL demonstrated sub-populations of CTL with low avidity for the target epitope. These clones released IFN-γ upon exposure to HLA matched target cells pulsed with high concentrations of relevant epitope, but did not release IFN-γ when exposed to the same target cells pulsed with lower concentrations of epitope. The low avidity of interaction with epitope-pulsed targets strongly correlated with inability to recognize HLA matched tumor target supposedly because of the lower surface epitope density naturally expressed by tumors. Overall, clonal analysis demonstrated that epitope-derived CTL cultures are extremely variable and only a minority of T cells with the highest avidity of TCR–epitope interactions can recognize tumor targets. This latter finding suggests that the expression of surface epitope in tumors may be below the threshold of recognition for some T cell populations elicited by the vaccination (Dudley *et al.*, 1999).

It is reasonable to postulate that CTL/TIL attracted to a tumor site and activated *in situ* by antigen-presenting cells or systemically by vaccination efforts may be incapable of recognizing tumor cells if the antigenic stimulation provided by the targets themselves is inadequate. Inadequacy of tumor cells includes loss of HLA (Ferrone and Marincola, 1995) and/or tumor antigens (Marincola *et al.*, 1996) and abnormalities in antigen processing (Restifo *et al.*, 1993). In general, such mechanisms are analyzed as ‘‘all-or-none’’ occurrences with little attention to quantitative aspects. It is possible, however, that in the natural environment, productive engagements between TCR and HLA–peptide complexes proceed to a point where balance between avidity for binding and availability of ligand is achieved. A recent analysis of HLA/MAA expression in cell lines showed that variation in HLA expression can occur in a limited but significant proportion of melanoma cell lines. This variability could have functional significance because it occurred within a range likely to affect recognition by T cells, particularly in situations of low MAA expression. Finally, decreased MAA expression was frequently observed in cell lines and was an independent factor determining target susceptibility to lysis by CTL (Cormier *et al.*,

1999). Based on the observation that CTL cultures have TCR repertoires with variable avidity for their target and the realization that several tumors may have sub-optimal epitope density, a new protocol was developed at the NCI, in which clones are developed from epitope-specific bulk cultures by limiting dilution. The clones are selected according to their avidity for the relevant epitope and recognition of HLA matched tumors, expanded with OKT3 and given to patients. This protocol has just been initiated. Although the strategy has proven feasible, no clinical data are yet available.

The main focus of adoptive therapy is to provide optimally activated T cell immune responses of a greater magnitude and breadth than those achievable *in vivo* by direct sensitization of circulating lymphocytes. However, the CTL to be used for adoptive transfer are quantitatively and qualitatively assessed by *in vitro* testing methods. All of these methods assume that the analyses performed *in vitro* are relevant to the *in vivo* environment. Many possible mechanisms, however, have been proposed for the inability of MAA-specific CTL to eliminate tumors *in vivo* (Table 5.3). Some have suggested that alteration in TCR and signal transduction molecules *in vivo* may lead to central immunosuppression of cancer patients (Zea *et al.*, 1995) which may affect selected sub-populations of tumor-specific T cells (Maccalli *et al.*, 1999), although its functional significance is controversial (Cardi *et al.*, 1997). It is also possible that the very nature of most MAA, which are non-mutated self-molecules, may be a reason for central tolerance (Kawakami *et al.*, 1995). Lack of CTL localization at the tumor site has been shown to correlate with lack of response to adoptive therapy with melanoma-specific CTL (Pockaj *et al.*, 1994). Furthermore, expression of apoptotic signals (Hahne *et al.*, 1996) has been reported to lead to tumor escape from immune recognition by elimination of tumor-reactive TIL. This mechanism, however, has been recently challenged by several investigators that either could not identify Fas-L expression by tumor cells (Chappell *et al.*, 1999) or could identify it only after treatment of the same with metalloprotease inhibitors (Rivoltini *et al.*, 1998). Furthermore, TIL appear to be resistant to Fas-L induced apoptosis (Rivoltini *et al.*, 1998). The tumor microenvironment is also characterized by the production of immunosuppressive cytokines either by tumor cells (Luscher *et al.*, 1994; Wojtowicz-Praga, 1997) or by TIL (Whiteside and Parmiani, 1994). As previously noted, loss of expression of HLA (Ferrone and Marincola, 1995) or target antigens (Cormier *et al.*, 1998). could lead to ineffectiveness of MAA-specific TIL. Finally it is possible that the conditions of antigen presentation exercised by tumors are not optimal to maintain relevant T cells in a status of activation at the tumor site (Fuchs and Matzinger, 1996; Gervois *et al.*, 1996). These multiple means of tumor tolerance should be considered in the future, particularly if the adoptive transfer of high avidity CTL clones fails to provoke the expected clinical responses.

ADOPTIVE IMMUNOTHERAPY IN HEMATOLOGICAL DISEASES

Adoptive immunotherapy is being successfully used in a particular clinical setting, namely in hematological diseases requiring allogeneic bone marrow transplantation. In fact, allogeneic stem cell transplants have been used in several hematological malignancies, including chronic myeloid leukemia (CML) and acute lymphoblastic B cell leukemia

(B-ALL) (O'Reilly, 1993). This therapeutic procedure may cause a graft vs. leukemia effect that is mediated by the donor T cells (see Antin, 1993). These cells represent a subpopulation of the whole T cells endowed with the capacity of recognizing the recipient-derived leukemic cells only and distinct from anti-allogeneic T lymphocytes (Mackinnon *et al.*, 1995).

The antigens recognized by the anti-leukemic T cells were also partially characterized as belonging to the ill-defined group of minor histocompatibility antigens known to be preferentially expressed by leukemic and EBV-transformed blasts (Den Haan *et al.*, 1995; Dolstra *et al.*, 1999). Therefore, clinical studies were carried out in which infusion of donors' T cells was shown to eradicate leukemic cells without compromising hematopoiesis of recipients during the chronic phase after allogeneic stem cell transplantation (Falkenburg *et al.*, 1993). More recently, even patients undergoing the accelerated phase of CML could achieve complete remission after adoptive immunotherapy with donor CTL recognizing CML precursor cells, such effectors being obtained after selection *in vitro* of T cells able to inhibit the *in vitro* growth of CML progenitors (Falkenburg *et al.*, 1999). Moreover, transplanted leukemic patients that develop EBV-induced B lymphomas upon immunosuppression, a potentially lethal complication, can also be cured by infusion of donor lymphocytes (Lucas *et al.*, 1996). Despite the fact that most of the therapeutic donor T cells are not directed against tumor antigens, these studies prove the principle that, in the presence of stably expressed antigens on target cells, infusion of T lymphocytes recognizing these antigens can result in a significant destruction of tumor cells.

CONCLUSIONS

Adoptive transfer of immune competent T cells has been instructive for tumor immunologists and the biomedical community at large. It has also suggested possible therapeutic benefits, although a definitive demonstration of its effectiveness is, contrary to murine models, still lacking in cancer patients. Thus the experimental nature of adoptive therapy for cancer needs to be emphasized at this point. Yet, it is likely that adoptive therapy will significantly contribute to the wealth of information accumulated by the exploitation of biological approaches for the treatment of cancer.

REFERENCES

Abrams, J.S., Rayner, A.A., Wiernik, P.H., Parkinson, D.R., Eisenberger, M., Aronson, F.R., Gucalp, R., Atkins, M.B., and Hawkins, M.J. (1990) High-dose recombinant interleukin-2 alone:a regimen with limited activity in the treatment of advanced renal cell carcinoma. *J. Natl. Cancer Inst. USA*, **82**, 1202–1206.

Aebersold, P., Kasid, A., and Rosenberg, S.A. (1990) Selection of gene-marked tumor infiltrating lymphocytes from post-treatment biopsies: a case study. *Hum. Gene Ther.*, **1**, 373–384.

Alexander, J., Sidney, J., Southwood, S., Ruppert, J., Oseroff, C., Maewal, A., Snoke, K., Serra, H.M., Kubbo, R.T., Sette, A., and Grey, H.M. (1994) Development of high potency universal DR-restricted helper epitopes by modification of high affinity DR-blocking peptides. *Immunity*, **1**, 751–761.

Angevin, E., Valteau-Couanet, D., Farace, F., Dietrich, P.Y., Lecesne, A., Triebel, F., and Escudier, B. (1995) Phase I study of prolonged low-dose subcutaneous recombinant interleukin-2 (IL-2) in patients with advanced cancer. *J. Immunother.*, **18**, 188–195.

Anichini, A., Maccalli, C., Mortarini, R., Salvi, S., Mazzocchi, A., Squarcina, P., Herlyn, M., and Parmiani, G. (1993) Melanoma cells and normal melanocytes share antigens recognized by HLA-A2-restricted cytotoxic T cell clones from melanoma patients. *J. Exp. Med.*, **177**, 989–998.

Anichini, A., Molla, A., Mortarini, R., Tragni, G., Bersani, I., Di Nicola, M., Gianni, M., Pilotti, S., Dunbar, R., Cerundolo, V., and Parmiani, G. (1999) An expanded peripheral T cell population to a cytotoxic T lymphocyte (CTL)-defined, melanocyte-specific antigen in metastatic melanoma patients impacts on generation of peptide-specific CTL, but does not overcome tumor escape from immune surveillance in metastatic lesions. *J. Exp. Med.*, **190**, 651–668.

Antin, J.H. (1993) Graft-versus-leukemia. No longer an epiphenomenon. *Blood*, **82**, 2273–2277.

Arienti, F., Belli, F., Rivoltini, L., Gambacorti-Passerini, C., Furlan, L., Mascheroni, L., Prada, A., Rizzi, M., Marchesi, E., Vaglini, M., Parmiani, G., and Cascinelli, N. (1993) Adoptive immunotherapy of advanced melanoma patients with interleukin-2 (IL-2) and tumor-infiltrating lymphocytes selected *in vitro* with low doses of IL-2. *Cancer Immunol. Immunother.*, **36**, 315–322.

Arienti, F., Belli, F., Napolitano, F., Sulé-Suso, J., Mazzocchi, A., Gallino, G.F., Cattelan, A., Sanantonio, C., Rivoltini, L., Melani, C., Colombo, M.P., Cascinelli, N., Maio, M., and Parmiani, G. (1999) Vaccination of melanoma patients with interleukin 4 gene-transduced allogeneic melanoma cells. *Hum. Gene Ther.*, **10**, 2907–2916.

Asher, A.L., Mulé, J.J., and Rosenberg, S.A. (1989) Recombinant human tumor necrosis factor mediates regression of a murine sarcoma *in vivo* via Lyt-2+ cells. *Cancer Immunol. Immunother.*, **28**, 153–156.

Ashley, D.M., Faiola, B., Nair, S., Hale, L.P., Bigner, D.D., and Gilboa, E. (1997) Bone marrow-generated dendritic cells pulsed with tumor extracts or tumor RNA induce antitumor immunity against central nervous system tumors. *J. Exp. Med.*, **186**, 1177–1182.

Atkins, M.B., Sparano, J., Fisher, R.I., Weiss, G.R., Margolin, K.A., Fink, K.I., Rubinstein, L., Louie, A., Mier, J.W., and Gucalp, R. (1993) Randomized phase II trial of high-dose interleukin-2 either alone or in combination with interferon-α-2b in advanced renal cell carcinoma. *J. Clin. Oncol.*, **11**, 661–670.

Atzpodien, J., Kirchner, H., Duensing, S., Lopez, H.E., Franzke, A., Buer, J., Probst, M., Anton, P., and Poliwoda, H. (1995a) Biochemotherapy of advanced metastatic renal-cell carcinoma: results of the combination of interleukin-2, alpha-interferon, 5-fluorouracil, vinblastine, and 13-cis-retinoic acid. *World J. Urol.*, **13**, 174–177.

Atzpodien, J., Lopez, H.E., Kirchner, H., Bodenstein, H., Pfreundschuh, M., Rebmann, U., Metzner, B., Illiger, H.J., Jakse, G., and Niesel, T. (1995b) Multiinstitutional home-therapy trial of recombinant human IL-2 and interferon-α-2 in progressive metastatic renal cell carcinoma. *J. Clin. Oncol.*, **13**, 497–501.

Bajetta, E., Del Vecchio, M., Mortarini, R., Nadeau, R., Rakhit, A., Rimassa, L., Fowst, C., Borri, A., Anichini, A., and Parmiani, G. (1998) Pilot study of subcutaneous recombinant human interleukin 12 in metastatic melanoma. *Clin. Cancer Res.*, **4**, 75–85.

Bajorin, D.F., Sell, K.W., Richards, J.M., Walther, P.J., O'Connell, M., Motzer, R., Vogelzang, N.J., Zeffren, J., and Levitt, D. (1990) A randomized trial of interleukin-2 plus lymphokine-activated killer cells versus il-2 alone in renal cell carcinoma. *Proc. Am. Ass. Cancer Res.*, **31**, A1106.

Banchereau, J., and Steinman, R.M. (1998) Dendritic cells and the control of immunity. *Nature*, **392**, 245–252.

Bartsch, H.H., Adler, M., Ringert, R.H., Boaziz, C., Symann, M., Humblet, Y., Bosly, A., Franks, C.R., Palmer, P., and Evers, M.P. (1990) Sequential therapy of recombinant interferon–alpha (IFN-α) and recombinant interleukin 2 (Il-2) in patients with advanced renal cell cancer (RCC). *Proc. Am. Soc. Clin. Oncol.*, **9**, A556.

Belldegrun, A., Tso, C.L., Kaboo, R., Pang, S., Pierce, W., deKernion, J.B., and Figlin, R. (1996) Natural immune reactivity-associated therapeutic response in patients with metastatic renal cell carcinoma receiving tumor-infiltrating lymphocytes and interleukin-2-based therapy. *J. Immunother. Emphasis Tumor Immunol.*, **19**, 149–161.

Belli, F., Arienti, F., Sulé-Suso, J., Clemente, C., Mascheroni, L., Cattelan, A., Sanantonio, C., Gallino, G.F., Melani, C., Rao, S., Colombo, M.P., Maio, M., Cascinelli, N., and Parmiani, G. (1997) Active immunization of metastatic melanoma patients with interleukin-2 transduced allogeneic melanoma cells: evaluation of efficacy and tolerability. *Cancer Immunol. Immunother.*, **44**, 197–203.

Bendandi, M., Gocke, C.D., Kobrin, C.B., Benko, F.A., Sternas, L.A., Pennington, R., Watson, T.M., Reynolds, C.W., Gause, B.L., Duffey, P.L., Jaffe, E.S., Creekmore, S.P., Longo, D.L., and Kwak, L.W. (1999) Complete molecular remissions induced by patient-specific vaccination plus granulocyte-monocyte colony-stimulating factor against lymphoma. *Nature Med.*, **5**, 1171–1177.

Bennett, S.R., Carbone, F.R., Karamalis, F., Flavell, R.A., Miller, J.F., and Heath, W.R. (1998) Help for cytotoxic-T-cell responses is mediated by CD40 signalling. *Nature*, **393**, 478–480.

Berd, D., and Mastrangelo, M.J. (1988) Effect of low dose cyclophosphamide on the immune system of cancer patients: depletion of CD4+, 2H4+ suppressor-inducer T-cells. *Cancer Res.*, **48**, 1671–1675.

Berd, D., Murphy, G., Maguire, H.C. Jr., and Mastrangelo, M.J. (1991) Immunization with haptenized, autologous tumor cells induces inflammation of human melanoma metastases. *Cancer Res.*, **51**, 2731–2734.

Bergmann, L., Weidmann, E., Mitrou, P.S., Runne, ·U., Keilholz, U., Bartsch, H.H., and Franks, C.R. (1990) Interleukin-2 in combination with interferon-alpha in disseminated malignant melanoma and advanced renal cell carcinoma. A phase I/II study. *Onkologie*, **13**, 137–140.

Bergmann, L., Fenchel, K., Weidmann, E., Enzinger, H.M., Jahn, B., Jonas, D., and Mitrou, P.S. (1993) Daily alternating administration of high-dose alpha-2b-interferon and interleukin-2 bolus infusion in metastatic renal cell cancer. A phase II study. *Cancer*, **72**, 1733–1742.

Besana, C., Tresoldi, M., Foppoli, M., Di Lucca, G., Fortis, C., Marcatti, M., Corti, C., Matteucci, P., Borri, A., and Tognella, S. (1993) Sequential therapy with recombinant interleukin-2 and alpha-interferon for advanced renal cell cancer: a preliminary report. *Proc. Am. Ass. Cancer Res.*, **34**, A2772.

Bettinotti, M., Kim, C.J., Lee, K.-H., Roden, M., Cormier, J.N., Panelli, M.C., Parker, K.C., and Marincola, F.M. (1998) Stringent allele/epitope requirements for MART-1/Melan A immunodominance: implications for peptide-based immunotherapy. *J. Immunol.*, **161**, 877–889.

Bindon, C., Czerniecki, M., Ruell, P., Edwards, A., McCarthy, W.H., Harris, R., and Hersey, P. (1983) Clearance rates and systemic effects of intravenously administered interleukin 2 (IL-2) containing preparations in human subjects. *Br. J. Cancer*, **47**, 123–133.

Boon, T., Coulie, P.G., and Van den Eynde, B. (1997) Tumor antigens recognized by T cells. *Immunol. Today*, **18**, 267–268.

Borysiewicz, L.K., Fiander, A., Nimako, M., Man, S., Wilkinson, G.W.G., Westmoreland, D., Evans, A.S., Adams, M., Stacey, S.N., Boursnell, M.E.G., Rutheford, E., Hickling, J.K., and Inglis, S.C. (1996) A recombinant vaccinia virus encoding human papillomavirus type 16 and 18, E6 and E7 protins as immunotherapy for cervical cancer. *Lancet*, **347**, 1523–1527.

Budd, G.T., Sergi, J., Finke, J., Tubbs, R., Murthy, S., Gibson, V., Medendorp, S., Bauer, L., Barna, B., and Boyett, J. (1990) Combination interleukin-2 and alpha-interferon therapy of metastatic renal cell carcinoma and malignant melanoma. *Proc. Am. Ass. Cancer Res.*, **31**, A1603.

Budd, G.T., Murthy, S., Finke, J., Sergi, J., Gibson, V., Medendorp, S., Barna, B., Boyett, J., and Bukowski, R.M. (1992) Phase I trial of high-dose bolus interleukin-2 and interferon alfa-2a in patients with metastatic malignancy. *J. Clin. Oncol.*, **10**, 804–809.

Bukowski, R.M., Olencki, T., Wang, Q., Peereboom, D., Budd, G.T., Elson, P., Sandstrom, K., Tuason, L., Rayman, P., Tubbs, R., McLain, D., Klein, E., Novick, A., and Finke, J. (1997) Phase II trial of interleukin-2 and interferon-alpha in patients with renal cell carcinoma: clinical results and immunologic correlates of response. *J. Immunother.*, **20**, 301–311.

Burnet, F.M. (1970) The concept of immunological surveillance. *Prog. Exp. Tumor Res.*, **13**, 1–27.

Carbone, F.R., Kurts, C., Bennett, S.R.M., Miller, J.F.A.P., and Heath, W.R. (1998) Cross-presentation: a general mechanism for CTL immunity and tolerance. *Immunol. Today*, **19**, 368–373.

Cardi, G., Heaney, J.A., Schned, A.R., Phillips, D.M., Branda, M.T., and Ernstoff, M.S. (1997) T-cell receptor zeta-chain expression on tumor-infiltrating lymphocytes from renal cell carcinoma. *Cancer Res.*, **57**, 3517–3519.

Cascinelli, N. (1995). Evaluation of efficacy of adjuvant rIFN alpha 2a in melanoma patients with regional node metastases. *Proc. Am. Soc. Clin. Oncol.*, **15**, 15.

Cassel, W.A., and Murray, D.R. (1992) A ten-year follow-up on stage II malignant melanoma patients treated postsurgically with Newcastle Disease Virus oncolysate. *Med. Oncol. Tumor Pharmacother.*, **9**, 169–171.

Castelli, C., Storkus, W.J., Maeurer, M.J., Martin, D.M., Huang, E.C., Pramanik, B.N., Nagabhushan, T.L., Parmiani, G., and Lotze, M.T. (1995) Mass spectrometric identification of a naturally processed melanoma peptide recognized by $CD8^+$ cytotoxic T lymphocytes. *J. Exp. Med.*, **181**, 363–368.

Cebon, J.S., Jaeger, E., Gibbs, P., Davis, I., Hopkins, W., Gibbs, S. *et al.* (1999) Phase I studies of immunization with Melan-A and IL-12 in HLA-A2+ positive patients with stage III and IV malignant melanoma. *Proc. Am. Soc. Clin. Oncol.*, **18**, 434a.

Celluzzi, C.M., and Falo, L.D. Jr. (1998) Physical interaction between dendritic cells and tumor cells results in an immunogen that induces protective and therapeutic tumor rejection. *J. Immunol.*, **160**, 3081–3085.

Chakraborty, N.G., Sporn, J.R., Tortora, A.F., Kurtzman, S.H., Yamase, H., Ergin, M.T., and Mukherji, B. (1998) Immunization with a tumor-cell-lysate-loaded autologous-antigen-presenting-cell-based vaccine in melanoma. *Cancer Immunol. Immunother.*, **47**, 58–64.

Chang, A.E., Cameron, M.J., Sondak, V.K., Geiger, J.D., and Vander, W.D. (1995) A phase II trial of interleukin-2 and interferon-alpha in the treatment of metastatic colorectal carcinoma. *J. Immunother.*, **18**, 253–262.

Chappell, D.B., Zaks, T.Z., Rosenberg, S.A., and Restifo, N.P. (1999) Human melanoma cells do not express Fas (APO-1/CD95) ligand. *Cancer Res.*, **59**, 59–62.

Chaux, P., Vantomme, V., Coulie, P., Boon, T., and van der Bruggen, P. (1998) Estimation of the frequencies of anti-MAGE-3 cytolytic T-lymphocyte precursors in blood from individuals without cancer. *Int. J. Cancer*, **77**, 538–542.

Chen, Y.-T., Stockert, E., Tsang, S., Coplan, K.E., and Old, L.J. (1995) Immunophenotyping of melanomas for tyrosinase: implications for vaccine development. *Proc. Natl. Acad. Sci. USA*, **92**, 8125–8129.

Chu, R.S., Targoni, O.S., Krieg, A.M., Lehmann, P.V., and Harding, C.V. (1997) CpG oligodeoxynucleotides act as adjuvants that switch on T helper 1 (Th1) immunity. *J. Exp. Med.*, **186**, 1623–1631.

Clemente, C.G., Mihm, M.C.J., Bufalino, R., Zurrida, S., Collini, P., and Cascinelli, N. (1996) Prognostic value of tumor infiltrating lymphocytes in the vertical growth phase of primary cutaneous melanoma. *Cancer*, **77**, 1303–1310.

Clemente, C., Rao, S., Lupetti, R., Tragni, G., Pisarra, P., Bersani, I., Parmiani, G., Mihm, M.C.J., and Sensi, M. (1998) Immunohistochemical analysis of the T-cell receptor beta-chain variable regions expressed by T lymphocytes infiltrating primary human melanoma. *Lab. Invest.*, **78**, 619–627.

Cole, D.J., Wilson, M.C., Baron, P.L., O'Brien, P., Reed, C., Tsang, K.Y., and Schlom, J. (1996) Phase I study of recombinant CEA vaccinia virus vaccine with post vaccination CEA peptide challenge. *Hum. Gene Ther.*, **7**, 1381–1394.

Cole, D.J., Wilson, M.C., Rivoltini, L., Custer, M., and Nishimura, M.I. (1997) T-cell receptor repertoire in matched MART-1 peptide-stimulated peripheral blood lymphocytes and tumor-infiltrating lymphocytes. *Cancer Res.*, **57**, 5320–5327.

Cole, D.E., Sanda, M.G., Yang, J.C., Schwartzentruber, D., Weber, J., Ettinghausen, S., Pockaj, B.A., Kim, H.I., Levin, R., Progrebniak, H.W., Balkissoon, J., Fenton, R., DeBarge, L.R., Kaye, J., Rosenberg, S.A., and Parkinson, D.R. (1998). Phase I trial of recombinant human macrophage colony-stimulating factor administered by continuous intravenous infusion in patients with metastatic cancer. *J. Natl. Cancer Inst. USA*, **86**, 39–45.

Cormier, J.N., Hurst, R., Vasselli, J., Lee, D., Kim, C.J., McKee, M., Venzon, D., White, D., Marincola, F.M., and Rosenberg, S.A. (1997a) A prospective randomized evaluation of the prophylactic use of low-dose dopamine in cancer patients receiving interleukin-2. *J. Immunother.*, **20**, 292–300.

Cormier, J.N., Salgaller, M.L., Prevette, T., Barracchini, K.C., Rivoltini, L., Restifo, N.P., Rosenberg, S.A., and Marincola, F.M. (1997b) Enhancement of cellular immunity in melanoma patients immunized with a peptide from MART-1/Melan A. *Cancer J. Sci. Am.*, **3**, 37–44.

Cormier, J.N., Hijazi, Y.M., Abati, A., Fetsch, P., Bettinotti, M., Steinberg, S.M., Rosenberg, S.A., and Marincola, F.M. (1998) Heterogeneous expression of melanoma-associated antigens (MAA) and HLA-A2 in metastatic melanoma *in vivo*. *Int. J. Cancer*, **75**, 517–524.

Cormier, J.N., Panelli, M.C., Hackett, J.A., Bettinotti, M., Mixon, A., Wunderlich, J., Parker, L., Restifo, N.P., Ferrone, S., and Marincola, F.M. (1999) Natural variation of the expression of HLA and endogenous antigen modulates CTL recognition in an *in vitro* melanoma model. *Int. J. Cancer*, **80**, 781–790.

Creagan, E.T., Dalton, R.J., Ahmann, D.L., Jung, S.H., Morton, R.F., Langdon, R.M.J., Kugler, J., and Rodrigue, L.J. (1995) Randomized, surgical adjuvant clinical trial of recombinant interferon alfa-2a in selected patients with malignant melanoma. *J. Clin. Oncol.*, **13**, 2776–2783.

Creekmore, S.P., Harris, J.E., Ellis, T.M., Braun, D.P., Cohen, I.I., Bhoopalam, N., Jassak, P.F., Cahill, M.A., Canzoneri, C.L., and Fisher, R.I. (1989) A phase I clinical trial of recombinant interleukin-2 by periodic 24-hour intravenous infusions. *J. Clin. Oncol.*, **7**, 276–284.

Culver, K., Cornetta, K., Morgan, R., Morecki, S., Aebersold, P., Kasid, A., Lotze, M., Rosenberg, S.A., Anderson, W.F., and Blaese, R.M. (1991) Lymphocytes as cellular vehicles for gene therapy in mouse and man. *Proc. Natl. Acad. Sci. USA*, **88**, 3155–3159.

Curti, B.D., Ochoa, A.C., Powers, G.C., Kopp, W.C., Alvord, W.G., Janik, J.E., Gause, B.L., Dunn, B., Kopreski, M.S., Fenton, R., Zea, A., Dansky-Ullmann, C., Strobl, S., Harvey, L., Nelson, E., Sznol, M., and Longo, D.L. (1998) Phase I trial of anti-CD3-stimulated $CD4^+$ T cells, infusional interleukin-2, and cyclophosphamide in patients with advanced cancer. *J. Clin. Oncol.*, **16**, 2752–2760.

DeBruyne, L.A., Chang, A.E., Cameron, M.J., Yang, Z., Gordon, D., Nabel, E.G., Nabel, G.J., and Bishop, D.K. (1996) Direct transfer of a foreign MHC gene into human melanoma alters T cell receptor V beta usage by tumor-infiltrating lymphocytes. *Cancer Immunol. Immunother.*, **43**, 49–58.

Demchak, P., Atkins, M., Sell, K., Givant, E., and Lipton, A. (1991a) Phase II study of interleukin-2 (IL-2) and interferon alpha-2a (IFN-Alpha) outpatient therapy for metastatic renal cancer. *Proc. Am. Soc. Clin. Oncol.*, **10**, A565.

Demchak, P.A., Mier, J.W., Robert, N.J., O'Brien, K., Gould, J.A., and Atkins, M.B. (1991b) IL-2 and high-dose cisplatin in patients with metastatic melanoma: a pilot study. *J. Clin. Oncol.*, **9**, 1821–1830.

Den Haan, J.M.M., Sherman, N.E., Blokland, E., Huczko, E., Koning, F., Drijfhout, J.W., Skipper, J., Shabanowitz, J., Hunt, D.F., Engelhard, V.H., and Goulney, E. (1995) Identification of a graft versus host disease-associated human minor histocompatibility antigen. *Science*, **268**, 1476–1480.

Disis, M.L., Gralow, J.R., Bernhard, H., Hand, S.L., Rubin, W.D., and Cheever, M.A. (1996) Peptide-based, but not whole protein, vaccines elicit immunity to HER-2/neu, an oncogenic self-protein. *J. Immunol.*, **156**, 3151–3158.

Doherty, P.C., Dunlop, M.B., Parish, C.R., and Zinkernagel, R.M. (1976) Inflammatory process in murine lymphocytic choriomeningitis is maximal in H-2K or H-2D compatible interactions. *J. Immunol.*, **117**, 187–190.

Dolstra, H., Fredrix, H., Maas, F., Coulie, P.G., Brasseur, F., Mensink, E., Adema, G.J., de Witte, T.M., Figdor, C.G., and van de Wiel-van Kemenade, E. (1999) A human minor histocompatibility antigen specific for B cell acute lymphoblastic leukemia. *J. Exp. Med.*, **189**, 301–308.

Dorval, T., Fridman, W.H., Mathiot, C., Sastre, X., and Pouillart, P. (1992) Treatment of metastatic malignant melanoma with interleukin-2. *Bull. Cancer*, **79**, 781–787.

Dranoff, G., Jaffee, E., Lazenby, A., Golumbek, P., Levitsky, H., Brose, K., Jackson, V., Hamada, H., Pardoll, D., and Mulligan, R.C. (1993) Vaccination with irradiated tumor cells engineered to secrete murine granulocyte-macrophage colony-stimulating factor stimulates potent, specific, and long-lasting anti-tumor immunity. *Proc. Natl. Acad. Sci. USA*, **90**, 3539–3543.

Dudley, M.E., Nishimura, M.I., Holt, A.K.C., and Rosenberg, S.A. (1999) Anti-tumor immunization with a minimal peptide epitope (G9-209-2M) leads to a functionally heterogeneous CTL response. *J. Immunother.*, **22**, 288–298.

Dunbar, P.R., Chen, J.L., Chao, D., Rust, N., Teisserenc, H., Ogg, G.S., Romero, P., Weynants, P., and Cerundolo, V. (1999) Cutting edge: rapid cloning of tumor-specific CTL suitable for adoptive immunotherapy of melanoma. *J. Immunol.*, **162**, 6959–6962.

Dutcher, J.P., Atkins, M., Fisher, R., Weiss, G., Margolin, K., Aronson, F., Sosman, J., Lotze, M., Gordon, M., Logan, T., and Mier, J. (1997) Interleukin-2-based therapy for metastatic renal cell cancer: the Cytokine Working Group experience, 1989–1997. *Cancer J. Sci. Am.*, **3**, S73–S78.

Elder, G.J., Hersey, P., and Branley, P. (1997) Remission of transplanted melanoma – clinical course and tumour cell characterisation. *Clin. Transplant.*, **11**, 565–568.

Ellerhorst, J.A., Sella, A., Amato, R.J., Tu, S.M., Millikan, R.E., Finn, L.D., Banks, M., and Logothetis, C.J. (1997) Phase II trial of 5-fluorouracil, interferon-alpha and continuous infusion interleukin-2 for patients with metastatic renal cell carcinoma. *Cancer*, **80**, 2128–2132.

Esche, C., Subbotin, V.M., Maliszewski, C., Lotze, M.T., and Shurin, M.R. (1998) FLT3 ligand administration inhibits tumor growth in murine melanoma and lymphoma. *Cancer Res.*, **58**, 380–383.

Escudier, B., Rossi, J.F., Ravaud, A., Douillard, J.Y., Negrier, S., Baume, D., Dorval, T., Chevreau, C., Mignot, L., and Pein, F. (1992) French experience of high-dose il2 on a two-days-a-week schedule in metastatic renal cell carcinoma: a multicentric study. *Proc. Am. Soc. Clin. Oncol.*, **11**, A651.

Eskander, E.D., Harvey, H.A., Givant, E., and Lipton, A. (1997) Phase I study combining tumor necrosis factor with interferon-alpha and interleukin-2. *Am. J. Clin. Oncol.*, **20**, 511–514.

Estin, C.D., Stevenson, U.S., Plowman, G.D., Hu, S.L., Sridhar, P., Hellstrom, I., Brown, J.P., and Hellstrom, K.E. (1988) Recombinant vaccinia virus vaccine against the human melanoma antigen p97 for use in immunotherapy. *Proc. Natl. Acad. Sci. USA*, **85**, 1052–1056.

Eton, O., Talpaz, M., Lee, K.H., Rothberg, J.M., Brell, J.M., and Benjamin, R.S. (1996) Phase II trial of recombinant human interleukin-2 and interferon-alpha-2a: implications for the treatment of patients with metastatic melanoma. *Cancer*, **77**, 893–899.

Falkenburg, J.H., Faber, L.M., van den Elshout, M., van Luxemburg-Heijs, S.A., Hooftman-den Otter, A., Smit, W.M., Voogt, P.J., and Willemze, R. (1993) Generation of donor-derived antileukemic cytotoxic T-lymphocyte responses for treatment of relapsed leukemia after allogeneic HLA-identical bone marrow transplantation. *J. Immunother.*, **14**, 305–309.

Falkenburg, J.H.F., Wafelman, A.R., Joosten, P., Smit, W.M., van Bergen, C.A.M., Bongaerts, R., Lurvink, E., van der Hoorn, M., Kluck, P., Landegent, J.E., Kluin-Nelemans, H.C., Fibbe, W.E., Willemze, R. (1999) Complete remission of accelerated phase chronic myeloid leukemia by treatment with leukemia-reactive cytotoxic T lymphocytes. *Blood*, **94**, 1201–1208.

Fenton, R.G., Keller, C.J., Hanna, N., and Taub, D.D. (1995) Induction of T-cell immunity against Ras oncoproteins by soluble protein or Ras-expressing Escherichia coli. *J. Natl. Cancer Inst. USA*, **87**, 1853–1861.

Ferrone, S., and Marincola, F.M. (1995) Loss of HLA class I antigens by melanoma cells: molecular mechanisms, functional significance and clinical relevance. *Immunol. Today*, **16**, 487–494.

Figlin, R.A., Pierce, W.C., Kaboo, R., Tso, C.L., Moldawer, N., Gitlitz, B., deKernion, J., and Belldegrun, A. (1997) Treatment of metastatic renal cell carcinoma with nephrectomy, interleukin-2 and cytokine-primed or CD8(+) selected tumor infiltrating lymphocytes from primary tumor. *J. Urol.*, **158**, 740–745.

Foon, K.A., Maluish, A.E., Abrams, P.G., Wrightington, S., Stevenson, H.C., Alarif, A., Fer, M.F., Overton, W.R., Poole, M., and Schnipper, E.F. (1986) Recombinant leukocyte A interferon therapy for advanced hairy cell leukemia. Therapeutic and immunologic results. *Am. J. Med.*, **80**, 351–356.

Freedman, R.S., and Platsoucas, C.D. (1996) Immunotherapy for peritoneal ovarian carcinoma metastasis using *ex vivo* expanded tumor-infiltrating lymphocytes. *Cancer Treat. Res.*, **82**, 115–146.

Freedman, R.S., Platsoucas, C.D., and Deisseroth, A.B. (1996) Use of a retroviral vector to study the trafficking patterns of purified ovarian tumor infiltrating lymphocytes (TIL) used in intraperitoneal adoptive immunotherapy of ovarian cancer patients. A pilot study. *Hum. Gene Ther.*, **7**, 1351–1365.

Fuchs, E.J., and Matzinger, P. (1996) Is cancer dangerous to the immune system? *Sem. Immunol.*, **8**, 271–280.

Fyfe, G., Fisher, R.I., Rosenberg, S.A., Sznol, M., Parkinson, D.R., and Louie, A.C. (1995) Results of treatment of 255 patients with metastatic renal cell carcinoma who received high-dose recombinant interleukin-2 therapy. *J. Clin. Oncol.*, **13**, 688–696.

Garrido, F., Ruiz-Cabello, F., Cabrera, T., Perez-Villar, J.J., Lopez-Nevot, M.A., Duggan-Keen, M., and Stern, P.L. (1997) Implications for immunosurveillance of altered HLA class I phenotypes in human tumours. *Immunol. Today*, **18**, 89–95.

Geertsen, P.F., Hermann, G.G., von der Maase, H., and Steven, K. (1992) Treatment of metastatic renal cell carcinoma by continuous intravenous infusion of recombinant interleukin-2: a single-center phase II study. *J. Clin. Oncol.*, **10**, 753–759.

Gervois, N., Guilloux, Y., Diez, E., and Jotereau, F. (1996) Suboptimal activation of melanoma infiltrating lymphocytes (TIL) due to low avidity of TCR/MHC-tumor peptide interactions. *J. Exp. Med.*, **183**, 2403–2407.

Gjertsen, M.K., and Gaudernack, G. (1998) Mutated Ras peptides as vaccines in immunotherapy of cancer. *Vox Sang.*, **74**, 489–495.

Gleave, M.E., Elhilali, M., Fradet, Y., Davis, I., Venner, P., Saad, F., Klotz, L.H., Moore, M.J., Paton, V., and Bajamonde, A. (1998) Interferon gamma-1b compared with placebo in metastatic renal-cell carcinoma. Canadian Urologic Oncology Group. *N. Engl. J. Med.*, **338**, 1265–1271.

Goey, S.H., Gratama, J.W., Primrose, J.N., Ward, U., Mertelsmann, R.H., Osterwalder, B., Verweij, J., and Stoter, G. (1996) Interleukin 2 and interferon alpha-2a do not improve anti-tumour activity of 5-fluorouracil in advanced colorectal cancer. *Br. J. Cancer*, **74**, 2018–2023.

Gold, P.J., Markowitz, D.R., Neumann, S., and Fefer, A. (1997). Metastatic renal cell carcinoma: long term survival after therapy with high-dose countinuous-infusion interleukin-2. *Cancer J. Sci. Am.*, **3**, S85–S91.

Grimm, E.A., Robb, R.J., Roth, J.A., Neckers, L.M., Lachman, L.B., Wilson, D.J., and Rosenberg, S.A. (1983) Lymphokine-activated killer cell phenomenon. III. Evidence that IL-2 is sufficient for direct activation of peripheral blood lymphocytes into lymphokine-activated killer cells. *J. Exp. Med.*, **158**, 1356–1361.

Guida, M., Latorre, A., Mastria, A., and De Lena, M. (1996) Subcutaneous recombinant interleukin-2 plus chemotherapy with cisplatin and dacarbazine in metastatic melanoma. *Eur. J. Cancer*, **32A**, 730–733.

Guilloux, Y., Viret, C., Gervois, N., Le Drean, E., Pandolfino, M.-C., Diez, E., and Jotereau, F. (1994) Defective lymphokine production by most $CD8^+$ and $CD4^+$ tumor-specific T cell clones derived from human melanoma-infiltrating lymphocytes in response to autologous tumor cells *in vitro*. *Eur. J. Immunol.*, **24**, 1966–1973.

Hahne, M., Rimoldi, D., Schroter, M., Romero, P., Schreier, M., French, L.E., Schneider, P., Bornand, T., Fontana, A., Liénard, D., Cerottini, J.-C., and Tschopp, J. (1996) Melanoma cell expression of Fas (Apo-1/CD95) ligand: Implications for tumor immune escape. *Science*, **274**, 1363–1366.

Helling, F., Zhang, S., and Shang, A. (1995) GM2-KLH conjugate vaccine: increased immunogenicity in melanoma patients after administration with immunological adjuvants QS-21. *Cancer Res.*, **55**, 2783–2788.

Henriksson, R., Nilsson, S., Colleen, S., Wersall, P., Helsing, M., Zimmerman, R., and Engman, K. (1998) Survival in renal cell carcinoma-a randomized evaluation of tamoxifen vs interleukin 2, alpha-interferon (leucocyte) and tamoxifen. *Br. J. Cancer*, **77**, 1311–1317.

Hersey, P., and Balch, C.M. (1984) Current status and future prospects for adjuvant therapy of melanoma. *Aust. N. Z. J. Surg.*, **54**, 303–315.

Hersey, P., Edwards, A., Coates, A., Shaw, H., McCarthy, W., and Milton, G. (1987) Evidence that treatment with vaccinia melanoma cell lysates (VMCL) may improve survival of patients with stage II melanoma. *Cancer Immunol. Immunother.*, **25**, 257–265.

Hersey, P., Coates, A., and McCarthy, W.H. (1996) Interim analysis of a randomized trial of immunotherapy with vaccinia melanoma cell lysates (VMCL) following surgical removal of high risk melanoma. *Proc. Am. Ass. Cancer Res.*, **37**, 489.

Hersey, P. (1997) Melanoma vaccines. Prospects for the treatment of melanoma. *Expert Op., Invest. Drugs*, **6**, 267–277.

Hersey, P. (1999) Impediments to successful immunotherapy. *Pharmacol. Ther.*, **81**, 111–119.

Hersh, E.M., Murray, J.L., Hong, W.K., Rosenblum, M.G., Reuben, J.M., Weilbaecher, R., Sarwal, A.N., Bradley, E.C., Konrad, M., and Arnett, F.C. (1989) Phase I study of cancer therapy with recombinant interleukin-2 administered by intravenous bolus injection. *Biotherapy*, **1**, 215–226.

Hishii, M., Andrews, D., Boyle, L.A., Wong, J.T., Pandolfi, F., Van den Elsen, P.J., and Kurnick, J.T. (1997) *In vivo* accumulation of the same anti-melanoma T cell clone in two different metastatic sites. *Proc. Natl. Acad. Sci. USA*, **94**, 1378–1383.

Hjelm, A.L., Ragnhammar, P., Fagerberg, J., Magnusson, I., Frodin, J.E., Svanstrom, R., Shetye, J., Mellstedt, H., and Wersall, J.P. (1995) Subcutaneous interleukin-2 and alpha-interferon in advanced colorectal carcinoma. A phase II study. *Cancer Biother.*, **10**, 5–12.

Hodge, J.W., McLaughlin, J.P., Kantor, J.A., and Schlom, J. (1997) Diversified prime and boost protocols using recombinant vaccinia virus and recombinant non-replicating avian pox virus to enhance T-cell immunity and antitumor responses. *Vaccine*, **15**, 759–768.

Hu, X., Chakraborty, N.G., Sporn, J.R., Kurtzman, S.H., Ergin, M.T., and Mukherji, B. (1996) Enhancement of cytolytic T lymphocyte precursor frequency in melanoma patients following immunization with the MAGE-1 peptide loaded antigen presenting cell-based vaccine. *Cancer Res.*, **56**, 2479–2483.

Huang, A.Y.C., Golumbek, P., Ahmadzadeh, M., Jaffee, E., Pardoll, D., and Levitsky, H. (1994) Role of bone marrow-derived cells in presenting MHC class I-restricted tumor antigens. *Science*, **264**, 961.

Ilson, D., Motzer, R., Kradin, R., Vogelzang, N., Bajorin, D., Scher, H., O'Moore, P., Zeffren, J., Marathias, K., and Lazarus, D. (1991) A phase II study of recombinant interleukin-2 and alpha interferon (Roferon) for patients with advanced renal cell cancer. Proc. *Am. Ass. Cancer Res.*, **32**, A1116.

Isaacs, A., and Lindenman, J. (1957) Virus interference. The interferon. *Proc. R. Soc. Lond. B. Biol. Sci.*, **147**, 258–267.

Itoh, K., Tilden, A.B., and Balch, C.M. (1986) Interleukin 2 activation of cytotoxic T-lymphocytes infiltrating into human metastatic melanomas. *Cancer Res.*, **46**, 3011–3017.

Jäger, E., Bernhard, H., Romero, P., Ringhoffer, M., Arand, M., Karbach, J., Ilsemann, C., Hagedorn, M., and Knuth, A. (1996a) Generation of cytotoxic T-cell responses with synthetic melanoma-associated peptides *in vivo*: implications for tumor vaccines with melanoma-associated antigens. *Int. J. Cancer*, **66**, 162–169.

Jäger, E., Ringhoffer, M., Dienes, H.P., Arand, M., Karbach, J., Jäger, D., Ilsemann, C., Hagedorn, M., Oesch, F., and Knuth, A. (1996b) Granulocyte-macrophage-colony-stimulating factor enhances immune responses to melanoma-associated peptides *in vivo*. *Int. J. Cancer*, **67**, 54–62.

Jäger, E., Ringhoffer, M., Karbach, J., Arand, M., Oesch, F., and Knuth, A. (1996c) Inverse relationship of melanocyte differentiation antigen expression in melanoma tissues and $CD8^+$ cytotoxic-T-cell responses: evidence for immunoselection of antigen-loss variants *in vivo*. *Int. J. Cancer*, **66**, 470–476.

Janik, J.E., Miller, L.L., Longo, D.L., Powers, G.C., Urba, W.J., Kopp, W.C., Gause, B.L., Curti, B.D., Fenton, R.G., Oppenheim, J.J., Conlon, K.C., Holmlund, J.T., Sznol, M., Sharfman, W.H., Steis, R.G., Creekmore, S.P., Alvord, W.G., Beauchamp, A.E., and Smith, J.W. (1996) Phase II trial of interleukin 1 alpha and indomethacin in treatment of metastatic melanoma. *J. Natl. Cancer Inst. USA*, **88**, 44–49.

Jayson, G.C., Middleton, M., Lee, S.M., Ashcroft, L., and Thatcher, N. (1998) A randomized phase II trial of interleukin 2 and interleukin 2-interferon alpha in advanced renal cancer. *Br. J. Cancer*, **78**, 366–369.

Johnston, S.R., Constenla, D.O., Moore, J., Atkinson, H., A'Hern, R.P., Dadian, G., Riches, P.G., and Gore, M.E. (1998) Randomized phase II trial of BCDT [carmustine (BCNU), cisplatin, dacarbazine (DTIC) and tamoxifen] with or without interferon alpha (IFN-alpha) and interleukin (IL-2) in patients with metastatic melanoma. *Br. J. Cancer*, **77**, 1280–1286.

Kammula, U.S., White, D.E., and Rosenberg, S.A. (1998) Trends in the safety of high dose bolus interleukin-2 administration in patients with metastatic cancer. *Cancer*, **83**, 797–805.

Karp, S.E. (1998) Low-dose intravenous bolus interleukin-2 with interferon-alpha therapy for metastatic melanoma and renal cell carcinoma. *J. Immunother.*, **21**, 56–61.

Kawakami, Y., Zakut, R., Topalian, S.L., Stotter, H., and Rosenberg, S.A. (1992) Shared human melanoma antigens. Recognition by tumor-infiltrating lymphocytes in HLA-A2.1-transfected melanomas. *J. Immunol.*, **148**, 638–643.

Kawakami, Y., Eliyahu, S., Sakaguchi, K., Robbins, P.F., Rivoltini, L., Yannelli, J.R., Appella, E., and Rosenberg, S.A. (1994) Identification of the immunodominant peptides of the MART-1 human melanoma antigen recognized by the majority of HLA-A2-restricted tumor infiltrating lymphocytes. *J. Exp. Med.*, **180**, 347–352.

Kawakami, Y., Eliyahu, S., Jennings, C., Sakaguchi, K., Kang, X., Southwood, S., Robbins, P.F., Sette, A., Appella, E., and Rosenberg, S.A. (1995) Recognition of multiple epitopes in the human melanoma antigen gp100 by tumor-infiltrating T lymphocytes associated with *in vivo* tumor regression. *J. Immunol.*, **154**, 3961–3968.

Keilholz, U., Scheibenbogen, C., Tilgen, W., Bergmann, L., Weidmann, E., Seither, E., Richter, M., Brado, B., Mitrou, P.S., and Hunstein, W. (1993) Interferon-alpha and interleukin-2 in the treatment of metastatic melanoma. Comparison of two phase II trials. *Cancer*, **72**, 607–614.

Kim, C.J., Taubenberger, J.K., Simonis, T.B., White, D.E., Rosenberg, S.A., and Marincola, F.M. (1996) Combination therapy with Interferon-gamma and Interleukin-2 for the treatment of metastatic melanoma. *J. Immunother.*, **19**, 50–58.

Kirkwood, J.M. (1995) Biologic therapy with interferon-α and β: clinical applications. Melanoma. In: V.T. DeVita, S. Hellman, and S.A. Rosenberg, (eds.), *Biologic Therapy of Cancer* (2nd edn), J.B. Lippincott Co., Philadelphia, pp. 388–411.

Kirkwood, J.M., Strawderman, M.H., Ernstoff, M.S., Smith, T.J., Borden, E.C., and Blum, R.H. (1996) Interferon alfa-2b adjuvant therapy of high-risk resected cutaneous melanoma: the Eastern Cooperative Oncology Group Trial EST 1684. *J. Clin. Oncol.*, **14**, 7–17.

Klinman, D.M., Yamshchikov, G., and Ishigatsubo, Y. (1997) Contribution of CpG motifs to the immunogenicity of DNA vaccines. *J. Immunol.*, **158**, 3635–3639.

Knuth, A., Danowski, B., Oettgen, H.F., and Old, L.J. (1984) T-cell-mediated cytotoxicity against autologous malignant melanoma: analysis with interleukin 2-dependent T-cell cultures. *Proc. Natl. Acad. Sci. USA*, **81**, 3511–3515.

Krigel, R.L., Padavic-Shaller, K., Toomey, C., Comis, R.L., and Weiner, L.M. (1995) Phase I study of sequentially administered recombinant tumor necrosis factor and recombinant interleukin-2. *J. Immunother.*, **17**, 161–170.

Kruit, W.H., Goey, S.H., Monson, J.R., Stahel, R.A., Calabresi, F., Mertelsmann, R., Holdener, E.E., Eggermont, A.M., Bolhuis, R.L., and De Mulder, P.H (1991) Clinical experience with the combined use of recombinant interleukin-2 (IL2) and interferon alfa-2a (IFN alpha) in metastatic melanoma. *Br. J. Haematol.*, **79**, 84–86.

Kruit, W.H., Punt, C.J., Goey, S.H., de Mulder, P.H., Gratama, J.W., Eggermont, A.M., Bolhuis, R.L., and Stoter, G. (1996) Dose efficacy study of two schedules of high-dose bolus administration of interleukin 2 and interferon alpha in metastatic melanoma. *Br. J. Cancer*, **74**, 951–955.

Kwak, L.W., Campbell, M.J., Czerwinski, D., Hart, S., Miller, R.A., and Levy, R. (1992) Induction of the immune response in patients with B-cell lymphoma against the surface immunoglobulin idiotype expressed by their tumors. *N. Engl. J. Med.*, **327**, 1209–1215.

Labarriere, N., Diez, E., Pandolfino, M.-C., Viret, C., Guilloux, Y., Le Guiner, S., Fonteneau, J.-F., Dreno, B., and Jotereau, F. (1997) Optimal T cell activation by melanoma cells depends on a minimal level of antigen transcription. *J. Immunol.*, **158**, 1238–1245.

Law, T.M., Motzer, R.J., Mazumder, M., Sell, K.W., Walther, P.J., O'Connell, M., Khan, A., Vlamis, V., Vogelzang, N.J., and Bajorin, D.F. (1995) Phase III randomized trial of interleukin-2 with or without lymphokine-activated killer cells in the treatment of patients with advanced renal cell carcinoma. *Cancer*, **76**, 824–832.

Lawrence, G.W., Saul, A., Giddy, A.J., Kemp, R., and Pye, D. (1997) Phase I trial in humans of an oil-based adjuvant SEPPIC MONTANIDE ISA 720. *Vaccine*, **15**, 176–178.

Lee, K., Talpaz, M., Legha, S., Plager, C., Papadopoulos, N., Benjamin, R., and Gutterman, J. (1989) Combination treatment of recombinant human interleukin-2 and recombinant interferon alpha-2a in patients with advanced melanoma. *Proc. Am. Soc. Clin. Oncol.*, **8**, A1129.

Lee, K.-H., Panelli, M.C., Kim, C.J., Riker, A., Roden, M., Fetsch, P.A., Abati, A., Bettinotti, M.P., Rosenberg, S.A., and Marincola, F.M. (1998) Functional dissociation between local and systemic immune response following peptide vaccination. *J. Immunol.*, **161**, 4183–4194.

Legha, S.S., Gianan, M.A., Plager, C., Eton, O.E., and Papadopoulous, N.E. (1996a) Evaluation of IL-2 administered by continuous infusion in patients with metastatic melanoma. *Cancer*, **77**, 89–96.

Legha, S.S., Ring, S., Bedikian, A., Plager, C., Eton, O., Buzaid, A.C., and Papadopoulos, N. (1996b) Treatment of metastatic melanoma with combined chemotherapy containing cisplatin, vinblastine and dacarbazine (CVD) and biotherapy using interleukin-2 and interferon-alpha. *Ann. Oncol.*, **7**, 827–835.

Li, W., Berencsi, K., Basak, S., Somasundaram, R., Ricciardi, R.P., Gonczol, E., Zaloudik, J., Linnenbach, A., Maruyama, H., Miniou, P., and Herlyn, D. (1997) Human colorectal cancer (CRC) antigen CO17-1A/GA733 encoded by adenovirus inhibits growth of established CRC cells in mice. *J. Immunol.*, **159**, 763–769.

Lipton, A., Harvey, H., Givant, E., Hopper, K., Lawler, J., Matthews, Y., Hirsh, M., and Zeffren, J. (1993) Interleukin-2 and interferon-alpha-2a outpatient therapy for metastatic renal cell carcinoma. *J. Immunother.*, **13**, 122–129.

Livingston, P.O. (1994) Improved survival in stage III melanoma patients with GM2 antibodies: a randomized trial of adjuvant vaccination with GM2. *J. Clin. Oncol.*, **12**, 1036–1044.

Livingston, P.O. (1995) Approaches to augmenting the immunogenicity of melanoma gangliosides: from whole melanoma cells to ganglioside-KLH conjugate vaccines. *Immunol. Rev.*, **145**, 147–166.

Livingston, B.D., Crimi, C., Grey, H., Ishioka, G., Chisari, F.V., Fikes, J., Chesnut, R.W., and Sette, A. (1997) The hepatitis B virus-specific CTL responses induced in humans by lipopeptide vaccination are comparable to those elicited by acute viral infection. *J. Immunol.*, **159**, 1383–1392.

Lotze, M.T., Frana, L.W., Sharrow, S.O., Robb, R.J., and Rosenberg, S.A. (1985) *In vivo* administration of purified human interleukin 2. I. Half-life and immunologic effects of the Jurkat cell line-derived interleukin 2. *J. Immunol.*, **134**, 157–166.

Lotze, M.T. (1991) Interleukin-2: Basic principles. In: V.T. DeVita, S. Hellman, and S.A. Rosenberg, (eds.), *Biologic Therapy of Cancer* (1st edn), J.B. Lippincott Co., Philadelphia, pp. 123–141.

Lotze, M.T., Storkus, W.J., Falo, L., Baar, J., Davis, I., Tueting, T., Esche, C., Whiteside, T.L., Elder, E.M., Kinzler, D.M., Paradise, C., and Kirkwood, J.M. (1997) Dendritic cells (DCs) and the immunotherapy of melanoma. *Melanoma Res.*, **7**, S4.

Lucas, K.G., Small, T.N., Heller, G., Dupont, B., and O'Reilly, R. (1996) The development of cellular immunity to Epstein-Barr virus after allogeneic bone marrow transplantation. *Blood*, **87**, 2594–2603.

Luscher, U., Filgueira, L., Juretic, A., Zuber, M., Luscher, N.J., Heberer, M., and Spagnoli, G.C. (1994) The pattern of cytokine gene expression in freshly excised human metastatic melanoma suggests a state of reversible anergy of tumor-infiltrating lymphocytes. *Int. J. Cancer*, **57**, 612–619.

Lynch, D.H., Andreasen, A., Maraskovsky, E., Whitmore, J., Miller, R.E., and Schuh, J.C.L. (1997) Flt3 ligand induces tumor regression and antitumor immune responses *in vivo*. *Nature Med.*, **3**, 625.

Maccalli, C., Farina, C., Sensi, M., Parmiani, G., and Anichini, A. (1997) TCR beta-chain variable region-driven selection and massive expansion of HLA-class I-restricted antitumor CTL lines from HLA-A*0201+ melanoma patients. *J. Immunol.*, **158**, 5902–5913.

Maccalli, C., Pisarra, P., Vegetti, C., Sensi, M., Parmiani, G., and Anichini, A. (1999) Differential loss of T cell signaling molecules in metastatic melanoma patients' T lymphocyte subsets expressing distinct TCR variable regions. *J. Immunol.*, **163**, 6912–6923.

Mackinnon, S., Papadopoulos, E.B., Carabasi, M.H., Reich, L., Collins, N.H., Boulad, F., Castro-Malaspina, H., Childs, B.H., Gillio, A.P., Kernan, N.A., Small, T.N., Young, J.W., and O'Reilly, R.J. (1995) Adoptive immunotherapy evaluating escalating doses of donor leukocytes for relapse of chronic myeloid leukemia after bone marrow transplantation: separation of graf-versus-leukemia from graft-versus-host disease. *Blood*, **86**, 1261–1268.

Manca, F., Fenoglio, D., Franchin, E., Saverino, D., Li, P.G., Buffa, F., Bignardi, D., Del Pup, L., and Palu, G. (1997) Anti-HIV genetic treatment of antigen-specific human CD4 lymphocytes for adoptive immunotherapy of opportunistic infections in AIDS. *Gene Ther.*, **4**, 1216–1224.

Marchand, M., van Baren, N., Weynants, P., Brichard, V., Dreno, B., Tessier, M.-H., Rankin, E., Parmiani, G., Arienti, F., Humblet, Y., Bourlond, A., Vanwijck, R., Lienard, D., Beauduin, M., Dietrich, P.-Y., Russo, V., Kerger, J., Masucci, G., Jäger, E., De Greve, J., Atzpodien, J., Brasseur, F., Coulie, P.G., van der Bruggen, P., and Boon, T. (1999) Tumor regressions observed in patients with metastatic melanoma treated with an antigenic peptide encoded by gene MAGE-3 and presented by HLA-A1. *Int. J. Cancer*, **80**, 219–230.

Marincola, F.M. (1994) Interleukin-2. *Biol. Ther. Cancer Updates*, **4**, 1–16.

Marincola, F.M., Shamamian, P., Alexander, R.B., Gnarra, J.R., Turetskaya, R.L., Nedospasov, S.A., Simonis, T.B., Taubenberger, J.K., Yannelli, J., Mixon, A., *et al.* (1994) Loss of HLA haplotype and B locus down-regulation in melanoma cell lines. *J. Immunol.*, **153**, 1225–1237.

Marincola, F.M., Shamamian, P., Rivoltini, L., Salgaller, M., Cormier, J., Restifo, N.P., Simonis, T.B., Venzon, D., White, D.E., and Parkinson, D.R. (1995a) HLA associations in the antitumor response against malignant melanoma. *J. Immunother.*, **18**, 242–252.

Marincola, F.M., White, D.E., Wise, A.P., and Rosenberg, S.A. (1995b) Combination therapy with interferon alpha-2a and interleukin-2 for the treatment of metastatic cancer. *J. Clin. Oncol.*, **13**, 1110–1122.

Marincola, F.M., Hijazi, Y.M., Fetsch, P., Salgaller, M.L., Rivoltini, L., Cormier, J., Simonis, T.B., Duray, P.H., Herlyn, M., Kawakami, Y., and Rosenberg, S.A. (1996) Analysis of expression of the melanoma associated antigens MART-1 and gp100 in metastatic melanoma cell lines and in *in situ* lesions. *J. Immunother.*, **19**, 192–205.

Marincola, F.M. (1997) The multiple ways to tumor tolerance. *J. Immunother.*, **20**, 178–179.

Marroquin, C.E., White, D.E., Steinberg, S., Rosenberg, S.A., and Schwartzentruber, D. (2000) Decreased tolerance to Interleukin-2 (IL-2) with repeated courses of therapy in patients with metastatic melanoma or renal cell cancer. *J. Immunother.*, in press.

McBride, G. (1997) New molecule under study: Flt3 ligand may mobilize dendritic cells. *J. Natl. Cancer Inst. USA*, **89**, 1257–1258.

McCabe, M.S., Stablein, D., and Hawkins, M.J. (1991) The modified group C experience-phase III randomized trials of il-2 vs IL-2/LAK in advanced renal cell carcinoma and advanced melanoma. *Proc. Am. Soc. Clin. Oncol.*, **10**, A714.

McMichael, A.J., and O'Callaghan, C.A. (1998) A new look at T cells. *J. Exp. Med.*, **187**, 1367–1371.

Melioli, G., Ratto, G.B., Ponte, M., Guastella, M., Semino, C., Fantino, G., Tassara, E., Pasquetti, W., Mereu, C., Merlo, F., Reggiardo, G., Morasso, G., Santi, L., and Moretta, L. (1996) Treatment of stage IIIB non-small-cell lung cancer with surgery followed by infusion of tumor infiltrating lymphocytes and recombinant interleukin-2: a pilot study. *J. Immunother.*, **19**, 224–230.

Mitchell, M.S., Harel, W., Kempf, R.A., Hu, E., Kan-Mitchell, J., Boswell, W.D., Dean, G., and Stevenson, L. (1990) Active-specific immunotherapy for melanoma. *J. Clin. Oncol.*, **8**, 856–869.

Mitchison, N.A. (1970) Immunologic approach to cancer. *Transplant. Proc.*, **2**, 92–103.

Mittelman, A., Huberman, M., Puccio, C., Fallon, B., Tessitore, J., Savona, S., Eyre, R., Gafney, E., Wick, M., and Skelos, A. (1990) A phase I study of recombinant human interleukin-2 and alpha-interferon-2a in patients with renal cell cancer, colorectal cancer, and malignant melanoma. *Cancer*, **66**, 664–669.

Morgan, D.A., Ruscetti, F.W., and Gallo, R.C. (1976) Selective *in vitro* growth of T-lymphocytes from normal bone marrow. *Science*, **193**, 1007–1008.

Morse, M.A., Lyerly, H.K., Gilboa, E., Thomas, E., and Nair, S.K. (1998) Optimization of the sequence of antigen loading and CD40-ligand-induced maturation of dendritic cells. *Cancer Res.*, **58**, 2965–2968.

Morton, D.L., Foshang, L.J., Hoon, D.S.B., Nizze, J.A., Wanek, L.A., Chang, C., Davtyan, D.G., Gupta, R.K., Elashoff, R., and Irie, R.F. (1992) Prolongation of survival in meatstatic melanoma after active specific immunotherapy with a new polyvalent melanoma vaccine. *Ann. Surg.*, **216**, 463–482.

Mosmann, T.R., and Sad, S. (1996) The expanding universe of T-cell subsets: Th1, Th2 and more. *Immunol. Today*, **17**, 138–146.

Motzer, R.J., Rakhit, A., Schwartz, L.H., Olencki, T., Malone, T.M., Sandstrom, K., Nadeau, R., Parmar, H., and Bukowski, R. (1998) Phase I trial of subcutaneous recombinant human interleukin-12 in patients with advanced renal cell carcinoma. *Clin. Cancer Res.*, **4**, 1183–1191.

Mukherji, B., Chakraborty, N.G., Yamasaki, S., Okino, T., Yamase, H., Sporn, J.R., Kurtzman, S.K., Ergin, M.T., Ozols, J., Meehan, J., and Mauri, F. (1995) Induction of antigen-specific cytolytic T cells in situ in human melanoma by immunization with synthetic peptide-pulsed autologous antigen presenting cells. *Proc. Natl Acad. Sci. USA*, **92**, 8078–8082.

Murphy, G.P., Tjoa, B.A., Simmons, S.J., Jarisch, J., Bowes, V.A., Ragde, H., Rogers, M., Elgamal, A., Kenny, G.M., Cobb, O.E., Ireton, R.C., Troychak, M.J., Salgaller, M.L., and Boynton, A.L. (1999) Infusion of dendritic ccells pulsed with HLA-A2-specific prostate-specific membrane antigen peptides: a phase II prostate cancer vaccine trial involving with hormone-refractory metastatic disease. *Prostate*, **38**, 73–78.

Negrier, S., Philip, T., Stoter, G., Fossa, S.D., Janssen, S., Iacone, A., Cleton, F.S., Eremin, O., and Israel, L. (1989) Interleukin-2 with or without lak cells in metastatic renal cell carcinoma: a report of a European multicentric study. *Eur. J. Cancer Clin. Oncol.*, **25**, S21–S28.

Negrier, S., Escudier, B., Lasset, C., Douillard, J.Y., Savary, J., Chevreau, C., Ravaud, A., Mercatello, A., Peny, J., Mousseau, M., Philip, T., and Tursz, T. (1998) Recombinant human interleukin-2, recombinant human interferon alfa-2a, or both in metastatic renal-cell carcinoma. Groupe Francais d'Immunotherapie. *N. Engl. J. Med.*, **338**, 1272–1278.

Nestle, F.O., Alijagic, S., Gilliet, M., Sun, Y., Grabbe, S., Dummer, R., Burg, G., and Schadendorf, D. (1998) Vaccination of melanoma patients with peptide- or tumor lysate-pulsed dendritic cells. *Nature Med.*, **4**, 328–332.

Nosten, F., Luxemburger, C., Kyle, D.E., Ballou, W.R., Wittes, J., Wah, E., Chongsuphajaisiddhi, T., Gordon, D.M., White, N.J., Sadoff, J.C., and Heppner, D.G. (1996) Randomised double-blind placebo-controlled trial of SPf66 malaria vaccine in children in northwestern Thailand. *Lancet*, **348**, 701–707.

O'Hagan, D.T., Ott, G.S., and Van Nest, G. (1997) Recent advances in vaccine adjuvants: the development of MF59 emulsion and polymeric microparticles. *Mol. Med. Today*, **3**, 69–75.

Old, L.J., and Chen, Y.T. (1998) New paths in human cancer serology. *J. Exp. Med.*, **187**, 1163–1167.

Oldham, R.K., Blumenschein, G., Schwartzberg, L., Birch, R., and Arnold, J. (1992) Combination biotherapy utilizing interleukin-2 and alpha interferon in patients with advanced cancer: a National Biotherapy Study Group Trial. *Mol. Biother.*, **4**, 4–9.

Ossendorp, F., Mengede, E., Camps, M., Filius, R., and Melief, C.J.M. (1998) Specific T helper cell requirement for optimal induction of cytotoxic T lymphocytes against major histocompatibility complex class II negative tumors. *J. Exp. Med.*, **187**, 693–702.

O'Sullivan, D., Arrhenius, T., Sidney, J., Del Guercio, M.-F., Albertson, M., Wall, M., Oseroff, C., Southwood, S., Colon, S.M., Gaeta, F.C.A., and Sette, A. (1991) On the interaction of promiscuous antigenic peptides with different DR alleles. *J. Immunol.*, **147**, 2663–2669.

Pandolfi, F., Boyle, L.A., Trentin, L., Kurnick, J.T., Isselbacher, K.J., and Gattoni-Celli, S. (1991) Expression of HLA-A2 antigen in human melanoma cell lines and its role in T-cell recognition. *Cancer Res.*, **51**, 3164–3170.

Panelli, M.C., Riker, A., Kammula, U., Wang, E., Lee, K.H., Rosenberg, S.A., and Marincola, F.M. (2000) Expansion of tumor-T cell pairs from fine needle aspirates of melanoma metastases. *J. Immunol.*, **164**, 495–504.

Pardoll, D.M. (1998) Cancer vaccines. *Nature Med.*, **4**, 525–531.

Parish, C.R. (1972) The relationship between humoral and cell-mediated immunity. *Transplant. Rev.*, **13**, 35–66.

Parish, C.R. (1996) Immune deviation: a historical perspective. *Immunol. Cell Biol.*, **74**, 449–456.

Parkhurst, M.R., Salgaller, M.L., Southwood, S., Robbins, P.F., Sette, A., Rosenberg, S.A., and Kawakami, Y. (1996) Improved induction of melanoma reactive CTL with peptides from the melanoma antigen gp100 modified at HLA-A*0201 binding residues. *J. Immunol.*, **157**, 2539–2548.

Parkinson, D.R., Abrams, J.S., Wiernik, P.H., Rayner, A.A., Margolin, K.A., Van Echo, D.A., Sznol, M., Dutcher, J.P., Aronson, F.R., and Doroshow, J.H. (1990) Interleukin-2 therapy in patients with metastatic malignant melanoma: a phase II study. *J. Clin. Oncol.*, **8**, 1650–1656.

Parmiani, G., Colombo, M.P., Melani, C., and Arienti, F. (1997) Cytokine gene transduction in the immunotherapy of cancer. *Adv. Pharmacol.*, **40**, 259–307.

Pectasides, D., Varthalitis, J., Kostopoulou, M., Mylonakis, A., Triantaphyllis, D., Papadopoulou, M., Dimitriadis, M., and Athanassiou, A. (1998) An outpatient phase II study of subcutaneous interleukin-2 and interferon-alpha-2b in combination with intravenous vinblastine in metastatic renal cell cancer. *Oncology*, **55**, 10–15.

Pehamberger, H., Soyer, H.P., Steiner, A., Kofler, R., Binder, M., Mischer, P., Pachinger, W., Aubock, J., Fritsch, P., Kerl, H., and Wolff, K. (1998) Adjuvant interferon alfa-2a treatment in resected primary stage II cutaneous melanoma. Austrian Malignant Melanoma Cooperative Group. *J. Clin. Oncol.*, **16**, 1425–1429.

Perez, E.A., Scudder, S.A., Meyers, F.A., Tanaka, M.S., Paradise, C., and Gandara, D.R. (1991) Weekly 24-hour continuous infusion interleukin-2 for metastatic melanoma and renal cell carcinoma: a phase I study. *J. Immunother.*, **10**, 57–62.

Player, M.A., Barracchini, K.C., Simonis, T.B., Rivoltini, L., Arienti, F., Castelli, C., Mazzocchi, A., Belli, F., and Marincola, F.M. (1996) Differences in frequency distribution of HLA-A2 sub-types between american and italian caucasian melanoma patients: relevance for epitope specific vaccination protocols. *J. Immunother.*, **19**, 357–363.

Pockaj, B.A., Sherry, R.M., Wei, J.P., Yannelli, J.R., Carter, C.S., Leitman, S.F., Carasquillo, J.A., Steinberg, S.M., Rosenberg, S.A., and Yang, J.C. (1994) Localization of 111indium-labeled tumor infiltrating lymphocytes to tumor in patients receiving adoptive immunotherapy. Augmentation with cyclophosphamide and correlation with response. *Cancer*, **73**, 1731–1737.

Ponnighaus, J.M., Fine, P.E.M., Sterne, J.A.C., Wilson, R.J., Msosa, E., Gruer, P.J.K., Jenkins, P.A., Lucas, S.B., Liomba, N.G., and Bliss, L. (1992) Efficacy of BCG vaccine against leprosy and tuberculosis in northern Malawi. *Lancet*, **339**, 636–639.

Poo, W.J., Fynan, T., Davis, C., Flynn, S., Durivage, H., and Todd, M. (1991) High-Dose Recombinant interleukin-2 alone in patients with metastatic renal cell carcinoma. *Proc. Am. Soc. Clin. Oncol.*, **10**, A557.

Puisieux, I., Bain, C., Merrouche, Y., Malacher, P., Kourilsky, P., Even, J., and Favrot, M. (1996) Restriction of the T-cell repertoire in tumor-infiltrating lymphocytes from nine patients with renal-cell carcinoma. Relevance of the CDR3 length analysis for the identification of *in situ* clonal T-cell expansions. *Int. J. Cancer*, **66**, 201–208.

Raff, M.C. (1973) T and B lymphocytes and immune responses. *Nature*, **242**, 19–23.

Ranieri, E., Kierstead, L.S., Zarour, H., Kirkwood, J.M., Lotze, M.T., Whiteside, T.and Storkus, W.J. (2000) Dendritic cell/peptide cancer vaccines: clinical responsiveness and epitope spreading. *Immunol. Invest.* **29**, 121–125.

Ratto, G.B., Zino, P., Mirabelli, S., Minuti, P., Aquilina, R., Fantino, G., Spessa, E., Ponte, M., Bruzzi, P., and Melioli, G. (1996) A randomized trial of adoptive immunotherapy with tumor-infiltrating lymphocytes and interleukin-2 versus standard therapy in the postoperative treatment of resected nonsmall cell lung carcinoma. *Cancer*, **78**, 244–251.

Ravaud, A., Audhuy, B., Gomez, F., Escudier, B., Lesimple, T., Chevreau, C., Douillard, J.Y., Caty, A., Geoffrois, L., Ferrero, J.M., Linassier, C., Drevon, M., and Negrier, S. (1998) Subcutaneous interleukin-2, interferon alfa-2a and continuous infusion of fluorouracil in metastatic renal cell carcinoma: a multicenter phase II trial. Groupe Francais d'Immunotherapie. *J. Clin. Oncol.*, **16**, 2728–2732.

Reddy, S.P., Harwood, R.M., Moore, D.F., Grimm, E.A., Murray, J.L., and Vadhan-Raj, S. (1997) Recombinant interleukin-2 in combination with recombinant interferon-gamma in patients with advanced malignancy: a phase 1 study. *J. Immunother.*, **20**, 79–87.

Restifo, N.P., Esquivel, F., Kawakami, Y., Yewdell, J.W., Mule, J.J., Rosenberg, S.A., and Bennink, J.R. (1993) Identification of human cancers deficient in antigen processing. *J. Exp. Med.*, **177**, 265–272.

Restifo, N.P., and Wunderlich, J.R. (1996) Principles of tumor immunity: biology of cellular immune responses. In: V.T. DeVita, S. Hellman, and S.A. Rosenberg, (eds.), *Biologic Therapy of Cancer* (1st edn), J.B. Lippincott Co., Philadelphia, pp. 3–21.

Rhodes, J. (1996) Covalent chemical events in immune induction: fundamental and therapeutic aspects. *Immunol. Today*, **17**, 436–441.

Richards, J.M., Bajorin, D.F., Vogelzang, N.J., Houghton, A.N., Seigler, H.F., Sell, K., Zeffrin, J., and Levitt, D. (1990) Treatment of metastatic melanoma with continuous intravenous (Civ) Il-2 +/- Lak cells: a randomized trial. *Proc. Am. Soc. Clin. Oncol.*, **9**, A1080.

Riddell, S.R., and Greenberg, P.D. (1994) Therapeutic reconstitution of human viral immunity by adoptive transfer of cytotoxic T lymphocyte clones. *Curr. Top. Microbiol. Immunol.*, **189**, 9–34.

Ridge, J.P., Di Rosa, F., and Matzinger, P. (1998) A conditioned dendritic cell can be a temporal bridge between a $CD4^+$ T-helper and a T-killer cell. *Nature*, **393**, 474–478.

Rivoltini, L., Baracchini, K.C., Viggiano, V., Kawakami, Y., Smith, A., Mixon, A., Restifo, N.P., Topalian, S.L., Simonis, T.B., Rosenberg, S.A., and Marincola, F.M. (1995a) Quantitative correlation between HLA Class I allele expression and recognition of melanoma cells by antigen specific cytotoxic T lymphocytes. *Cancer Res.*, **55**, 3149–3157.

Rivoltini, L., Kawakami, Y., Sakaguchi, K., Southwood, S., Sette, A., Robbins, P.F., Marincola, F.M., Salgaller, M., Yannelli, J.R., Appella, E., and Rosenberg, S.A. (1995b) Induction of tumor reactive CTL from peripheral blood and tumor infiltrating lymphocytes of melanoma patients by *in vitro* stimulation with an immunodominant peptide of the human melanoma antigen MART-1. *J. Immunol.*, **154**, 2257–2265.

Rivoltini, L., Radrizzani, M., Accornero, P., Squarcina, P., Chiodoni, C., Mazzocchi, A., Castelli, C., Tarsini, P., Viggiano, V., Belli, F., Colombo, M.P., and Parmiani, G. (1998) Human melanoma-reactive $CD4^+$ and $CD8^+$ CTL clones resist Fas ligand-induced apoptosis and use Fas/Fas ligand-independent mechanisms for tumor killing. *J. Immunol.*, **161**, 1220–1230.

Rivoltini, L., Squarcina, P., Loftus, D.J., Castelli, C.,Tarsini, P., Mazzocchi, A., Rini, F., Viggiano, V., Belli, F., and Parmiani, G. (1999) A superagonist variant of peptide MART-1/Melan A27–35 elicits anti-melanoma CD8+ T cells with enhanced functional characteristics. Implication for more effective immunotherapy. *Cancer Res.*, **59**, 301–306.

Rogge, L., Barberis-Maino, L., Biffi, M., Passini, N., Presky, D.H., Gubler, U., and Sinigaglia, F. (1997) Selective expression of an interleukin-12 receptor component by human T helper 1 cells. *J. Exp. Med.*, **185**, 825–831.

Romero, P., Gervois, N., Schneider, J., Escobar, P., Valmori, D., Pannetier, C., Steinle, A., Wolfel, T., Lienard, D., Brichard, V., van Pel, A., Jotereau, F., and Cerottini, J.-C. (1997) Cytolytic T lymphocyte recognition of the immunodominant HLA-A*0201-restricted melan-A/MART-1 antigenic peptide in melanoma. *J. Immunol.*, **159**, 2366–2374.

Romero, P., Dunbar, P.R., Valmori, D., Pittet, M., Ogg, G.S., Rimoldi, D., Chen, J.-L., Liénard, D., Cerottini, J.-C., and Cerundolo, V. (1998). Ex vivo staining of metastatic lymph nodes by class I major histocompatibility complex tetramers reveals high numbers of antigen-experienced tumor-specific cytolytic T lymphocytes. *J. Exp. Med.*, **188**, 1641–1650.

Rosenberg, S.A., Mulé, J.J., Spiess, P.J., Reichert, C.M., and Schwarz, S.L. (1985) Regression of established pulmonary metastases and subcutaneous tumor mediated by the systemic administration of high-dose recombinant interleukin 2. *J. Exp. Med.*, **161**, 1169–1188.

Rosenberg, S.A., Spiess, P., and Lafreniere, R. (1986) A new approach to the adoptive immunotherapy of cancer with tumor-infiltrating lymphocytes. *Science*, **233**, 1318–1321.

Rosenberg, S.A., Packard, B.S., Aebersold, P.M., Solomon, D., Topalian, S.L., Toy, S.T., Simon, P., Lotze, M.T., Yang, J.C., Seipp, C.A., Simpson, C., Carter, C., BLock, S., Schwartzentruber, D.J., Wei, J.P., and White, D.E. (1988) Use of tumor-infiltrating lymphocytes and interleukin-2 in the immune therapy of patients with metastatic melanoma. A preliminary report. *N. Engl. J. Med.*, **319**, 1676–1680.

Rosenberg, S.A., Aebersold, P., Cornetta, K., Kasid, A., Morgan, R.A., Moen, R., Karson, E.M., Lotze, M.T., Yang, J.C., and Topalian, S.L. (1990) Gene transfer into humans – immunotherapy of patients with advanced melanoma, using tumor-infiltrating lymphocytes modified by retroviral gene transduction. *N. Engl. J. Med.*, **323**, 570–578.

Rosenberg, S.A., Anderson, W.F., Blaese, M., Hwu, P., Yannelli, J.R., Yang, J.C., Topalian, S.L., Schwartzentruber, D.J., Weber, J.S., Ettinghausen, S.E. (1993a) The development of gene therapy for the treatment of cancer. *Ann. Surg.*, **218**, 455–63.

Rosenberg, S.A., Lotze, M.T., Yang, J.C., Topalian, S.L., Chang, A.E., Schwartzentruber, D.J., Aebersold, P., Leitman, S., Linehan, W.M., and Seipp, C.A. (1993b) Prospective randomized trial of high-dose interleukin-2 alone or in conjunction with lymphokine-activated killer cells for the treatment of patients with advanced cancer. *J. Natl. Cancer Inst. USA*, **85**, 622–632.

Rosenberg, S.A., Yang, J.C., Topalian, S.L., Schwartzentruber, D.J., Weber, J.S., Parkinson, D.R., Seipp, C.A., Einhorn, J.H., and White, D.E. (1994a) Treatment of 283 consecutive patients with metastatic melanoma or renal cell cancer using high-dose bolus interleukin 2. *JAMA*, **271**, 907–913.

Rosenberg, S.A., Yannelli, J.R., Yang, J.C., Topalian, S.L., Schwartzentruber, D.J., Weber, J.S., Parkinson, D.R., Seipp, C.A., Einhorn, J.H., and White, D.E. (1994b) Treatment of patients with metastatic melanoma with autologous tumor-infiltrating lymphocytes and IL-2. *J. Natl. Cancer Inst. USA*, **86**, 1159–1166.

Rosenberg, S.A. (1997a) Cancer vaccines based on the identification of genes encoding cancer regression antigens. *Immunol. Today*, **18**, 175–182.

Rosenberg, S.A. (1997b) Keynote address: perspective on the use of Interleukin-2 in cancer treatment. *Cancer J. Sci. Am.*, **3**, S2–S6.

Rosenberg, S.A., Yang, J.C., Schwartzentruber, D., Hwu, P., Marincola, F.C., Topalian, S.L., Restifo, N.P., Dufour, E., Schwartzberg, L., Spiess, P., Wunderlich, J., Parkhurst, M.R., Kawakami, Y., Seipp, C., Einhorn, J.H., and White, D. (1998a) Immunologic and therapeutic evaluation of a synthetic tumor associated peptide vaccine for the treatment of patients with metastatic melanoma. *Nature Med.*, **4**, 321–327.

Rosenberg, S.A., Zhai, Y., Yang, J.C., Schwartzentruber, D.J., Hwu, P., Marincola, F.M., Topalian, S.L., Restifo, N.P., Seipp, C.A., Einhorn, J.H., Roberts, B., and White, D.E. (1998b) Immunizing patients with metastatic melanoma using recombinant adenoviruses encoding MART-1 or gp100 melanoma antigens. *J. Natl Cancer Inst. USA*, **90**, 1894–1900.

Rosenberg, S.A., Yang, J.C., Schwartzentruber, D.J., Hwu, P., Marincola, F.M., Topalian, S.L., Restifo, N.P., Sznol, M., Schwarz, S.L., Spiess, P.J., Wunderlich, J.R., Seipp, C.A., Einhorn, J.H., Rogers-Freezer, L., and White, D.E. (1999a) Impact of cytokine administration on the generation of antitumor reactivity in patients with metastatic melanoma receiving a peptide vaccine. *J. Immunol.*, **163**, 1690–1695.

Rosenberg, S.A., Yang, J.C., Schwartzentruber, D.J., Hwu, P., Marincola, F.M., Topalian, S.L., Seipp, C.A., Einhorn, J.H., White, D.E., and Steinberg, S.M. (1999b) Prospective randomized trial of the treatment of patients with metastatic melanoma using chemotherapy with cisplatin, dacarbazine and tomoxifen alone or in combination with interleukin-2 and alpha-interferon. *J. Clin. Oncol.*, **17**, 968–975.

Royal, R.E., Steinberg, S.M., Krouse, S.E., Heywood, G., White, D.E., Hwu, P., Marincola, F.M., Parkinson, D.R., Schwartzentruber, D.J., Topalian, S.L., Yang, J.C., and Rosenberg, S.A. (1996) Correlates of response to il-2 therapy in patients treated for metastatic renal cancer and melanoma. *Cancer J. Sci. Am.*, **2**, 91–98.

Rusciani, L., Petraglia, S., Alotto, M., Calvieri, S., and Vezzoni, G. (1997) Postsurgical adjuvant therapy for melanoma. Evaluation of a 3-year randomized trial with recombinant interferon-alpha after 3 and 5 years of follow-up. *Cancer*, **79**, 2354–2360.

Salgaller, M.L., Marincola, F.M., Cormier, J.N., and Rosenberg, S.A. (1996) Immunization against epitopes in the human melanoma antigen gp100 following patient immunization with synthetic peptides. *Cancer Res.*, **56**, 4749–4757.

Savary, J. (1995) Biologic Therapy with interferon-α and β: clinical applications. Renal cell cancer. In: DeVita, V.T., Hellman, S., and Rosenberg, S.A., (Eds.) *Biologic Therapy of Cancer* (2 edn), pp. 373–387. Philadelphia: J.B. Lippincott Co.

Scalzo, A.A., Elliott, S.L., Cox, J., Gardner, J., Moss, D.J., and Suhrbier, A. (1995) Induction of protective cytotoxic T cells to murine cytomegalovirus by using a nonapeptide and a human-compatible adjuvant (Montanide ISA 720). *J. Vir.*, **69**, 1306–1309.

Schmittel, A., Keilholz, U., Max, R., Thiel, E., and Scheibenbogen, C. (1999) Induction of tyrosinase-reactive T cells by treatment with dacarbazine, cisplatin, interferon-alpha $+/-$ interleukin-2 in patients with metastatic melanoma. *Int. J. Cancer*, **80**, 39–43.

Schreurs, M.W., de Boer, A.J., Figdor, C.G., and Adema, G.J. (1998) Genetic vaccination against the melanocyte lineage-specific antigen gp100 induces cytotoxic T lymphocyte-mediated tumor protection. *Cancer Res.*, **58**, 2509–2514.

Schuler, M., Bruntsch, U., Spath-Schwalbe, E., Schrezenmeier, H., Peschle, C., Farber, L., Burger, K.J., Leissner, J., Huber, C., and Aulitzky, W.E. (1998) Lack of efficacy of recombinant human interleukin-6 in patients with advanced renal cell cancer: results of a phase II study. *Eur. J. Cancer*, **34**, 754–756.

Schwartzentruber, D.J., Topalian, S.L., Mancini, M., and Rosenberg, S.A. (1991) Specific release of granulocyte-macrophage colony-stimulating factor, tumor necrosis factor-alpha, and IFN-gamma by human tumor-infiltrating lymphocytes after autologous tumor stimulation. *J. Immunol.*, **146**, 3674–3681.

Seder, R.A., and Le Gros, G.G. (1995) The functional role of CD8$^+$ T helper type 2 cells. *J. Exp. Med.*, **181**, 449–451.

Sensi, M., Farina, C., Maccalli, C., Anichini, A., Berd, D., and Parmiani, G. (1998) Intralesional selection of T cell clonotypes in the immune response to melanoma antigens occurring during vaccination. *J. Immunother.*, **21**, 198–204.

Sinigaglia, F., and Hammer, J. (1995) Motifs and supermotifs for MHC class II binding peptides. *J. Exp. Med.*, **181**, 449–451.

Soiffer, R., Lynch, T., Mihm, M., Jung, K., Rhuda, C., Schmollinger, J.C., Hodi, F.S., Liebster, L., Lam, P., Mentzer, S., Singer, S., Tanabe, K.K., Cosimi, A.B., Duda, R., Sober, A., Bhan, A., Daley, J., Neuberg, D., Parry, G., Rokovich, J., Richards, L., Drayer, J., Berns, A., Clift, S., and Dranoff, G. (1998) Vaccination with irradiated autologous melanoma cells engineered to secrete human granulocyte-macrophage colony-stimulating factor generates potent antitumor immunity in patients with metastatic melanoma. *Proc. Natl. Acad. Sci. USA*, **95**, 13141–13146.

Sorio, R., Galligioni, E., Sacco, C., Morassut, S., Freschi, A., Quaia, M., Spada, A., Favaro, D., Santarosa, M., and Boccalon, M. (1992) Dose level and response in 30 patients with renal cell cancer (RCC) treated with recombinant interleukin-2 (RIL-2). *Proc. Am. Soc. Clin. Oncol.*, **11**, A658.

Sparano, J.A., Fisher, R.I., Sunderland, M., Margolin, K., Ernest, M.L., Sznol, M., Atkins, M.B., Dutcher, J.P., Micetich, K.C., Weiss, G.R., *et al.* (1993) Randomized phase III trial of treatment with high-dose interleukin-2 either alone or in combination with interferon alfa-2a in patients with advanced melanoma. *J. Clin. Oncol.*, **11**, 1969–1977.

Spiess, P.J., Yang, J.C., and Rosenberg, S.A. (1987) *In vivo* antitumor activity of tumor-infiltrating lymphocytes expanded in recombinant interleukin-2. *J. Natl. Cancer Inst. USA*, **79**, 1067–1075.

Stadler, W.M., Rybak, M.E., and Vogelzang, N.J. (1995) A phase II study of subcutaneous recombinant human interleukin-4 in metastatic renal cell carcinoma. *Cancer*, **76**, 1629–1633.

Stadler, W.M., Kuzel, T., Dumas, M., and Vogelzang, N.J. (1998) Multicenter phase II trial of interleukin-2, interferon-alpha, and 13-cis-retinoic acid in patients with metastatic renal-cell carcinoma. *J. Clin. Oncol.*, **16**, 1820–1825.

Stockert, E., Jäger, E., Chen, Y.T., Scanlan, M.J., Gout, I., Karbach, J., Arand, M., Knuth, A., and Old, L.J. (1998) A survey of the humoral immune response of cancer patients to a panel of human tumor antigens. *J. Exp. Med.*, **187**, 1349–1354.

Sznol, M., Mier, J.W., Sparano, J., Gaynor, E.R., Margolin, K.A., Bar, M.H., and Hawkins, M.J. (1990) A phase I study of high-dose interleukin-2 in combination with interferon-alpha 2b. *J. Biol. Resp. Mod.*, **9**, 529–537.

Talpaz, M., Kantarjian, H.M., McCredie, K., Trujillo, J.M., Keating, M.J., and Gutterman, J.U. (1986) Hematologic remission and cytogenetic improvement induced by recombinant human interferon alpha A in chronic myelogenous leukemia. *N. Engl. J. Med.*, **314**, 1065–1069.

Tepper, R.I., and Mulé, J.J. (1994) Experimental and clinical studies of cytokine gene-modified tumor cells. *Hum. Gene Ther.*, **5**, 153–164.

Thomas, W.D., and Hersey, P. (1998) TRAIL induces apoptosis in Fas ligand resistant melanoma cells and mediates CD4 T cell killing of target cells. *J. Immunol.*, **161**, 2195–2200.

Thompson, J.A., Lee, D.J., Lindgren, C.G., Benz, L.A., Collins, C., Levitt, D., and Fefer, A. (1988) Influence of dose and duration of infusion of interleukin-2 on toxicity and immunomodulation. *J. Clin. Oncol.*, **6**, 669–678.

thor Straten, S.P., Becker, J.C., Seremet, T., Brocker, E.B., and Zeuthen, J. (1996) Clonal T cell responses in tumor infiltrating lymphocytes from both regressive and progressive regions of primary human malignant melanoma. *J. Clin. Invest.*, **98**, 279–284.

Thurner, B., Haendle, I., Roder, C., Dieckmann, D., Keikavoussi, P., Jonuleit, H., Bender, A., Maczek, C., Schreiner, D., von den Driesch, P., Brocker, E.B., Steinman, R.M., Enk, A., Kampgen, E., and Schuler, G. (1999) Vaccination with mage-3A1 peptide-pulsed mature, monocyte-derived dendritic cells expands specific cytotoxic T cells and induces regression of some metastases in advanced stage IV melanoma. *J. Exp. Med.*, **190**, 1669–1678.

Tjandrawan, T., Martin, D.M., Maeurer, M.J., Castelli, C., Lotze, M.T., and Storkus, W.J. (1998) Autologous human dendriphages pulsed with synthetic or natural tumor peptides elicit tumor-specific CTLs *in vitro*. *J. Immunother.*, **21**, 149–157.

Toes, R.E.M., Blom, R.J.J., Offringa, R., Kast, W.M., and Melief, C.J.M. (1996) Enhanced tumor outgrowth after peptide vaccination. *J. Immunol.*, **156**, 3911–3918.

Tourani, J.M., Lucas, V., Mayeur, D., Dufour, B., DiPalma, M., Boaziz, C., Grise, P., Varette, C., Pavlovitch, J.M., Pujade-Lauraine, E., Larregain, D., Ecstein, E., Untereiner, M., Vuillemin, E., Merran, S., and Andrieu, J.M. (1996) Subcutaneous recombinant interleukin-2 (rIL-2) in out-patients with metastatic renal cell carcinoma. Results of a multicenter SCAPP1 trial. *Ann. Oncol.*, **7**, 525–528.

Tourani, J.M., Pfister, C., Berdah, J.F., Benhammouda, A., Salze, P., Monnier, A., Paule, B., Guillet, P., Chretien, Y., Brewer, Y., Di Palma, M., Untereiner, M., Malaurie, E., Tadrist, Z., Pavlovitch, J.M., Hauteville, D., Mejean, A., Azagury, M., Mayeur, D., Lucas, V., Krakowski, I., Larregain-Fournier, D., Abourachid, H., Andrieu, J.M., and Chastang, C. (1998) Outpatient treatment with subcutaneous interleukin-2 and interferon alfa administration in combination with fluorouracil in patients with metastatic renal cell carcinoma: results of a sequential nonrandomized phase II study. Subcutaneous administration propeukin program cooperative group. *J. Clin. Oncol.*, **16**, 2505–2513.

Townsend, A.R., Rothbard, J., Gotch, F.M., Bahadur, G., Wraith, D., and McMichael, A.J. (1986) The epitopes of influenza nucleoprotein recognized by cytotoxic T lymphocytes can be defined with short synthetic peptides. *Cell*, **44**, 959–968.

Tuting, T., Wilson, C.C., Martin, D.M., Kasamon, Y.L., Rowles, J., Ma, D.I., Slingluff, C.L. Jr., Wagner, S.N., van der Bruggen, P., Baar, J., Lotze, M.T., and Storkus, W.J. (1998) Autologous human monocyte-derived dendritic cells genetically modified to express melanoma antigens elicit primary cytotoxic T cell responses *in vitro*: enhancement by cotransfection of genes encoding the Th1-biasing cytokines IL-12 and IFN-alpha. *J. Immunol.*, **160**, 1139–1147.

Valmori, D., Lienard, D., Waanders, G., Rimoldi, D., Cerottini, J.-C., and Romero, P. (1997) Analysis of MAGE-3-specific cytolytic T lymphocytes in human leukocyte antigen-A2 melanoma patients. *Cancer Res.*, **57**, 735–741.

Vaughan, H.W. (1914) Cancer vaccine and anti-cancer globulin as an aid in the surgical treatment of malignancy. *J. Am. Med. Ass.*, **63**, 1258–1268.

Vierboom, M.P.M., Nijman, H.W., Offringa, R., Van Der Voort, E.I.H., van Hall, T., van den Broek, L., Fleuren, G.J., Kenemans, P., Kast, W.M., and Melief, C.J.M. (1997) Tumor eradication by Wild-type p53-specific cytotoxic T lymphocytes. *J. Exp. Med.*, **186**, 695–704.

Vitiello, A., Ishioka, G., Gray, H.M., Rose, R., Farness, P., LaFond, R., Yuan, L., Chisari, F.V., Furze, J., Bartholomeuz, R., and Chesnut, R.W. (1995) Development of a lipopeptide-based therapeutic vaccine to treat chronic HBV infection. *J. Clin. Invest.*, **95**, 341–349.

Vlasveld, L.T., Rankin, E.M., Heckman, A., Rodenhuis, S., Beijnen, J.H., Hilton, A.M., Dubbelman, A.C., Vyth-Dreese, F.A., and Melief, C.W. (1992) A phase I study of prolonged continuous infusion of low dose recombinant interleukin-2 in melanoma and renal cell cancer. Part I: clinical aspects. *Br. J. Cancer*, **65**, 744–750.

Vokes, E.E., Figlin, R., Hochster, H., Lotze, M., and Rybak, M.E. (1998) A phase II study of recombinant human interleukin-4 for advanced or recurrent non-small cell lung cancer. *Cancer J. Sci. Am.*, **4**, 46–51.

Walker, R.E. (1996) A phase I/II pilot study of the safety of the adoptive transfer of syngeneic gene-modified cytotoxic T lymphocytes in HIV-infected identical twins. *Hum. Gene Ther.*, **7**, 367–400.

Wallack, M.K., Sivanandham, M., Balch, C.M., Urist, M.M., Bland, K.I., Murray, D., Robinson, W.A., Flaherty, L., Richards, J.M., Bartolucci, A.A., and Rosen, L. (1998) Surgical adjuvant active specific immunotherapy for patients with stage III melanoma: the final analysis of data from a phase III, randomized, double-blind, multicenter vaccinia melanoma oncolysate trial. *J. Am. Coll. Surg.*, **187**, 69–77.

Wang, F., Bade, E., Kuniyoshi, C., Spears, L., Jeffery, G., Marty, V., Groshen, S., and Weber, J. (1999) Phase I trial of a MART-1 peptide vaccine with incomplete Freund's adjuvant for resected high-risk melanoma. *Clin. Cancer Res.*, **10**, 2756–2765.

Weber, J.S., Hua, F.L., Spears, L., Marty, V., Kuniyoshi, C., and Celis, E. (1999) A phase I trial of an HLA-A1 restricted MAGE-3 epitope peptide with incomplete Freund's adjuvant in patients with resected high-risk melanoma *J. Immunother.*, **22**, 431–440.

Weiss, G.R., Margolin, K.A., Sznol, M., Atkins, M.B., Oleksowicz, L., Isaacs, R., Sosman, J.A., Doroshow, J.H., Trehu, E.G., and Dutcher, J.P. (1995) A phase II study of the continuous intravenous infusion of interleukin-6 for metastatic renal cell carcinoma. *J. Immunother.*, **18**, 52–56.

West, W., Schwartzberg, L., Blumenchein, G., Barth, N., Dillman, R., Birch, R., and Oldham, R. (1990) Continuous infusion interleukin-2 (IL-2) plus sc interferon alpha 2b (IFN) in advanced malignancy. *Proc. Am. Soc. Clin. Oncol.*, **9**, A738.

White, R.L.J., Schwartzentruber, D., Guleria, A.S., McFarlane, M.P., White, D.E., Ucker, E., and Rosenberg, S.A. (1994) Cardiopulmonary toxicity of treatment with high-dose interleukin-2 in 199 consecutive patients with metastatic melanoma or renal cell carcinoma. *Cancer*, **74**, 3212–3222.

Whitehead, R.P., Kopecky, K.J., Samson, M.K., Costanzi, J.J., Natale, R.B., Feun, L.G., Hersh, E.M., and Rinehart, J.J. (1991) Phase II study of intravenous bolus recombinant interleukin-2 in advanced malignant melanoma: Southwest Oncology Group study. *J. Natl. Cancer. Inst. USA*, **83**, 1250–1252.

Whitehead, R.P., Figlin, R., Citron, M.L., Pfile, J., Moldawer, N., Patel, D., Jones, G., Levitt, D., and Zeffren, J. (1993) A phase II trial of concomitant human interleukin-2 and interferon-alpha-2a in patients with disseminated malignant melanoma. *J. Immunother.*, **13**, 117–121.

Whitehead, R.P., Wolf, M.K., Solanki, D.L., Hemstreet, G.P., Benedetto, P., Richman, S.P., Flanigan, R.C., and Crawford, E.D. (1995) A phase II trial of continuous-infusion recombinant interleukin-2 in patients with advanced renal cell carcinoma: a Southwest Oncology Group study. *J. Immunother.*, **18**, 104–114.

Whiteside, T.L., and Parmiani, G. (1994) Tumor-infiltrating lymphocytes: their phenotype, functions and clinical use. *Cancer Immunol. Immunother.*, **39**, 15–21.

Witte, R.S., Leong, T., Ernstoff, M.S., Krigel, R.L., Oken, M.M., Harris, J., Tormey, D.C., and Trump, D.L. (1995) A phase II study of interleukin-2 with and without beta-interferon in the treatment of advanced renal cell carcinoma. *Invest. N. Drugs*, **13**, 241–247.

Woglom, W.H. (1929) Immunity to transplantable tumours. *Cancer Rev.*, **4**, 129–140.

Wojtowicz-Praga, S. (1997) Reversal of tumor-induced immunosuppression: a new approach to cancer therapy. *J. Immunother.*, **20**, 165–177.

Yang, J.C., Topalian, S.L., Schwartzentruber, D.J., Parkinson, D.R., Marincola, F.M., Weber, J.S., Seipp, C.A., White, D.E., and Rosenberg, S.A. (1995) The use of polyethylene glycol-modified interleukin-2 (PEG-IL-2) in the treatment of patients with metastatic renal cell carcinoma and melanoma. A phase I study and a randomized prospective study comparing IL-2 alone versus IL-2 combined with PEG-IL-2. *Cancer*, **76**, 687–694.

Yang, J.C., and Rosenberg, S.A. (1997) An ongoing prospective randomized comparison of interleukin-2 regimens for the treatment of metastatic renal cell cancer. *Cancer J. Sci. Am.*, **3**, S79–S84.

Yannelli, J.R., McConnell, S., Parker, L., Nishimura, M., Robbins, P., Yang, J., el Gamil, M., and Kawakami, Y. (1995) Melanoma tumor-infiltrating lymphocytes derived from four distinct anatomic sites obtained from a single patient: comparison of functional reactivity and melanoma antigen recognition. *J. Immunother. Emphasis Tumor Immunol.*, **18**, 263–271.

Yee, C., Gilbert, M.J., Riddell, S.R., Brichard, V.G., Fefer, A., Thompson, J.A., Boon, T., and Greenberg, P.D. (1996) Isolation of tyrosinase-specific CD8+ and CD4+ T cell clones from the peripheral blood of melanoma patients following *in vitro* stimulation with recombinant vaccinia virus. *J. Immunol.*, **157**, 4079–4086.

Yee, C., Savage, P.A., Lee, P.P., Davis, M.M., and Greenberg, P.D. (1999) Isolation of high avidity melanoma-reactive CTL from heterogeneous populations using peptide-MHC tetramers. *J. Immunol.*, **162**, 2227–2234.

Yewdell, J.W., and Bennink, J.R. (1990) The binary logic of antigen processing and presentation to T cells. *Cell*, **62**, 203–206.

Zaks, T.Z., and Rosenberg, S.A. (1998) Immunization with a peptide epitope (p369–377) from HER-2/neu leads to peptide-specific cytotoxic T lymphocytes that fail to recognize HER-2/neu + tumors. *Cancer Res.*, **58**, 4902–4908.

Zea, A.H., Curti, B.D., Longo, D.L., Alvord, W.G., Strobl, S.L., Mizoguchi, H., Creekmore, S.P., O'Shea, J.J., Powers, G.C., Urba, W.J., and Ochoa, A.C. (1995) Alterations in T cell receptor and signal transduction molecules in melanoma patients. *Clin. Cancer Res.*, **1**, 1327–1335.

Zinkernagel, R.M. (1996) Immunology taught by viruses. *Science*, **271**, 173–178.

6 Tumor Evasion of Immune System

Francisco Ruiz-Cabello and Federico Garrido

ABBREVIATIONS

Ad-2, -12	Adenovirus-2, -12
APC	Antigen-presenting cells
β2m	Beta2-microglobulin
CT	Computerized tomography
CTL	Cytotoxic T lymphocytes
EBV	Epstein-Barr virus
ER	Endoplasmic reticulum
HLA	Human leukocyte antigen
HNPCC	Hereditary non-polyposis colorectal cancer
IFN-γ	Interferon gamma
IL-...	Interleukin-2, -7, -10, -12
KIRs	Killing inhibitory receptors
mAb	Monoclonal antibodies
NK	Natural killer
PTK	Protein tyrosine kinases
RE	Regulatory elements
TAPs	Transporter associated with peptide
TCR	T cell receptors
TGF-β	Transforming growth factor beta
TH	T helper
TIL	Tumor-infiltrating lymphocytes
TNF-α	Tumor necrosis factor alpha

Tumor evasion of immune system

Evasion of immune response by tumor cells can be due to several factors, which affect tumor cells and/or the host immune system. The following mechanism play an important role in the selection of the appropiate tumor escape variants.

1. **HLA expression of neoplastic cells can be downregulated, or completely lacking, as a result of genetic alterations of genes encoding the heavy or light (β_2-microglobulin) chains of the MHC molecule, or abnormalities in transcription or in protein processing. This occurs in many types of tumors, particularly in metastatic lesions.**
2. **Oncogenic viruses (e.g. adenovirus, HPV, EBV) have evolved mechanisms by which they interfere with HLA expression in infected cells.**
3. **Tumor antigen expression can be significantly reduced by T-cell specific host immune reactions during tumor growth, and the most immunogenic tumor cells eliminated in favor of non-immunogenic counterparts.**
4. **NK cells can be activated by HLA loss-variant tumor cells since HLA are ligands for killer inhibitory receptors expressed by these effectors and by a subpopulation of T cells.**
5. **Immunosuppressive cytokines (e.g. TGFβ, IL-10, GM-CSF, VEGF) can be released by neoplastic cells, or other cells in the tumor microenvironment, thus blocking lymphocyte function.**
6. **Expression of FasL by tumor cells may induce apoptosis of Fas+, activated lymphocytes (tumor counterattack).**
7. **The presence of tumor cells can alter the signal transduction machinery of patients' T cells, particularly of those infiltrating metastatic lesions.**

INTRODUCTION

Over the past few years, there have been many studies elucidating mechanisms implicated in the low immunogenicity of tumor cells. This phenomenon is relatively common in most spontaneous tumors, despite the more than likely existence of numerous proteins that could function as potential targets for the immune system. Characterization of the mechanisms implicated in low immunogenicity could be important in cancer immunotherapy, since some recently developed strategies depend on the correct functioning of the entire antigenic processing machinery in order to enhance immunologic recognition. Some of these alterations in the capacity of antigenic presentation are irreversible when they affect structural genes but not when they affect regulatory processes, which may be sensitive to cytokine treatment. Knowledge of the exact mechanisms by which cancer can elude the immune system is important, because it can assist decision-making on changes in vaccination strategy or therapeutic approach.

In fact, tumor cells express new antigens as a result of multiple genetic alterations that participate in cell transformation. These antigens can originate variously: from oncogene products, including fusion proteins (i.e., mutations in Ras proteins, Bcr/Abl fusion proteins); mutated tumor-suppressor gene products; self-proteins of embryonic origin or expressed in immune privileged sites, such as components of the MAGE family; finally, foreign proteins from viral gene products or of idiotypic origin (see Chapter 1 in this book).

Although tumors can express some of these antigens that are susceptible to recognition as foreign by the tumor host, and while immunosurveillance can influence the growth of some tumors, the immune system does not achieve control over the growth of most human malignant tumors. This is due to a combination of factors that allow the tumor cells to be tolerated by the effector cells of the immune system. Indeed, it has been demonstrated that the humoral and cell components that fight against antigens derived from viral infections or intracellular bacteria are the same ones that attack neoplastic cells. In both situations, cells are sometimes efficiently recognized and the immune system is activated while on other occasions a tolerance is produced and the cells are simply ignored.

The ability of virus-infected and tumor cells to put themselves into an immune privileged situation depends on many factors, some of which can be understood as the result of a passive process: reduced or absent antigenic expression due to defects in the antigenic processing or presentation machinery, or lack of expression of the tumor antigens themselves or of molecules that participate in the triggering of T-cell induced apoptosis. In contrast, other mechanisms may imply an active process: secretion of suppressor cytokines, appearance of cell surface molecules that modulate the activity of T and NK cells, the induction of abnormalities in the signal transduction of T cells, etc. In the following sections we shall elucidate some of these mechanisms.

MODIFICATION OF TUMOR CELLS THAT INDUCE IMMUNOLOGIC IGNORANCE

Several mechanisms have been described to explain the poor immunogenicity or immune escape of tumor cells (Table 6.1). While this feature also exists in non-malignant diseases such as viral infection, it may enhance tumor growth. Amongst different reasons for the poor immunogenicity of tumor cells, the most frequent is the

TABLE 6.1
Mechanisms of immune escape

Mechanisms	*Effect*
Structural and regulatory HLA gene defects	Loss of CTL recognition
Defects in antigen-processing machinery	Loss of CTL recognition
Loss or decrease of tumor antigen expression	Loss of CTL recognition
Expression of HLA class Ib molecules	Inhibition of NK and KIR-CTLs
Production of immunosuppressive cytokines by tumor cells	Inhibition of APC function, inhibition of CTL responses
Loss of Fas in tumor cells	Absence of T-cell induced apoptosis
Expression of FasL on tumor cells	Induction of apoptosis in Fas+ CTLs

downregulation of the expression of major histocompatibility complex molecules, of importance because it prevents the presentation of tumor antigen peptides to T cells. In this section we also consider processes that lead to the loss of other molecules implicated in antigenic processing and presentation and those that give rise to the appearance of antigen-loss variants. One of these mechanisms, or the simultaneous combination of several, leads to a lack of adequate antigenic signals due to a low level of tumor antigen presentation.

EVASION BY MHC ALTERED GENE AND CELL SURFACE EXPRESSION

Human HLA class I downregulation is a widespread phenomenon in tumor biology (Festenstein, 1987; Garrido *et al.*, 1993; Garrido *et al.*, 1997) and probably reflects a mechanism by which tumor cells can escape immune response because of the role of HLA molecules in presenting immunogenic peptides to T cells (Branch *et al.*, 1995).

There have been many studies of mechanisms that lead to a low cell surface expression of HLA molecules (Festenstein and Garrido, 1986). It has been demonstrated that all the biosynthetic stages of these molecules are suitable targets for this strategy during tumorigenesis (Figure 6.1). The result is the attenuation of expression of one, various, or all of the HLA alleles, which gives a selective advantage because the cells are then invisible to CTLs. This strategy, acquired in a relatively short period of time during tumor progression, is also used by viruses for immune evasion but in their case as a consequence of evolution (Ploegh, 1998). Alterations in the expression of HLA are not a sporadic phenomenon, as could be deduced from the first immunohistologic studies performed with mAb (López-Nevot *et al.*, 1989), and may affect from 39% to 88% of tumors derived from HLA+ epithelia (Table 6.2). On one hand, this is even likely to be an underestimate due to the limited panel of mAbs that define HLA alleles and can be used in tissue sections (Cabrera *et al.*, 1996, 1998). On the other hand, a recent analysis suggests a more complex picture where the large proportion of the various HLA epitopes were relatively preserved in early passage cell line/PBMC pairs (Giacomini *et al.*, 1999). In any event, a large number of studies provide the basis for defining various phenotypes in tumor cells (Garrido *et al.*, 1995) (see Figure 6.2), as indicated below.

Phenotype I: total HLA loss (Figure 6.2a). Tumor cells may exhibit a complete loss of expression of HLA antigens. This is a relatively frequent phenotype (9–52%), readily detected in human tumors with mAbs. It can be associated with defects in β2 m, synthesis or transporter-associated processing.

Phenotype II: HLA haplotype loss (Figure 6.2b). Loss of an HLA haplotype has been shown in cervix melanoma, pancreas, larynx and in colon tumor cell lines. Loss of a full chromosome 6 or deletion of a large genomic region has been found in the majority of cases, as shown by immunohistochemistry in Figure 6.3 (Jimenez *et al.*, 1999). Recent data indicate that this HLA phenotype is detected with a high frequency when microdissected tumor samples are used (Ramal *et al.*, 2000).

Phenotype III: HLA locus loss (Figure 6.2c). Loss of class I locus expression of HLA-A (range 3–19%) or HLA-B (5–19%) has been documented in several tumors. The

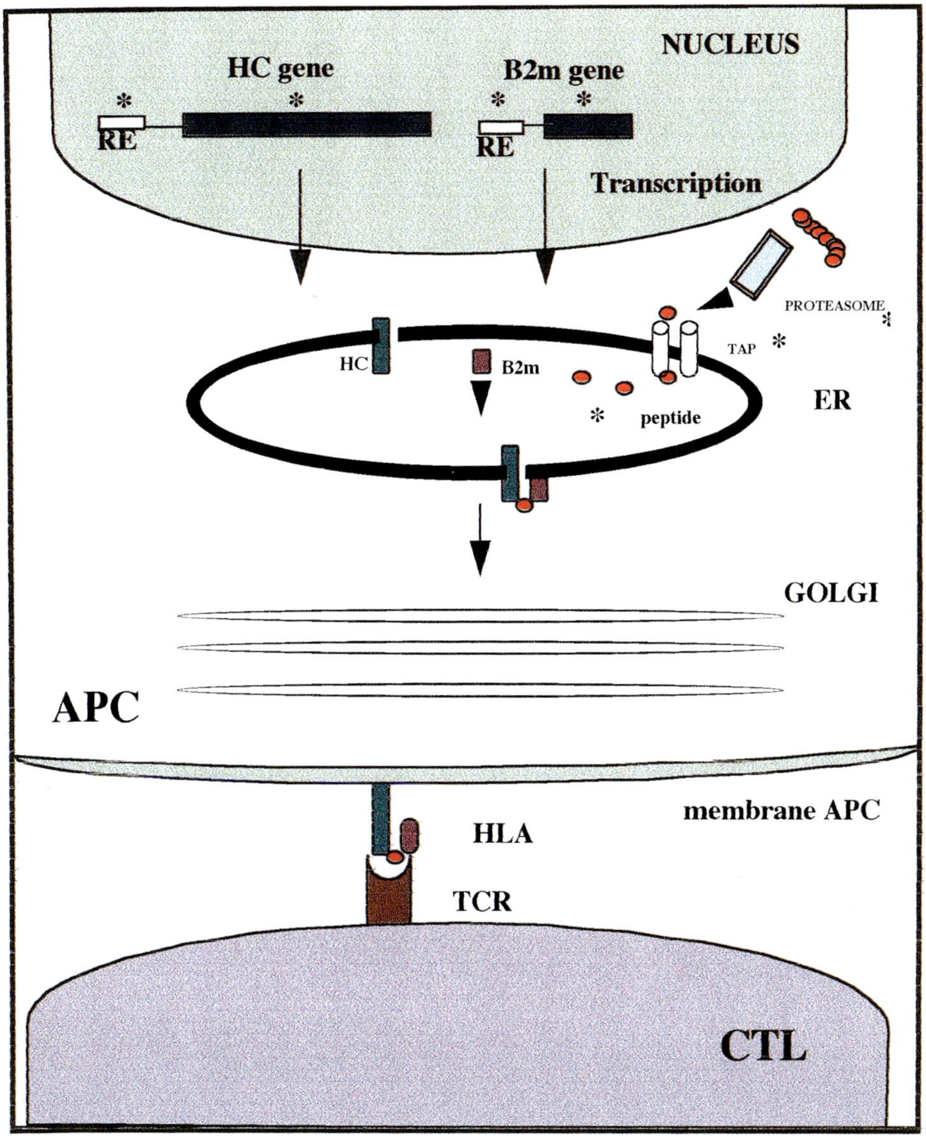

Figure 6.1 Trafficking pathways of MHC class I molecules. Cytotoxic T cells recognize antigen peptides presented by antigen-presenting cells in the context of MHC class I molecules. Asterisks indicate points where HLA class I cell surface expression is blocked.

mechanisms of locus-specific downregulation may be transcriptional since there are differences in HLA class I locus promoter sequences and in mRNA levels for some alleles in tumors vs. normal cells. Furthermore, in some tumors such as melanomas, the selective downregulation of HLA-B locus has been related to oncogenic products.

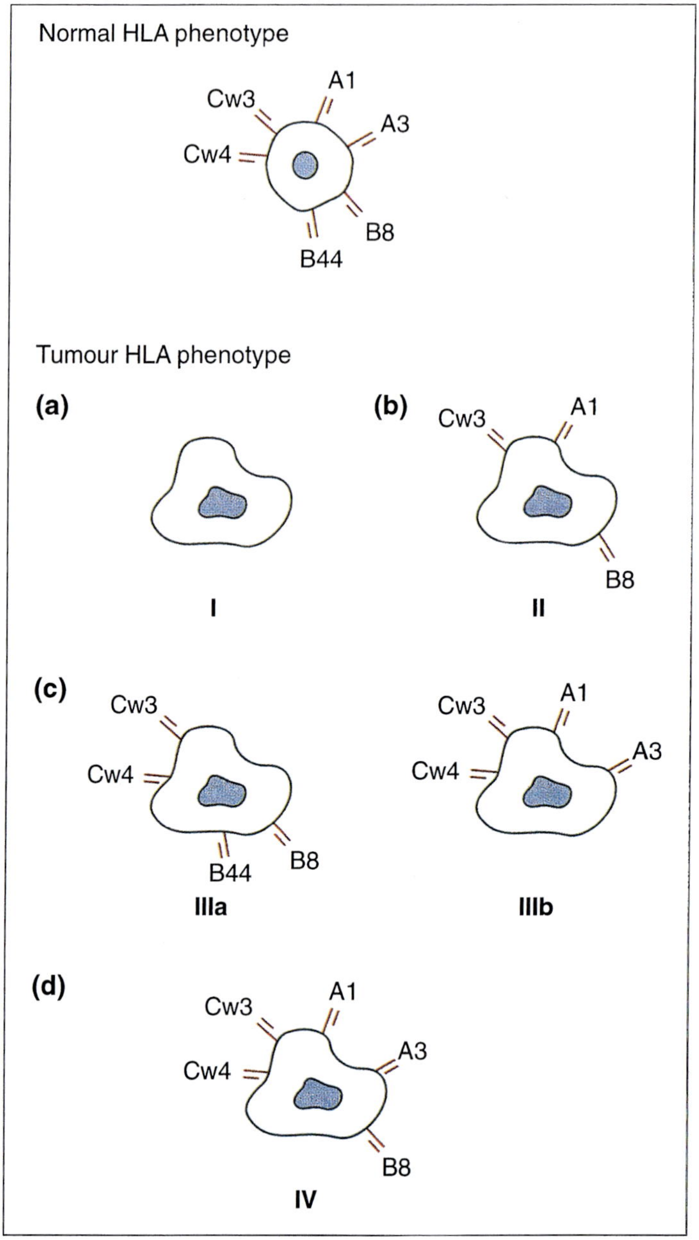

Figure 6.2 Altered HLA class I phenotypes in invasive tumors. Graphic representation of the different HLA class I phenotypes already identified in human tumors (from phenotype I–IV). (a) phenotype I corresponds with HLA class I total losses; (b) II with HLA haplotype losses; (c) IIIa and IIIb with HLA-A and -B locus-specific losses, respectively; (d) phenotype IV with HLA allelic losses (A, B, and C). There is no information about the frequency of HLA-C locus losses in tumors since there are no monoclonal antibodies capable of defining these alterations. The HLA-C-locus deficient phenotype is not included. A hypothetical patient with the HLA typing of A1, A3, B8, B44, Cw1, Cw3 is shown. Figure reproduced from Garrido *et al.*, 1997.

TABLE 6.2
Frequency (%) of HLA Class I altered phenotypes in invasive tumors (see Garrido *et al.*, 1997).

Tumor type	*Loss of*					*Total*
	HLA-ABC	*HLA-A*	*HLA-B*	*HLA-AB*	*HLA-allelic*	
Breast	52	4	8	9	15	88
Cervix	22	7	19	8	34	90
Colon	23	8	7	7	36	81
Larynx	9	19	16	9	26	79
Melanoma	16	3	5	2	25	51
Pancreas	12	19	8	not determined	not determined	39
Prostate	34	not determined	not determined	not determined	51	85

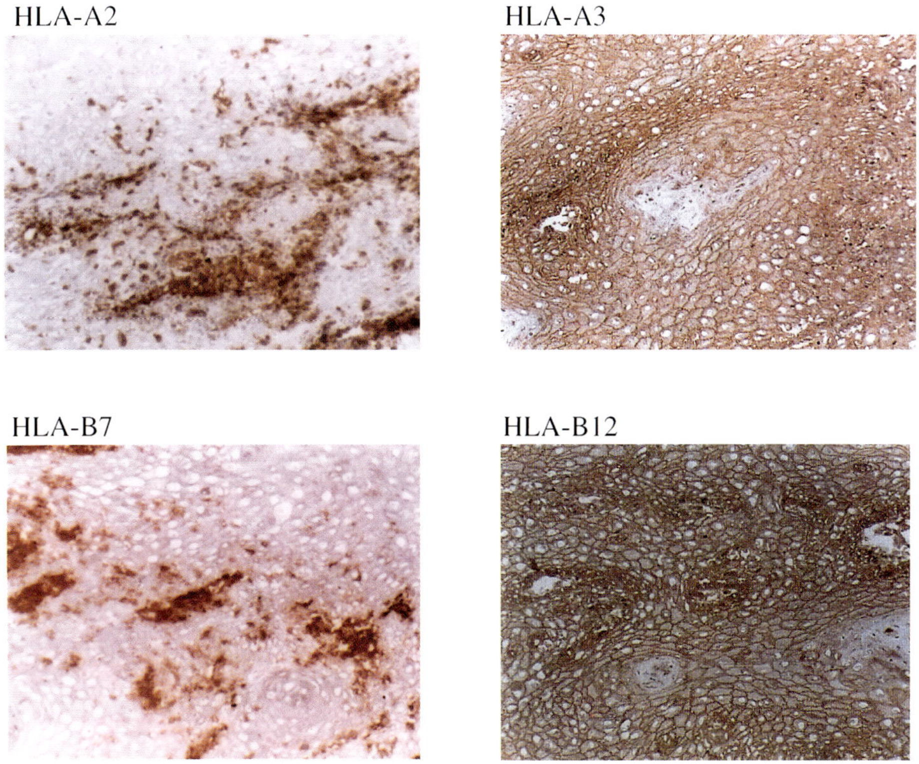

Figure 6.3 Immunoperoxidase staining of cryostatic sections showing selective loss of HLA class I A2 and B7 alleles. Stromal cells and lymphocytes are used as positive controls. Anti HLA-A3 and anti HLA-B12 show a positive staining of both the stromal and tumor cells. × 400.

Phenotype IV: HLA allelic loss (Figure 6.2d). It is difficult to define the precise frequency of tumors which show the loss of only one HLA allele because of defects in the repertoire of allele-specific antibodies. The allelic loss might result from point mutations or partial deletions of HLA class I genes.

Some tumors display complex HLA class I phenotypes that do not fit into categories I–V and might reflect multiple events that occur during tumor progression. For instance, we recently defined a compound phenotype in a melanoma cell line in which HLA haplotype loss and HLA-B locus downregulation generate a cell with the expression of a single allele (Real *et al.*, 1998). Other support for this idea comes from evidence of an increased incidence of HLA class I downregulation in cervical carcinoma lymph node metastases compared to the primary cancers and in metastatic lesions obtained at different times from the same patients (Lehmann *et al.*, 1995). These observations are consistent with the selection of HLA class I-defective cell variants during tumor progression that may influence clinical outcome. In this sense, HLA tumor loss can be a dynamic process (Figure 6.4) that is likely produced as a consequence of selective pressure by antitumor T and NK cell responses (Garrido and Ruiz-Cabello, 1991; Lehmann *et al.*, 1995; Ikeda *et al.*, 1997). In the following sections we describe some of the mechanisms that produce HLA underexpression in tumor cells and discuss how the level of HLA class I expression can modulate T and NK-cell responses.

Altered MHC Class I Antigen Presentation

The accumulation of defects in antigen processing and presentation may be selected because they represent an advantage for tumor growth through the reduced recognition and destruction of malignant cells by the immune system. The classical MHC class I pathway requires the presentation to CTLs of peptides derived from intracellular synthesized proteins. The correct assembly of MHC class I/peptide complexes is

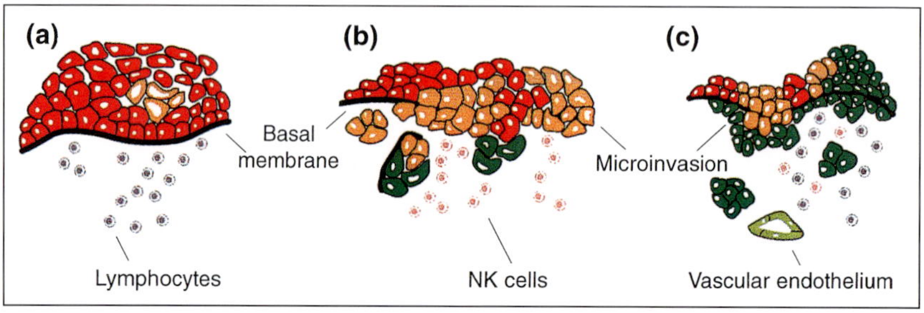

Figure 6.4 HLA changes occur during tumor progression to generate T and NK resistant cell variants (reproduced from Garrido *et al.*, 1997). (a) A hypothetical patient with the HLA phenotype A1, B3, B8, B44, Cw1, Cw3 contains a tumor that is HLA class I positive (red = stop). This tumor generates an HLA-deficient variant that is T-cell resistant but NK susceptible (orange = ready to go) (phenotype I). (b) At this stage the tumor generates a new variant (green = can go) that has lost HLA-A1 antigen but retains the other HLA alleles (phenotype IV). This variant remains T-cell resistant since A1 is the restriction element for antitumor CTLs but also escapes NKs owing to the inhibitory effect of the remaining HLA alleles on p58, p70 and p140 NK receptors. (c) The tumor escapes T and NK cell attack. The green population (phenotype IV) takes over the others.

required for the stable expression of HLA class I molecules. This assembly occurs in the ER, where newly synthesized MHC class I heavy chain and β2m form dimers (Pamer and Cresswell, 1998). The peptides that are generated from cytosolic proteins by a multisubunit protease called proteasome are translocated to the lumen of the ER by the transporting proteins (TAPs) (Figure 6.1). TAP is a heterodimer with two subunits TAP1 and TAP2 encoded by genes in the class II region of the MHC and is also polymorphic. TAP proteins are physically linked to class I molecules through association with tapasin, an ER-resident protein. When the class I molecule is correctly assembled and loaded with peptide it is released from ER and enters the secretory pathway to the cell surface (see also Chapter 2).

The identification of antigen-processing mutant cells was an important event in the characterization of all the machinery necessary to process endogenously synthesized proteins. In mutant cell lines that do not express TAP proteins, empty heavy chain-β2 m complexes do not acquire peptides and are unstable. Consequently, such cells express very little MHC class I on the cell surface and are unable to present peptides to CTLs. An inherent human deficiency in the TAP transporter has been identified in two siblings suffering from recurrent respiratory bacterial infections. TAP2 null allele was a consequence of truncation proteins and the cell surface expression of class I proteins was very low in these patients. This mechanism is a relatively common finding in human tumors and, as we shall see later on, is not the only one that can originate totally negative cells, because mutations that affect the β2 m chain give rise to the same phenotype. Restifo *et al.* (1993) identified a deficiency in antigen processing in small cell lung carcinoma cell lines derived from solid tumors and found low levels of mRNA for proteasome components and peptide transporters. Loss of TAP-1 expression has also been found in a high percentage of human cervical and renal cell carcinomas and is associated with tumor progression in breast cancer (Vitale *et al.*, 1998). Among the mechanisms implicated in the low expression of TAP genes stand out the presence of mutations or deletion of coding sequences that produce truncated protein through the appearance of a premature stop codon. This situation can especially occur in tumors with the mutator phenotype, where the possibility of a knock-out of both alleles appears more likely. However, an experimental study of transformed fibroblasts with *ras* demonstrated that the neoplastic transformation mechanisms themselves may be implicated in the destruction of antigen presentation machinery (Seliger *et al.*, 1998). The end result is similar to the double knock-out out of the β2 m gene observed in colon carcinoma cell lines with the mutator phenotype, which gives rise to tumors with a nearly total deficit of HLA molecules on the surface (see later). As in TAP-negative mutant cell lines, the tumor cells have very low cell-surface expression of MHC class I antigens. However, not all the alleles are equally affected in TAP-deficient cells, and peptides that enter the lumen of the ER independently of TAP can stabilize specific HLA allele expression. For example, such a pathway is used by HLA-A2 molecules that can associate with the peptides from the leader segment proteins (Bai and Forman, 1997). TAP defects provide malignant cells with a mechanism for escaping CTL lysis, but they also become susceptible to NK-cell clones. This phenotype could be restored after the gene transduction of peptide transporter genes (Salcedo *et al.*, 1994). This could be a rational strategy to enhance the immunogenicity of malignant tumors that express high levels of tumor antigen target but show functional defects in the endogenous processing of CTL epitopes and are poorly recognized by specific T lymphocytes (White *et al.*, 1998).

Structural Defects of β_2-Microglobulin Gene

As mentioned above, β2 m and peptide are essential for the conformation and transport of class I HLA to the cell surface (Figure 6.1). In this sense it is reasonable to think that mutations affecting this gene may substantially modify the expression of all HLA class I molecules. The main feature of this alteration is that it is an irreversible process resistant to treatment with IFN, and class I HLA expression can only be restored by somatic cell fusion assays, or by transfection of the β2-m gene.

Different molecular mechanisms have been shown to induce class I HLA down-regulation through a β2-m defect. Total loss of expression of β2 m was seen in tumor cell lines homozygous for one mutation or heterozygous for two mutations, whereas reduced expression correlated with a mutation in one allele of β2 m (Browning *et al.*, 1996). The first data showing the importance of this chain in the control of class I antigen expression were obtained in Daudi, a Burkitt's lymphoma B cell line. Daudi fails to express HLA because of the presence of a mutation in the initiation codon that results in the synthesis of an abnormal mRNA with low efficiency in its binding to ribosomes and does not involve translation (Rosa *et al.*, 1983).

Following this initial finding in a cell line, different defects ranging from point mutation to large deletions have been described. For example, in the melanoma cell line FO-1 defects in transcription of the β2-m gene result from a deletion involving the first exon of the 5′ flanking region and a segment of the first intron (D'Urso *et al.*, 1991). In the melanoma cell line SK-MEL-33, lack of β2-m expression is caused by a guanosine deletion in the β2 m gene involving a frame shift and the introduction of a stop codon. This molecular alteration represents a somatic mutation acquired during tumor progression, since it is also detected in the autologous melanoma tissue (Wang *et al.*, 1993).

In many reported cases, the mutation is localized in a 8-base-pair CT repeat region of exon 1, indicating that this region could be a hot spot for mutations (Perez *et al.*, 1999). Sequence repeats are very abundant in the genome and are frequently found to be mutated in processes related to DNA repair enzyme defects (Linch's Syndrome). As expected, the mutator phenotype has been encountered in most colon cell-lines found to be mutated for the β2-m gene (Branch *et al.*, 1995). Mutations in genes that encode DNA repair enzymes are the molecular basis of hereditary non-polyposis colorectal cancer (HNPCC), but this type of tumor represents a very small proportion of colon cancers. What happens in most spontaneous tumors? We recently analyzed a large number of phenotype I colon and larynx tumors and observed that structural mutations in the β2-m gene causing defective MHC class I expression are rare (data not shown). These data suggest that the underlying problem in cancer cells may be regulatory rather than structural, or that other proteins involved in antigen processing and presentation are affected (see below). However, structural defects in the β_2-m gene can be of particular relevance in melanoma lesions without detectable HLA class I molecules (Hicklin *et al.*, 1998), in comparison with other tumors (Chen *et al.*, 1996; Fernandez and Garrido, unpublished results). However, the relationship between β_2-m gene mutations and the oncogenic mechanism in melanoma is not fully defined.

Finally, our group demonstrated the negative impact of β_2-m gene mutations on the T-cell-based immunotherapy of melanoma. In order to discover why their tumors progressed despite immunization with MAGE peptides, two melanoma patients were studied and found to be resistant to HLA-A1-restricted MAGE-encoded peptide immunization and to have clinically evident metastases. No tumor regression was observed, in contrast to several other patients with significant regressions of metastatic lesions after receiving the same treatment. Mutations in the β2-m gene were observed in the tumor tissues, in one case an altered initiation codon, and in the other mutations in the exon 2 producing a premature stop codon. A phenotype with a complete loss of HLA class I alleles was detected in both metastatic lesions because another independent event (deletion of the other β2-m gene) was observed in both cases (Benitez *et al.*, 1998).

Abnormalities that Affect Class I MHC Heavy Chain

At least six different class I HLA genes are constitutively expressed in most cells. For this reason it seems unlikely that structural genes are affected in tumors with total lack of HLA molecules, because this would imply the existence of multiple mutations. Because of the relatively high frequency of total HLA antigen loss in tumors, it seems unlikely that mutations or deletions exist in coding regions of genes for the heavy chain. It is therefore improbable that the total loss of HLA antigens is the result of mutations (large deletions) in both chromosomes. This possibility was considered in initial studies but was soon ruled out (Esteban *et al.*, 1989; Ruiz-Cabello *et al.*, 1991). Thus, it is easy to understand that the mechanisms that directly affect the heavy chain and participate in a downregulation of all the antigens (phenotype I), or of one locus (phenotype III), are essentially regulatory.

MHC class I molecule expression on virtually all nucleated cells is cell-type and developmentally regulated (Singer and Maguire, 1990). These regulations occur mainly at the transcriptional level through conserved *cis*-acting regulatory elements, although they are also influenced by DNA methylation and probably by chromatin structure. Most of the *cis*-acting elements are located at 5′ position within 200 bp of the transcription initiation site. These sequences have been shown to bind trans-acting protein factors associated with MHC class I expression and related to HLA alterations. Some of these elements are present in the β-2 m gene and in the heavy chain gene promoters. In fact, the expression of altered binding of NFκB/Rel regulatory factor to a class I enhancer sequence has been described in cell lines lacking class I HLA (Henseling *et al.*, 1990; Blanchet *et al.*, 1991). Therefore, reduced or absent MHC class I and β2-m gene expression is accounted for by an inability to detect low factor binding activity in the regulatory elements (RE) of these genes (Figure 6.1). This mechanism would give rise to tumor cells with the phenotype I with a low expression of heavy chain and β_2-m, as observed in the human neuronal cell, neuroblastoma cell-lines and some HLA class I deficient tumor cell-lines (Blanchet *et al.*, 1991; Drew *et al.*, 1993). This phenotype can be reversible and TNF-α and IFN-γ can increase the expression of both chains on tumor cells.

An additional mechanism affecting expression of HLA-A2 allele in melanoma has been recently described that involves selective loss of this allele caused by aberrant pre-mRNA splicing which results in the translation of a truncated HLA-A2 without the $\alpha 1$ domain (Wang *et al.*, 1999).

The presence of additional locus-specific sequences also suggests that the different HLA-A, -B, -C loci are regulated in a locus-specific manner. Transcriptional locus-specific factors have also been implicated in tumor cell lines with defective locus expression (Soong and Hui, 1992). HLA-B locus downregulation is frequently observed in melanoma tumor cell lines and appears to be mediated by sequences near the transcription initiation site. This phenotype can also be reversible with cytokine stimuli. Furthermore, it can also be associated with c-*myc* oncogene expression, indicating that this alteration could be derived from the process of neoplastic transformation in melanomas (Peltenburg and Schrier, 1994). However, this mechanism of selective HLA-B locus suppression by oncogenes is not completely elucidated and is not observed in other tumors (Redondo *et al.*, 1991).

In contrast to the above regulatory defects that often are reversible, somatic mutations in HLA genes also occur in human cancer and cannot be compensated for with IFN-γ treatment.

Loss of genetic material occurs frequently during carcinogenesis and is associated with the development and progression of tumors. Genomic losses that affect a single allele (phenotype IV) or a complete haplotype (phenotype II) have been observed in melanoma and colon tumor cell-lines and other tumor tissues (Torres *et al.*, 1996; Wang *et al.*, 1998). Chromosomal non-disjunction or mitotic recombination might underlie this HLA haplotype loss.

Modulation of MHC Class I Expression by Viral Infection

Viruses can interfere with antigen presentation by altering the surface expression of cell membrane proteins involved in the recognition of antigens by T cells. Through elimination of class I HLA molecules from the cell surface, the infected cells become temporarily invisible to CTLs and the pathogen has time to proliferate (Ploegh, 1998). Infected cells can be targeted for destruction by NK and T cells. However, viruses have evolved strategies to inhibit both effector cells simultaneously, and these are widespread in viruses that produce persistent infection. A clear example is HIV which can selectively downregulate HLA-A, -B without affecting HLA-C or -E, thus allowing infected cells (or tumor cells harboring the virus) to avoid both T and NK recognition (Cohen *et al.*, 1999). We describe here just some of the strategies used by viruses with oncogenic potential.

Downregulation of MHC class I expression has been reported to occur at both transcriptional and post-transcriptional levels. Many DNA viruses frequently affect the assembly and transport of class I molecules to the cell surface. The transport of class I molecules to the cell surface depends on assembly in the ER with the peptides generated in the cytosol (Figure 6.1). The E3 region of Ad2 encodes the protein E3/19 K, which inhibits transport to the cell surface through the binding of class I peptides that then remain in this form in the ER (Andersson *et al.*, 1985).

In Ad12 infected cells, MHC class I downregulation is caused by at least two different mechanisms: a) reduction of the mRNA levels of TAP, and b) impaired transcription of MHC class I genes, likely by inhibition of the maturation of the transcriptional factors NF-kB that interact with enhancer A of the class I HLA regulatory promoter.

EBV provides an excellent example of the multiple strategies that favor the long-term survival of virus-infected cells in immunocompetent hosts. The inability to generate CTLs against the viral protein EBNA-1 confers several advantages to the virus, including persistence (Wiertz *et al.*, 1997). It seems that the inability to be recognized by CTLs resides in an N-terminal polymorphic segment that consists of Gly-Ala units. Possibly these units impede an effective degradation by the proteasome and thus insufficient amounts of peptides are generated (Figure 6.1). Moreover, EBV expresses a late protein, the BCRF1 gene product, that is similar in sequence to human interleukin-10. This protein induces downregulation of TAP-1, as does hIL-10, resulting in a reduction of surface MHC class I molecules on B lymphocytes (Zeidler *et al.*, 1997).

Finally, the development of cervical carcinoma is strongly associated with specific types of human papilloma virus (HPVs). Seventy-three per cent of cervical carcinomas show alterations in HLA expression in one or more alleles related to TAP expression (Cromme *et al.*, 1994). Recently, this figure raised to 95% (Koopman *et al.*, 2000). The process of HPV integration is apparently related to the repression of HLA expression (Bartholomew *et al.*, 1997). Another mechanism for tumor escape may be a variation in the sequence of the viral antigen (see also in the next section). For example, a consistent variation in the HPV16E6 oncoprotein sequence has been observed in HLA-B7 patients with cervical cancer, altering the HLA-B7 peptide binding epitope in a way likely to influence immune recognition by CTLs (Ellis *et al.*, 1997).

LOSS OF TUMOR ANTIGEN EXPRESSION

During tumor progression each step may involve activation, mutation or loss of different genes. New cell variants arise and those with growth advantage over earlier forms are selected. Whether an antigenic loss is advantageous to the tumor or not depends on the particular tumor antigen. For instance, human solid tumors appear to maintain mutant oncoproteins uniformly throughout their course. It is very likely that the expression of tumor antigen derived from such oncoproteins in tumor tissue is homogeneous, because tumor cells require the continued presence of this protein to maintain their transformed phenotype. In fact, only tumor cells that have acquired mutant copies of the protein become malignant. The clearest example of these antigens is the oncogenic DNA viruses that carry their own transforming genes. For this reason, the appearance of antigen loss variants in these neoplasms occur less frequently. However, tumor antigens derived from many other proteins (tumor-specific shared antigens, differentiation antigens, etc.) that are not intrinsically involved in cell transformation mechanisms can be lost in the course of tumor progression. Some of these antigens are being used in clinical trials of peptide-derived vaccines (MAGE, tyrosinase, gp100, Melan A/MART-1) and the selection of antigen-loss variants is being encountered often in non-responsive patients, even in the presence of antigen-specific CTLs (Jäger *et al.*, 1997; Thurner *et al.*, 1999).

Immunoselection of Mutated Peptides that Evade Antigen Presentation

Many of the relevant proteins involved in neoplastic transformation and tumor growth are intracellular mutant oncoproteins that can generate individual tumor antigens recognized by T cells. Peptides derived from this mutant intracellular protein can be presented by class I HLA. However, what would happen if the mutations in these oncogene products were located outside the consensus binding motif for a given HLA haplotype? Logically, cancer cells might develop and grow unrestrained by the immune system only when these mutations occur outside a MHC binding motif or in cells that acquire antigen processing and presentation defects. This could be expected to occur only as a process of selection during the development of cancer and it would thus be possible that the immune system selects those oncoprotein-derived mutated peptides that cannot be presented by the host's MHC molecules. This hypothesis was tested by Wiedenfeld *et al.* (1994) in lung carcinomas bearing p53 missense mutations. They found that the p53 mutations fell within the HLA A0201 motif less often than would be expected, likely due to the selection of tumor clones with mutant forms of p53 that do not bind to MHC. Furthermore, those tumors that did contain missense mutations within the motif had lost the HLA A0201 allele (Figure 6.5). A similar finding was reported by Nisticò *et al.* (1997) for breast cancer patients overexpressing ErbB-2 molecules.

EXPRESSION OF MOLECULES THAT INHIBIT T AND NK RESPONSE

It is possible that tumor cells use strategies like those of viruses to inhibit NK and T cells at the same time. It could be speculated that the use of a "stealth strategy" alone would be inadequate to evade the immune response. If cancer cells can successfully alter MHC class I expression to escape from T cell responses, how do they then evade NK attack?

The consequences for the inhibition of T and NK cells vary depending on the HLA phenotype of the tumor cell (Ikeda *et al.*, 1997; Ruiz-Cabello and Garrido, 1998). NK cells are normally inhibited from killing their target by inhibitory signals via NK-cell receptors that recognize their own HLA class I molecules (Figure 6.6a). In this way, the failure to express MHC molecules may render a tumor susceptible to NK-mediated lysis. Killing inhibitory receptors (KIRs) have been also found to be expressed on a subset of activated T cells (Speiser *et al.*, 1999), and T cells that rely on KIR for inhibition can then detect the loss of specific MHC class I gene products (Ikeda *et al.*, 1997) (Figure 6.6b). However, tumor cells with defects in the expression of single alleles evade specific T cell responses but do not necessarily generate an NK-cell-susceptible target (Table 6.3). Some viruses, such as the human cytomegalovirus, have evolved different strategies to interfere with T and NK recognition. They synthesize a number of "stealth proteins" that inhibit cell surface expression of HLA class I antigens (Ploegh, 1998), and at the same time use a "decoy strategy" by synthesizing their own class I HLA homologues to inhibit NK lysis (Farrell *et al.*, 1997; Reyburn *et al.*, 1997). Can a similar mechanism be effective in human tumors? Several reports have shown that nonclassical HLA-G is expressed ectopically in tumors. This non-classical class I HLA is expressed in extravillus trophoblasts and has been postulated to

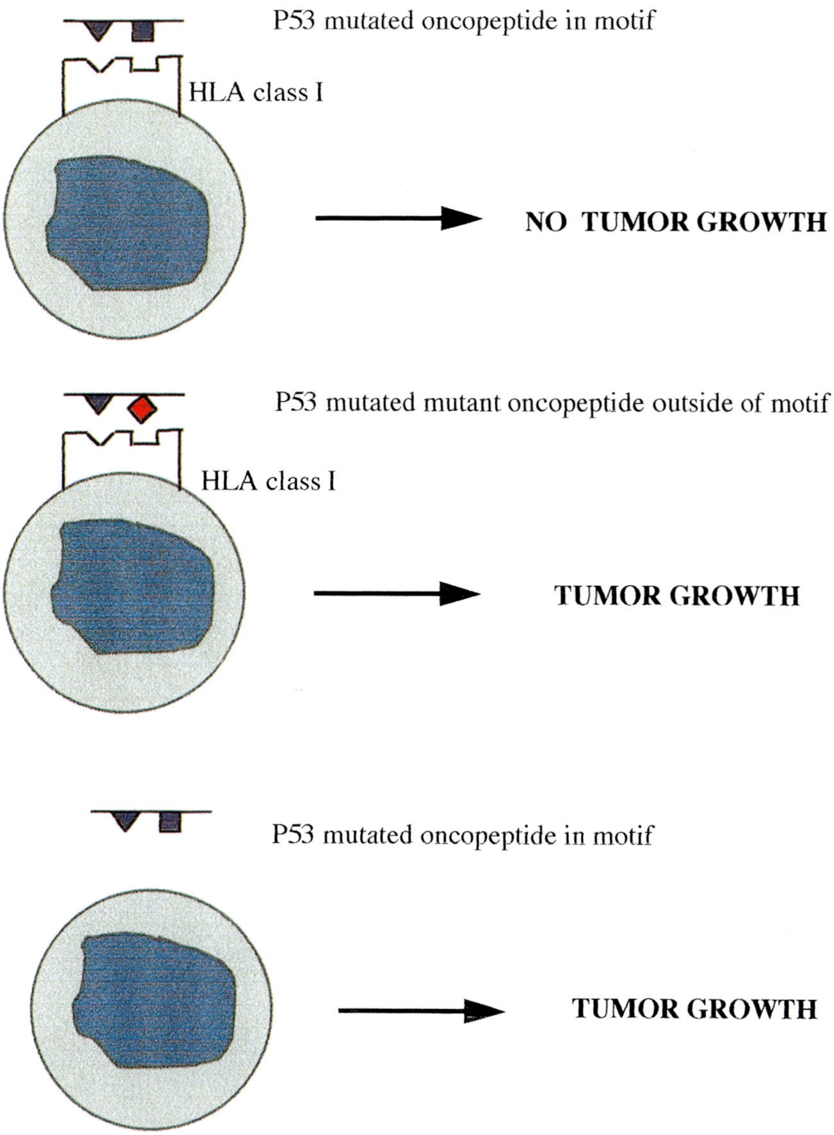

Figure 6.5 Modification of target peptides as model for tumor progression. In A, mutant oncopeptide is presented in the context of HLA class I allele and the tumor cell is eliminated by CTLs. In B, tumor cells escape because the peptide consensus motif is mutated and is not presented effectively. In C, tumor escape is produced by the absence of HLA class I allele (Widenfeld *et al.*, 1994).

play a key role in protecting the placenta from decidual-associated but not peripheral blood NK cell-mediated damage and thus favor human placental implantation (Ponte *et al.*, 1999). Thus, the lack of classical HLA molecules would prevent allorecognition and lysis by maternal T lymphocytes while expression of HLA-G would evade attack by NK

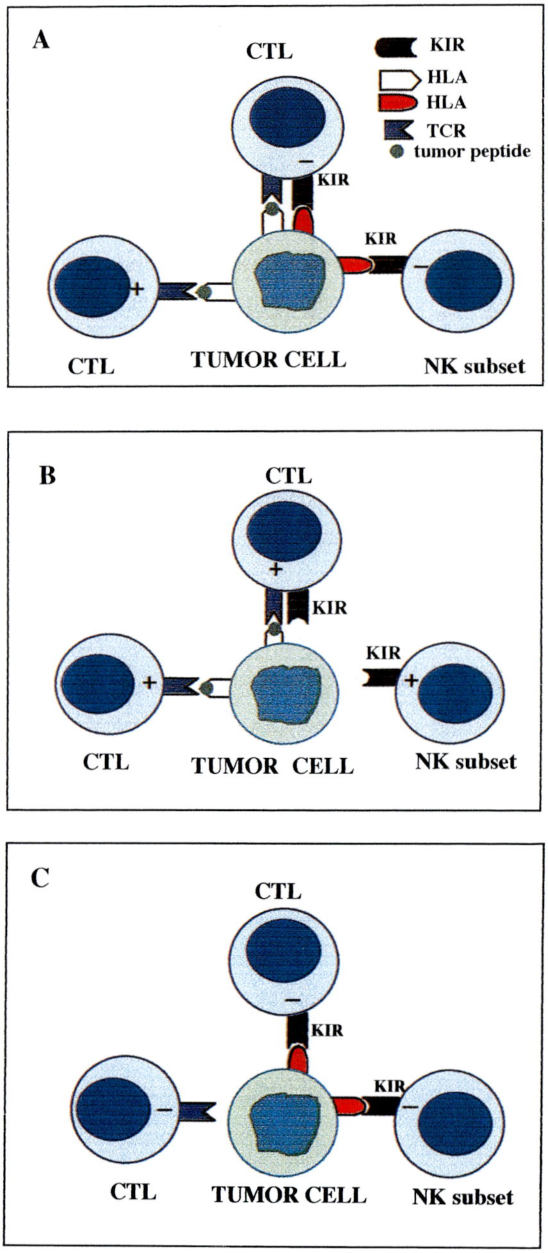

Figure 6.6 Biological effects of KIR expression in NK and CTL activation. (A) Classical cytotoxic T lymphocytes without KIR expression recognize tumor cells expressing normal HLA phenotype. NK and CTL expressing KIR are inhibited by the same or different HLA class I alleles. (B) Tumor cells with selective HLA losses might be efficiently recognized by CTLs expressing KIR or NK cells. (C) However, tumor cells expressing only HLA class I like molecules or non-HLA class I restrictive elements inhibit CTL and NK cell activation.

TABLE 6.3
Consequences of HLA loss for potential susceptibility to NK subsets (see Garrido *et al.*, 1997).

Tumor phenotype	*HLA*	*KIR p70 BW4*	*KIR p58.1 Cw2,4,5,6**	*KIR p58.2 + Cw1,3,7,8*[†]	*KIR p70/140 + A3,11*
Normal	A1,2 – B8,44 – Cw3,4	not susceptible	not susceptible	not susceptible	not susceptible
I	Total loss	susceptible	susceptible	susceptible	susceptible
II	Haplotype loss A3, B44, Cw3	susceptible	not susceptible	susceptible	susceptible
III	Locus loss A1, A3	not susceptible	not susceptible	not susceptible	susceptible
III	Locus loss B8, B44	susceptible	not susceptible	not susceptible	not susceptible
IV	Allele loss A3	not susceptible	not susceptible	not susceptible	susceptible
IV	Allele loss B44	susceptible	not susceptible	not susceptible	not susceptible
IV	Allele loss Cw4	not susceptible	susceptible	not susceptible	not susceptible

* Also blanks which contain Asn 77 and Lys 80.
[†] Also blanks which contain Ser 77 and Asn 80.

cells. Thus, the consequence of abnormal HLA-G expression in tumor cells that have lost the restricted element for CTLs should allow a simultaneous escape from NK cells (Figure 6.6c) (Paul *et al.*, 1998). We explored this possibility in a large series of human tumors (Real *et al.*, 1999a, b), and our results suggest that this immunosurveillance evasion strategy is playing a minor role, if any, in our tumor series. For this reason it is at present impossible to assess the biological relevance of this phenomenon, which could in turn be one more manifestation of the aberrant genetic expression of tumors. Nevertheless, further studies are required to establish whether other non-classical molecules (HLA-E, HLA-F) that bind with NK cell receptors and confer resistance to cell mediated lysis (Braud *et al.*, 1998) participate in the tumor escape to NK recognition.

IMMUNOSUPPRESSION INDUCED BY TUMOR CELLS

IMMUNOSUPPRESSIVE CYTOKINES

Apart from alterations in the antigen processing and presentation machinery, low immunogenicity can be caused by the production of immunosuppressive cytokines that also contribute to immunologic escape. Some of them may act in an autocrine pathway and confer growth advantage to tumor cells.

The constitutive production of cytokines by tumor cells has been demonstrated, and may play an important role not only in tumor growth but also in angiogenesis through their effect on neovascularization (Herlyn *et al.*, 1990; Jong *et al.*, 1998). These cytokines were found in the supernatant of tumor cell cultures, with TGF-β and IL-10 among those found to have a strong immunosuppressive activity.

TGF-β was first identified for its ability to transform normal fibroblasts and to inhibit tumor and normal epithelial cells. TGF-β is frequently expressed in many tumor cells *in vivo* (Derynck *et al.*, 1987) and also in immune privileged sites, and suppresses inflammatory T-cell responses and cell-mediated immunity. This cytokine exerts a potent immunosuppressive activity through inhibition of the production and activity of other cytokines (i.e. IL-2, IFN-γ)

by blocking the signal transduction pathway induced. Thus, TGF-β inhibits the differentiation of CTLs likely by inhibition of IL-12, a cytokine produced by APC that is crucial for the generation of protective cell-mediated antitumor responses.

IL-10 is spontaneously secreted by many human tumors, including 38% of melanoma lines and 70% of colon carcinomas (Gastl *et al.*, 1993; Luscher *et al.*, 1994). Moreover, as with TNF-β, IL-10 can be identified in serum and ascitic fluid due to release by tumor cells. This cytokine is normally produced by TH2 cells and may shift immune responses towards the humoral component by the inhibition of cytokines involved in cell-mediated responses. The end result is the inhibition of the tumoricidal function of T cells, NK cells and macrophages. IL-10 inhibits cytokine synthesis by TH1 cells, but not directly. IL-10 acts on monocytes and macrophages, preventing the surface display of MHC class II antigens by inhibiting recruitment from intracellular compartments to the cell surface (Koppelman *et al.*, 1997). IL-10 then inhibits the production by macrophages of IL-12, a cytokine that promotes IFN-γ production and interferes with the development of the TH1 subset (Figure 6.7a). Finally, IL-10 may also contribute to the downregulation of MHC class I antigens in human tumors, perhaps as an indirect consequence of an inhibition of the antigen processing machinery (Matsuda *et al.*, 1994; Zeidler *et al.*, 1997). Finally, *in vivo* evidence that IL-10 released by host immune cells upon their interaction with tumor cells can prevent generation of TH1 immune response has been provided (Halak *et al.*, 1999). All these effects indicate that the local production of IL-10 by tumor cells could modulate the immune response by making tumor cells insensitive to CTL cytotoxicity.

Another cytokine involved in modulating antitumor activity of the host is GM-CSF, which was shown to be produced by several human cancers (Trutman *et al.*, 1998). Animal models show that *in vivo* release of GM-CSF by tumor cells may result in inhibition of $CD8^+$ T cell responses through a disregulation of APC (Bronte *et al.*, 1999).

Other tumor-derived products have been reported to inhibit the antitumor immune response by different mechanisms, like gangliosides (McKallip *et al.*, 1999), MUC1 (Chan *et al.*, 1999) and vascular endothelial growth factor (Gabrilovich *et al.*, 1996). The latter is specifically able, when released by tumor cells, to block DC maturation, thus preventing presentation of tumor antigens to host's T cells.

EXPRESSION OF MOLECULES THAT OPERATE ON THE APO-FAS PATHWAY

FAS (CD95) is among the most important molecules involved in delivering the death signal that triggers apoptosis. In the immune system, CD95 and the perforin-granzyme system mediate T-cell cytotoxicity. Cross-linking of FAS on one cell and Fas ligand (FasL, CD95L) on the other cell induces programmed cell death (apoptosis) in the Fas-bearing cell (Figure 6.8a). Apoptosis is a homeostatic mechanism and an active termination of T-cell immune response pathway is delivered in order to limit the proliferation of the immune cells. Thus, although T cells use FASL to kill their target cells, they also use the FAS pathway to downregulate the immune response. In fact, the activation of T cells leads to the coexpression of CD95 and CD95L and induces death in the cell as well as in neighboring cells (Parijs and Abbas, 1998). Failure in this system may result in autoimmunity. Whereas a wide range of tissues constitutively express FAS on their cell surfaces, FASL was initially thought to

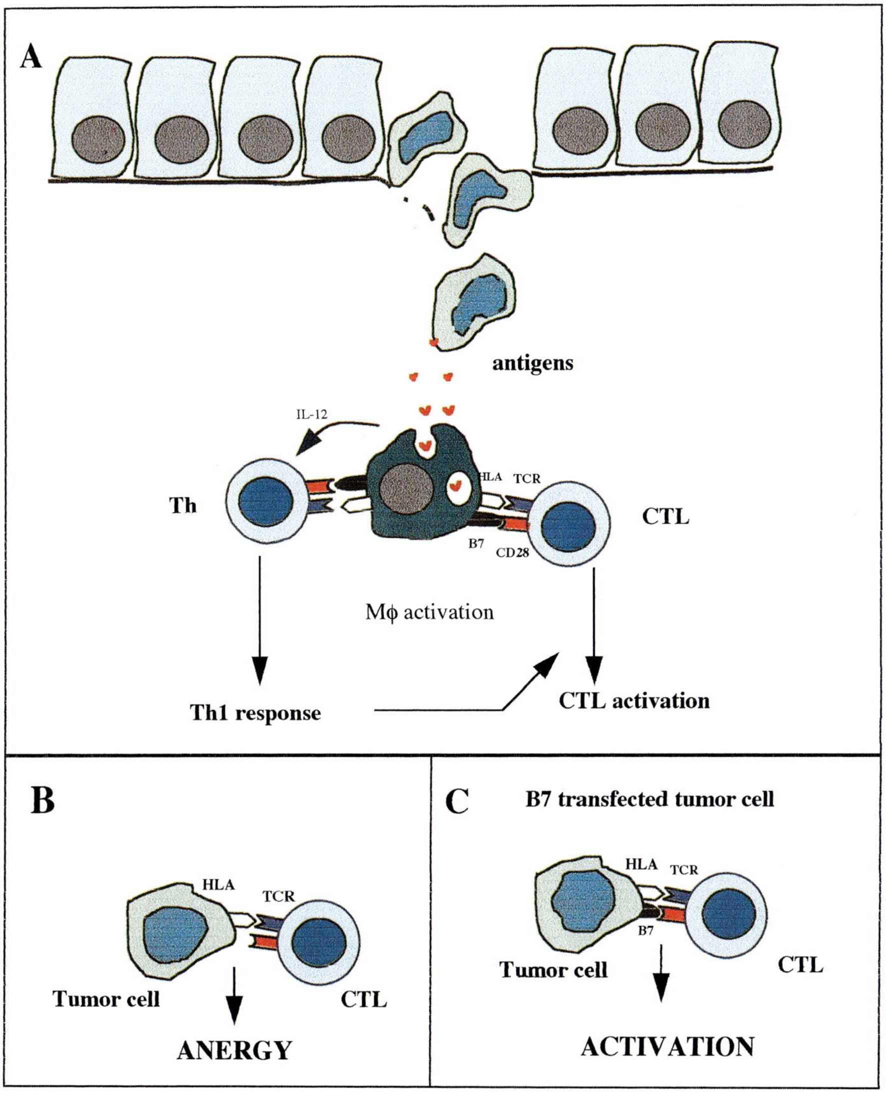

Figure 6.7 Schematic representation of interactions of tumor cells and the T cell effector arms. (A) Recognition of tumor cells by cytotoxic T cells is dependent on the processing and presentation of tumor antigens by APCs. Tumor antigens released by secretion, shedding or tumor lysis are captured by antigen-presenting cells that express co-stimulatory molecules such as B7; T lymphocyte activation is induced. (B) T cell that recognizes directly tumor cells that do not express co-stimulatory molecules; T cell anergy is induced. (C) B7-transfected tumor cells act as antigen-presenting cells and T lymphocyte activation is induced.

be restricted to activated T lymphocytes, but the ligand is also expressed on non-lymphoid cells from immune privileged sites. In these sites, allogeneic and xenogeneic tissue grafts enjoy

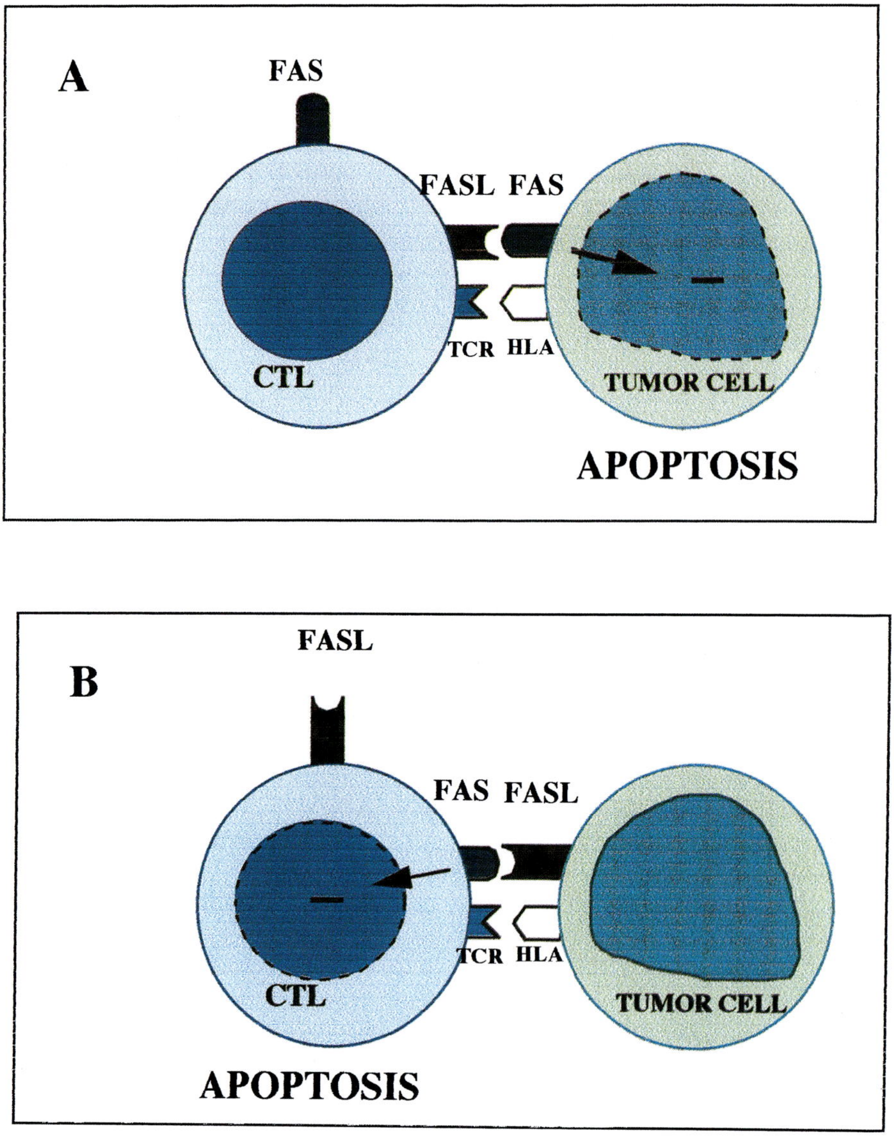

Figure 6.8 Proposed mechanism for CTL depletion in cancer. (A) FASL expression in the effector T cell, target FAS molecule and induces tumor cell apoptosis. (B) Loss of FAS expression and simultaneous appearance of FASL on the tumor cell might induce T cell apoptosis.

unusually high acceptance rates. High levels of FASL expression have been observed in the eye and testis, suggesting that FASL expression forms a barrier surrounding the organs (Griffith and Ferguson, 1997). Any activated T cells expressing FAS that enter these sites encounter cells expressing FASL and receive a death signal. Tumor cells may use these mechanisms to form an immune privileged site (limiting the cell surface expression of HLA class I molecules, secreting soluble inhibitory cytokines and expressing FasL). In theory, tumors that express CD95L can actively kill CD95$^+$ T cells (Figure 6.8b). However, as it occurs in lymphocytes, the simultaneous expression of CD95 and CD95L in the same cell leads to death. Hahne *et al.* (1996) showed that tumor cells expressed CD95L but not CD95; in this way the tumor cells delivered the death signal to activated T lymphocytes bearing Fas but could not receive a death signal. The loss of CD95 expression has been described in hepatocellular carcinomas in comparison with normal or diseased liver tissues, which display a homogeneous expression of CD95. The tumor cells acquire non-responsiveness towards CD95 stimulation, then express CD95L and act as effector cells by actively destroying lymphocytes via the CD95 pathway (Strand *et al.*, 1996). However, the *in vivo* relevance of T-cell destruction *via* Fas/FasL remains controversial, since anti-melanoma-specific T-cell clones are resistant to such a tumor counterattack (Rivoltini *et al.*, 1998), and other factors may be involved in modulation of Fas signals in tumor cells (see O'Connell *et al.*, 1999).

ABNORMALITIES IN SIGNAL TRANSDUCTION OF T CELLS

A critical number of TCR molecules engaged with peptide–MHC is required for T-cell activation to be triggered. Moreover, an optimal stimulus for T-cell response to a peptide–MHC complex needs a second signal delivered by antigen-presenting cells. Depending on the nature of the stimulus, T cells may be either fully activated or anergized (Figure 6.7b). In fact, the interaction of TCR alone often results in the induction of tolerance, characterized by a lack of IL-2 production that leads the T cell to a state of ignorance, anergy or even apoptosis. Thus, even when tumor cells express the appropriate tumor-associated antigens they may not be immunogenic when the second signal cannot be delivered. In contrast, the presence of adequate cytokine production and professional APC expressing co-stimulatory molecules such as B7 promotes a correct T-cell activation (Figure 6.7b). The ability of tumors to induce this state of tolerance to specific neoantigens has recently been demonstrated (Staveley-O'Carrol *et al.*, 1998). The molecular bases for tumor cells being poor stimulators of the immune response may perhaps be interrelated, because the normal cells from which they derive are unable to produce cytokines and surface molecules whose expression is restricted to professional APCs. In fact, most tumors derived from parenchymal or mesenchymal cells do not express B7 and are unlikely to induce an effective immunologic response. In summary, the mechanisms that induce peripheral tolerance to prevent deleterious autoimmune responses are those that then contribute to the lack of appropriate co-stimulation against tumor cells. These mechanisms are the inadequate production of IL-2 as a second signal for T-cell activation and proliferation and also as a cytokine that inhibits tumor-induced anergy, and the absence of B7 as an inhibitor of TCR-induced apoptosis. For this reason, immunogene therapy is focusing many efforts on the direct activation of cytolytic T cells. The transfection of genes encoding members of the B7 co-stimulatory family (B7-1 or B7-2) into tumor cells appears to inhibit apoptosis of CTL (Figure 7c), and restore T-cell activation above all when B7 genes are used in combination with the appropriate cytokines (IL-2, IL-7) (Farzaneh *et al.*, 1998).

Furthermore, it has been shown that the long-term presence of tumors can alter the function of key molecules of the T cells, thereby disrupting T-cell internal signals and leading to immunosuppression (Mizoguchi *et al.*, 1992). It has long been known that progressive tumor growth is associated with a state of immunosuppression. Many of the mechanisms we have analyzed contribute to this state, i.e. the loss of antigens or the secretion of inhibitory cytokines. However, why the T cells of cancer patients respond poorly to mitogenic stimuli in *in vitro* reactions is not known. The mechanism of this T-cell dysfunction has been elucidated in the past few years, and alterations in the TCR and in the pathways of signal transduction in T cells have been described. T cells from mice bearing the MCA-38 colon carcinoma line were deficient in the expression of TCRζ chain of the TCR-CD3 complex and in two protein tyrosine kinases (PTK), $p56^{lck}$ and $p59^{fyn}$. Similar defects were also found in tumor-infiltrating lymphocytes (TILs) from patients with melanoma or renal carcinoma. These alterations were present mostly in TILs and much less or not in peripheral blood leukocytes from the same patients, indicating that the defects are induced by exposure to the tumor (Finke *et al.*, 1993). Tumor may also cause a direct degradation of T cell ζ-chain by caspase (Gastman *et al.*, 1999). Moreover, it appears that the extent of TCR signaling molecule loss in T cells of metastatic patients can be variable depending on the TCRV region and that tumor-derived soluble HLA class I molecules may contribute to induce such alterations (Maccalli *et al.*, 1999). It is of note that defects of signal transduction of T cells can be corrected by administration of IL-2 even *in vivo* (Rabinowich *et al.*, 1996) or by *in vitro* exposure to TCR and CD28 (Maccalli *et al.*, 1999). However, these alterations in signal transduction are reversible and might not depend directly on tumor cells. In fact, it has recently been reported that H_2O_2 production by tumor-infiltrating macrophages can effectively alter signal transduction in T and NK cells and that some of these defects can be reversed by cytokines (Kono *et al.*, 1996). It has also been reported that impairment in ζ-chain expression in T cells at tumor site can correlate with poor survival in at least some cancer patients (e.g. oral carcinoma) (Reichert *et al.*, 1998). These findings indirectly suggest a potential role of the immune system in controlling tumor growth and progression.

CONCLUSIONS

In recent years, there has been a great improvement in our understanding of escape mechanisms used by tumor cells to avoid immunosurveillance. One of the most important of these mechanisms is the alteration of HLA on tumor cell membranes.

T lymphocytes and NK cells see class I HLA differently: for T cells, HLA class I molecules associate to a particular peptide and induce an activation signal, generating a clonal expansion of the appropriate effector T cell; in contrast, for NK cells, HLA are inhibitory molecules that constantly modulate NK cell function, and their absence triggers NK cell cytotoxicity.

Cancer cells derived from HLA positive epithelia escape T-cell killing by losing all or some HLA class I molecules. T cells are then blind and cannot see the tumor antigen. This phenomenon is associated with invasion and metastasis. As a second step, the deficient tumor cells are theoretically susceptible to be killed by a particular NK cell clone. The question is why these cancer cells are not eliminated. An unknown NK escape mechanism is selected by tumor cells, which produce NK cell escape tumor variants.

In this chapter we have also described other escape mechanisms employed by tumor cells to avoid immunosurveillance, but their relevance and use are as yet unknown. Identification of the escape strategies used by a particular tumor in a particular patient should improve therapeutic decision-making by clinical oncologists.

ACKNOWLEDGMENTS

This work was supported by the Fondo de Investigaciones Sanitarias and Plan Andaluz de Investigación, Spain.

REFERENCES

Andersson, M., Paabo, S., Nilsson, T., and Peterson, P.A. (1985) Impaired intracellular transport of class I MHC antigens as a possible means for adenoviruses to evade immune surveillance. *Cell*, **43**, 215–222.

Bai, A., and Forman, J. (1997) The effect of the proteasome inhibitor lactacystin on the presentation of transporter associated with antigen processing (TAP)-dependent and TAP-independent peptide epitopes by class I molecules. *J. Immunol.*, **159**, 2139–2146.

Bartholomew, J.S., Glenville, S., Sarkar, S., Burt, D.J., Stanley, M.A., Ruiz-Cabello, F., Chengan, J., Garrido, F., and Stern, P.L. (1997) Integration of high-risk human papillomavirus DNA is linked to the down-regulation of class I human leukocyte antigens by steroid hormones in cervical tumor cells. *Cancer Res.*, **57**, 937–942.

Benitez, R, Godelaine, D., Lopez Nevot, M., Brasseur, F., Marchand, M., Cabrera, T., van Baren, N., Andry, G., Jimenez P., Landry, C., Ruiz-Cabello, F., Boon, T., and Garrido, F. (1998) Mutations of β2-microglobulin gene result in lack of HLA class I molecules on melanoma cells of two patients immunized with MAGE peptides. *Tissue Antigens*, **52**, 520–529.

Blanchet, O., Bourge, J.F., Zinszer, H., Tatari, Z., Degos, L., and Paul, P. (1991) DNA binding of regulatory factors interacting with MHC-class-I gene enhancer correlates with MHC class I transcriptional level in class I defective cell lines. *Int. J. Cancer*, **6**, 138–145.

Branch, P., Bicknell, D.C., Rowan, A., Bodmer, W.F., and Karran, P. (1995) Immune surveillance in colorectal carcinoma. *Nature Genetics*, **9**, 231–232.

Braud, V.M., Allan, D.S., O'Callaghan, C.A., Söderström, K., D'Anrea, A., Ogg, G.S., Lazetic, S., Young, N.T., Bell, J.I., Phillips, J.H., Lanier, L.L., and McMichael, A. (1998) HLA-E binds to natural killer cell receptors CD94/NKG2A, B and C. *Nature*, **391**, 795–799.

Bronte, V., Chappell, D.B., Apolloni, E., Cabrelle, A., Wang, M., Hwu, P., and Restifo, N P. (1999) Unopposed production of granulocyte-macrophage colony-stimulating factor by tumors inhibits CD8+ T cell responses by dysregulating antigen-presenting cell maturation. *J. Immunol.*, **162**, 5728–5737.

Browning, M.J., Petronzelli, F., Bicknell, D.C., Krausa, P., Rowan, A., Tonks, S., Murray, N., and Bodmer, W.F. (1996) Mechanisms of loss of HLA class I expression on colorectal tumor cells. *Tissue Antigens*, **47**, 364–371.

Cabrera, T., Fernandez, M.A., Sierra, A., Garrido, A., Herruzo, A., Escobedo, A., Fabra, A., and Garrido, F. (1996) High frequency of altered HLA class I phenotypes in invasive breast carcinomas. *Hum. Immunol.*, **50**, 127–134.

Cabrera, F., Collado, A., Fernandez, A., Ferron, A., Sancho, F., Ruiz-Cabello, F., and Garrido, F. (1998) High frequency of altered HLA class I phenotypes in invasive colorectal carcinomas. *Tissue Antigens.*, **52**, 114–123.

Chan, A.K., Lockhart, D.C., von Bernstorff, W., Spanjaard, R.A., Joo, H. G., Eberlein, T.J., and Goedegebuure, P.S. (1999) Soluble MUC1 secreted by human epithelial cancer cells mediates immune suppression by blocking T-cell activation. *Int. J. Cancer*, **82**, 721–726.

Chen, H.L., Gabrilovich, D., Virmani, A., Ratnani, I., Girgis, K.R., Nadaf-Rahrov, S., Fernandez-Viña, M., and Carbone, P. (1996) Structural and functional analysis of β2 microglobulin abnormalities in human lung and breast cancer. *Int. J. Cancer*, **67**, 756–763.

Cohen, G.B., Gandhi, R.T., Davis, D.M., Mandelboim, O., Chen, B.K., Strominger, J.L., and Baltimore, D. (1999) The selective downregulation of class I major histocompatibility complex proteins by HIV-1 protects HIV-infected cells from NK cells. *Immunity*, **10**, 661–671.

Cromme, F.V., Airley, J., Heemels, M.T., Ploegh, H.L., Keating, P.J., Stern, P.L., Meijer, C.J., and Walboomers, J.M. (1994) Loss of transporter protein, encoded by the TAP-1 gene, is highly correlated with loss of HLA expression in cervical carcinomas. *J. Exp. Med.*, **179**, 335–340.

Derynck, R., Goeddel, D.V. Ullrich, A., Gutterman, J.U., Willians, R.D., Bringman, T.S., and Berger, W.H. (1987) Synthesis of mRNAs for transforming growth factors-α and -β and the epidermal growth factor receptor by human tumors. *Cancer Res.*, **47**, 707–712.

Drew, P.D., Lonergan, M., Goldstein, M.E., Lampson, L.A., Ozato, K., and McFarlin, D.E. (1993). Regulation of MHC class I and β2-microglobulin gene expression in human neuronal cells. *J. Immunol.*, **150**, 3300–3310.

D'Urso, C.M., Wang, Z., Cao, Y., Tatake, R., Zeff, R.A., and Ferrone, S. (1991) Lack of HLA class I antigen expression by cultured melanoma cells FO-1 due to a defect in B2m gene expression. *J. Clin. Invest.*, **87**, 284–290.

Ellis, J.R., Keating, P.J., Baird, J., Hounsell, E.F., Renouf, D.V., Rowe, M., Hopkins, D., Duggan-Keen, M.F., Bartholomew, J.S., Young, L.S., and Stern, P.L. (1997) The association of an HPV16 oncogene variant with HLA-B7 has implications for vaccine design in cervical cancer. *Nature Med.*, **1**, 464–470.

Esteban, F., Concha, A., Huelin, C., Sanchez Rozas, F., Pedrinaci, S., Ruiz-Cabello, and Garrido, F. (1989) Histocompatibility antigens in primary and metastatic squamous cell carcinoma of the larynx. *Int. J. Cancer*, **43**, 436–442.

Farrell, H.E., Hally, H., Lynch, D.M., Fleming, P., Shellam, G.R., Scalzo, A.A., and Davis-Poynter, N.J. (1997) Inhibition of natural killer cells by a cytomegalovirus MHC class I homologue *in vivo*. *Nature*, **386**, 510–514.

Farzaneh, F., Trefzer, U., Sterry, W., and Walden, P. (1998) Gene therapy in cancer. *Immunol. Today*, **19**, 294–296.

Festenstein, H. (1987) The biological consequences of altered MHC expression on tumours. *Br. Med. Bull.*, **43**, 217–227.

Festenstein, H., and Garrido, F. (1986) MHC antigens and malignancy. *Nature.*, **322**, 502–503.

Finke, H., Zea, A.H., Stanley, J., Longo, D.L., Mizoguchi, H., Tubbs, R.R., Wiltrout, R.H., O'Shea, J.J., Kudoh, S., Klein, E., Bukowski, R.M., and Ochoa, A.C. (1993) Loss of T-cell receptor, chain and p56^{lck} in T cells infiltrating human renal cell carcinoma. *Cancer Res.*, **56**, 5613–5616.

Gabrilovich, D.I., Chen, H.L., Girgis, K.R., Cunningham, H.T., Meny, G. M., Nadaf, S., Kavanaugh, D., and Carbone, D.P. (1996) Production of vascular endothelial growth factor by human tumors inhibits the functional maturation of dendritic cells (Published erratum appears in Nature Med 1996, 2, 1267). *Nature Med.*, **2**, 1096–1103.

Garrido, F., and Ruiz-Cabello, F. (1991) MHC expression on human tumors. Its relevance for local tumor growth and metastasis. *Sem. Cancer Biol.*, **2**, 3–10.

Garrido, F., Cabrera, T., Concha, A., Glew, S., Ruiz-Cabello, F., and Stern, P. (1993) Natural history of HLA expression during tumor development. *Immunol. Today*, **14**, 491–493.

Garrido, T., Cabrera, T., López Nevot, M.A., and Ruiz-Cabello, F. (1995) HLA class I antigens in human tumors. *Adv. Cancer Res.*, **67**, 155–195.

Garrido, F., Ruiz-Cabello, F., Cabrera, T., Perez-Villar, J.J., Lopez-Botet. M.A., Duggan-Keen, M., and Stern, P. (1997) Implications for immunosurveillance of altered HLA class I phenotypes in human tumors. *Immunol. Today*, **18**, 89–95.

Gastl, G.A., Abrams, J.S., Nanus, D.M., Oosterkamp, R., Siver, J., Liu, F., Chen, M., Albino, A.P., and Bander, N.H. (1993) Interleukin-10 production by human carcinoma cell lines and its relationship to interleukin-6 expression. *Int. J. Cancer*, **55**, 96–103.

Gastman, B.R., Johnson, D.E., Whiteside, T.L., and Rabinowich, H. (1999) Caspase-mediated degradation of T-cell receptor zeta-chain. *Cancer Res.*, **59**, 1422–1427.

Giacomini, P., Giorda, E., Fraioli, R., Nicotra, M.R., Vitale, N., Setini, A., Delfino, L., Morabito, A., Benevolo, M., Venturo, I., Mottolese, M., Ferrara, G. B., and Natali, P.G. (1999) Low prevalence of selective human leukocyte antigen (HLA)-A and HLA-B epitope losses in early-passage tumor cell lines. *Cancer Res.*, **59**, 2657–2667.

Griffith, T.S., and Ferguson, T.A. (1997) The role of FasL induced apoptosis in immune privilege. *Immunol. Today*, **18**, 240–244.

Hahne, M, Rimoldi, D., Schröter, M., Romero, P., Schreier, M., French, L.E., Schneider, P., Bornand, T., Fontana, A., Liénard, D., Cerottini, J.C., and Tschopp, J. (1996) Melanoma cell expression of Fas(Apo-1/CD95) ligand: implications for tumor escape. *Science*, **274**, 1363–1366.

Halak, B.K., Maguire, H.C. Jr, and Lattime, E.C. (1999) Tumor-induced interleukin-10 inhibits type 1 immune responses directed at a tumor antigen as well as a non-tumor antigen present at the tumor site. *Cancer Res.*, **59**, 911–917.

Henseling, U., Schmidt, W., Scholer, H.R., Gruss, P., and Hatzopoulos, A.K. (1990) A transcription factor interacting with the class I gene enhancer is inactive in tumorigenic cell lines which suppress major histocompatibility complex class I genes. *Mol. Cell Biol.*, **10**, 4100–4109.

Herlyn, M., Kath, R., Williams, N., Valyi-Nagy, I., and Rodeck, U. (1990) Growth-regulatory factors for normal, premalignant, and malignant human cells *in vitro*. *Adv. Cancer Res.*, **54**, 213–234.

Hicklin, D.J., Wang, Z., Arienti, F., Rivoltini, L., Parmiani, G., and Ferrone, S. (1998) Beta2-Microglobulin mutations, HLA class I antigen loss, and tumor progression in melanoma. *J. Clin. Invest.*, **101**, 2720–2729.

Ikeda, H., Lethe, B., Lehman, F., van Baren, N., Baurain, J.F., de Smet, C., Chambost, H., Vitale, M., Moretta, A., Boon, T., and Coulie, P. (1997) Characterization of an antigen that is recognized on a melanoma showing partial HLA loss by CTL expressing and NK inhibitory receptor. *Immunity*, **6**, 199–208.

Jäger, E., Ringhoffer, M., Altmannsberger, M., Arand, M., Karbach, J., Jäger, D., Oesch, F., and Knuth, A. (1997). Immunoselection *in vivo*: independent loss of MHC class I and melanocyte differentiation antigen expression in metastatic melanoma. *Int. J. Cancer*, **71**, 142–147.

Jimenez, P., Canton, J., Collado, A., Cabrera, T., Serrano, A., Real, L. M., Garcia, A., Ruiz-Cabello, F., and Garrido, F. (1999) Chromosome loss is the most frequent mechanism contributing to HLA haplotype loss in human tumors. *Int. J. Cancer*, **83**, 91–97.

Jong, J.S., van Diest, P.J., van der Valk, P., and Baak, J.P. (1998) Expression of growth factors, growth-inhibiting factors, and their receptors in invasive breast cancer. II: Correlations with proliferation and angiogenesis. *J. Path.*, **184**, 53–57.

Kono, K., Salazar-Onfray, F., Hansson, P.M., Masucci, G., Wasserman, K., Nakazawa, T., Anderson, P., and Kiessling, R. (1996) Hydrogen peroxide secreted by tumor-derived macrophages dow-modulates signal transducing zeta molecules and inhibits tumor-specific T cell- and natural killer cell-mediated cytotoxicity. *Eur. J. Immunol.*, **26**, 1308–1313.

Koopman, L., Corver, W., van der Slik, A., Giphart, M., and Fleuren, G. (2000) Multiple genetic alterations cause frequent and heterogeneous human histocompatibility leukocyte antigen class I loss in cervical cancer. *J. Exp Medicine.*, **20**, 961–975.

Koppelman, B., Neefjes, J.J., de Vries, J.E., and de Waal Malefyt, R. (1997) Interleukin-10 down-regulates MHC class II alpha beta peptide complexes at the plasma membrane of monocytes by affecting arrival recycling. *Immunity*, **7**, 861.

Lehmann, F., Marchand, M., Hainaut, P., Pouillart, P., Sastre, X., Ikeda, H., Boon, T., and Coulie, P.G. (1995) Differences in the antigens recognized by cytolytic T cells on two successive metastases of a melanoma patient are consistent with immune selection. *Eur. Immunol.*, **25**, 340–347.

López Nevot, M.A., Esteban, F., Ferron, A., Ruiz-Cabello, F., and Garrido, F. (1989) HLA class I gene expression on human primary tumours and autologous metastases: demostration of selective losses of HLA antigens on colorectal, gastric and laryngeal carcinomas. *Br. J. Cancer*, **59**, 221–226.

Luscher, U., Filgueira, L., Juretic, A., Zuber, M., Luscher, N.J., Heberer, M., and Spagnoli, G.C. (1994) The pattern of cytokine gene expression in freshley excised human metastatic melanoma suggests a state of reversible anergy of tumor-infiltrating lymphocytes. *Int. J. Cancer*, **57**, 612–619.

Maccalli, C., Pisarra, P., Vegetti, C., Sensi, M., Parmiani G, and Anichini, A. (1999) Differential loss of T cell signaling molecules in metastatic melanoma patients' T lymphocyte subsets expressing distinct TCR variable regions. *J. Immunol.*, **163**, 6912–6923.

Matsuda, M., Salzar, F., Petersson, M., Masucci, G., Hansson, J., Pisa, P., Zang Q.J., Masucci, M.G., and Kiessling, R. (1994) Interleukin 10 pretreatment protects target cells from tumor and allo-specific cytotoxic T cells and downregulates HLA class I expression. *J. Exp. Med.*, **180**, 2371–2376.

McKallip, R., Li, R., and Ladisch, S. (1999) Tumor gangliosides inhibit the tumor-specific immune response. *J. Immunol.*, **163**, 3718–3726.

Mizoguchi, H., O'Shea, J.J., Longo, D.L., Loefler, C.M., McVicar, D.W., and Ochoa, A.C. (1992) Alterations in signal transduction molecule in T lymphocytes from tumor-bearing mice. *Science*, **258**, 1795–1798.

Nisticò, P., Mottolese, M., Mammi, C., Benevolo, M., Del Bello, D., Gentile, P., Botti, C., Venturo, I., and Natali, P.G. (1997) Low frequency of ErbB-2 proto-oncogene overexpression in human leukocyte antigen-A2-positive breast cancer patients. *J. Natl. Cancer Inst. USA*, **89**, 319–321.

O'Connell, J., Bennett, M.W., O'Sullivan, G.C., Collins, J.K., and Shanahan, F. (1999) The Fas counterattack: cancer as a site of immune privilege. *Immunol. Today*, **20**, 46–52.

Parijs, L.V., and Abbas, A.K. (1998) Homeostasis and self-tolerance in the immune system: turning lymphocytes off. *Science*, **280**, 243–248.

Pamer, E., and Cresswell, P. (1998) Mechanisms of MHC class I restricted antigen processing. *Annu. Rev. Immunol.*, **16**, 323–358.

Paul, P., Rouas-Freiss, N., Khalil-Daher, I., Moreau, P., Riteau, B., Le Gal, F.A., Avril, M.R., Dausset, J., Guillet, J.G., and Carosella, E.D. (1998) HLA-G expression in melanoma: a way for tumor cells to escape from immunosurveillance. *Proc. Natl. Acad. Sci. USA*, **95**, 4510–4515.

Peltenburg, L.T.C., and Schrier, P.I. (1994) Transcriptional suppression of HLA-B expression by c-Myc is mediated through the core promoter elements. *Immunogenetics*, **40**, 54–61.

Perez, B., Benitez, R., Fernandez, M.A., Oliva, M.R., Soto, J.L., Serrano, S., Lopez-Nevot, M.A., and Garrido, F. (1999) A new $\beta 2$ microglobuline mutation found in a melanoma tumor cell line. *Tissue Antigens.*, **53**, 569–572.

Ploegh, H.L. (1998) Viral strategies of immune evasion. *Science*, **280**, 248–253.

Ponte, M., Cantoni, C., Biassoni, R., Tradori-Cappai, A., Bentivoglio, G., Vitale, C., Bertone, S., Moretta, A., Moretta, L., and Mingari, M.C. (1999) Inhibitory receptors sensing HLA-G1 molecules in pregnancy:

decidua-associated natural killer cells express LIR-1 and CD94/NKG2A and acquire p49, an HLA-G1-specific receptor. *Proc. Natl Acad. Sci. USA*, **96**, 5674–5679.

Rabinowich, H., Banks, M., Reichert, T.E., Logan, T.F., Kirkwood, J.M., and Whiteside, T.L. (1996) Expression and activity of signaling molecules in T lymphocytes obtained from patients with metastatic melanoma before and after interleukin 2 therapy. *Clin. Cancer Res.*, **2**, 1263–1274.

Ramal, L.M., Fenstra, M., van der Zwan, A., Collado, A., Lopez-Nevot, M.A., Tilanus, M., Garrido, F. (2000) Criteria to define HLA haplotype loss in human solid tumors. *Tissue Antigens.*, **55**, 443–440.

Real, L.M., Jimenez, P., Cantón, J., Kirkin, A.F., García, A., Abril, E., Zeuthen, A., Ruiz-Cabello, F., and Garrido, F. (1998) *In vivo* and *in vitro* generation of a new altered HLA phenotype in melanoma-tumor cell variants expressing a single HLA class I allele. *Int. J. Cancer*, **75**, 317–323.

Real, L.M., Cabrera, T., Ruiz-Cabello, F., and Garrido, F. (1999a) The expression of HLA-G in human tumors is not a frequent event. *Int. J. Cancer*, **81**, 512–518.

Real, L.M., Cabrera, T., Canton, J., Oliva, R., Ruiz-Cabello, F., and Garrido, F. (1999b) Looking for HLA-G expression in human tumours. *J. Rep. Immunol.*, **43**, 263–73.

Redondo, M., Ruiz-Cabello, F., Concha, A., Cabrera, T., Pérez, M., Oliva, M.R., and Garrido, F. (1991) Altered HLA class I expression in NSCLC is independent of c-myc activation. *Cancer Res.*, **51**, 2463–2468.

Reichert, T.E., Day, R., Wagner, E.M., and Whiteside, T.L. (1998) Absent or low expression of the zeta chain in T cells at the tumor site correlates with poor survival in patients with oral carcinoma. *Cancer Res.*, **58**, 5344–5347.

Restifo, N.P., Esquivel, F., Kawakami, Y., Yewdell, J., Mulé J.J., and Rosenberg, S.A. (1993) Identification of human cancers deficient in antigen processing. *J. Exp. Med.*, **177**, 265–272.

Reyburn, H.T., Mandelboim, O., Valès Gomez, M., Davis, D.M., Pazmani, L., and Strominger, J.L. (1997) The class I MHC homologue of human cytomegalovirus inhibits attack by natural killer cells. *Nature*, **386**, 514–516.

Rivoltini, L., Radrizzani, M., Accornero, P., Squarcina, P., Chiodoni, C., Mazzocchi, A., Castelli, C., Tarsini, P., Viggiano, V., Belli, F., Colombo, M.P., and Parmiani, G. (1998) Human melanoma-reactive CD4+ and CD8+ CTL clones resist Fas ligand-induced apoptosis and use Fas/Fas ligand-independent mechanisms for tumor killing. *J. Immunol.*, **161**, 1220–1230.

Rosa, F., Berissi, H., Weissenbach, J., Maroteaux, L., Fellous, M., and Revel, M. (1983) The beta-2-microglobulin mRNA in human Daudi cells has a mutated initiation codon but is still inducible by interferon. *EMBO J.*, **2**, 239–243.

Ruiz-Cabello, F., Pérez-Ayala, M., Gomez, O., Redondo, M., Concha, A., Cabrera, A., and Garrido, F. (1991) Molecular analysis of MHC class I alterations in human tumor cell lines. *Int. J. Cancer*, **6**, S123–130.

Ruiz-Cabello, F., and Garrido, F. (1998) HLA and cancer: from research to clinical impact. *Immunol. Today*, **19**, 539–542.

Salcedo, M., Momburg, F., Hämmerling, G., and Ljunggren, H.G. (1994) Resistance to natural killer cell lysis conferred by TAP1/2 genes in human antigen-processing mutant cells. *J. Immunol.*, **152**, 1702–1708.

Seliger, B., Harders, C., Lohmann, S., Momburg, F., Urliger, S., Tampe, R., and Huber, C. (1998) Down-regulation of the MHC class I antigen-processing machinery after oncogenic transformation of murine fibroblasts. *Eur. J. Immunol.*, **28**, 122–133.

Singer, D.S., and Maguire, J.E. (1990) Regulation of the expression of class I MHC genes. *Crit. Rev. Immunol.*, **10**, 235–237.

Soong, T.W., and Hui, K.M. (1992) Locus-specific transcriptional control of HLA genes. *J. Immunol.*, **149**, 2008–2014.

Speiser, D.E., Pittet, M.J., Valmori, D., Dunbar, R., Rimoldi, D., Liénard, D., MacDonald, H.R., Cerottini, J.C., Cerundolo, V., and Romero, P. (1999) *in vivo* expression of natural killer cell inhibitory receptors by human melanoma-specific cytolytic T lymphocytes. *J. Exp. Med.*, **190**, 775–782.

Staveley-O'Carroll, K., Sotomayor, E., Montgomery, J., Borrello, I., Hwang, L., Fein, S., Pardoll, D., and Levitsky, H. (1998) Induction of antigen-specific T cell anergy: an early event in the course of tumor progression. *Proc. Natl. Acad. Sci. USA*, **95**, 1178–1183.

Strand, S., Hofmann, W.J., Hug, H., Müller, M, Otto, G., Strand, D., Mariani, S.M., Stremmel, W., Krammer, P.H., and Galle, P.R. (1996) Lymphocyte apoptosis induced by CD95 (Apo-1/Fas) ligand-expressing tumor cells. A mechanism of immune evasion? *Nature Med.*, **2**, 1361–1366.

Thurner, B., Haendle, I., Roder, C., Dieckmann, D., Keikavoussi, P., Jonuleit, H., Bender, A., Maczek, C., Schreiner, D., von den Driesch, P., Brocker, E.B., Steinman, R.M., Enk, A., Kampgen, E., and Schuler, G. (1999) Vaccination with MAGE-3A1 peptide-pulsed mature, monocyte-derived dendritic cells expands specific cytotoxic T cells and induces regression of some metastases in advanced stage IV melanoma. *J. Exp. Med.*, **190**, 1669–1678.

Torres, M., Ruiz-Cabello, F., Skoudy, A., Berrozpe, G., Serrano, A., Jimenez, P., Real F.X., and Garrido, F. (1996) Loss of an HLA haplotype in pancreas cancer tissue and its corresponding tumor derived cell line. *Tissue Antigens*, **47**, 372–381.

Trutmann, M., Terracciano, L., Noppen, C., Kloth, J., Kaspar, M., Peterli, R., Tondelli, P., Schaeffer, C., Zajac, P., Heberer, M., and Spagnoli, G.C. (1998) GM-CSF gene expression and protein production in human colorectal cancer cell lines and clinical tumor specimens. *Int. J. Cancer*, **77**, 378–385.

Vitale, M. Rezzani, R., Zauli, L., Grigolato, P., Cadei, M., Hicklin, D. J., and Ferrone, S. (1998) HLA class I antigen transporter associated with antigen processing (TAP1 and TAP2) down-regulation in high-grade primary breast carcinomas lesions. *Cancer Res.*, **58**, 737–742.

Wang, Z., Cao, Y., Albino, A.P., Zeff, R.A., Houghton, A., and Ferrone, S. (1993) Lack of HLA class I antigen expression by melanoma cells SK-MEL-33 caused by a reading frameshift in beta 2-microglobulin messenger RNA. *J. Clin. Invest.*, **91**, 684.

Wang, Z., Seliger, B., Mike, N., Momburg, F., Knuth, A., and Ferrone, S. (1998) Molecular analysis of the HLA-A2 antigen loss by melanoma cells SK-MEL-29-1.22 and SK-MEL-29.1.2.29. *Cancer Res.*, **58**, 2149–2157.

Wang, Z., Marincola, F.M., Rivoltini, L., Parmiani, G., and Ferrone, S. (1999) Selective histocompatibility leukocyte antigen (HLA)-A2 loss caused by aberrant pre-mRNA splicing in 624MEL28 melanoma cells. *J. Exp. Med.*, **190**, 205–215.

Wiedenfield, E.A., Fernandez-Vina, M., Berzofsky, J.A., and Carbone, D.P. (1994). Evidence for selection against human cancers bearing p53 missense mutations which occur within the HLA A*0201 peptide consensus motif. *Cancer Res.*, **54**, 1175–1177.

Wiertz, E.J., Mukherjee, S., and Ploegh, H.L. (1997) Viruses use stealth technology to escape from the host immune system. *Mol. Med. Today*, **3**, 116–123.

White, C.A., Thomson, S.A., Cooper, L., van Endert, P.M., Tampe, R., Coupar, B., Qiu, L., Parsons, P.G., Mos, D.J., and Khanna, R. (1998) Constitutive transduction of peptide transporter and HLA genes restores antigen processing function and cytotoxic T cell-mediated immune recognition of human melanoma cells. *Int. J. Cancer*, **75**, 590–595.

Zeidler, R., Eissner, G., Meissner, P., Uebel, S., Tampe, R., Lazis, S., and Hammerschmidt, W. (1997) Downregulation of TAP1 and B lymphocytes by cellular and Epstein-Barr virus-encoded interleukin-10. *Blood*, **90**, 2390–2396.

Index